# OUR OVERWEIGHT CHILDREN

CALIFORNIA STUDIES IN FOOD AND CULTURE

*Darra Goldstein, Editor*

# OUR OVERWEIGHT CHILDREN

WHAT PARENTS, SCHOOLS,
AND COMMUNITIES
CAN DO TO CONTROL
THE FATNESS EPIDEMIC

## SHARRON DALTON

UNIVERSITY OF CALIFORNIA PRESS

BERKELEY   LOS ANGELES   LONDON

University of California Press
Berkeley and Los Angeles, California

University of California Press, Ltd.
London, England

The poem "You Can Only Demonstrate," from William C.
Martin, *The Parent's Tao Te Ching,* © 1999 by William
Martin, appears by permission of the publisher, Marlowe &
Company.

Library of Congress Cataloging-in-Publication Data

Dalton, Sharron.
    Our overweight children : what parents, schools, and
communities can do to control the fatness epidemic /
Sharron Dalton.
        p.    cm. — (California studies in food and culture ; 13)
    Includes bibliographical references and index.
    ISBN 0-520-22574-0 (cloth : alk. paper)
    1. Overweight children—United States.    2. Obesity
in children—United States. [DNLM:   1. Obesity—
prevention & control—Child.    WD 210 D1520 2004]
I. Title.   II. Series.
RJ399.C6D358   2004
618.92'398—dc22                                    2003026339

Manufactured in the United States of America
13   12   11   10   09   08   07   06   05   04
10   9   8   7   6   5   4   3   2   1

The paper used in this publication is both acid-free
and totally chlorine-free (TCF). It meets the minimum
requirements of ANSI/NISO z39.48-1992 (R 1997)
*(Permanence of Paper).*

*To Dennis, my spouse, who for four decades has given very little advice, much assistance, and abundant role modeling of healthy living to me, our children and grandchildren, and to his thousands of students*

NOTHING IN EXCESS.

*Oracle at ancient Delphi*

# CONTENTS

---------------------------------------------------------------

# OUR OVERWEIGHT KIDS

---------------------------------------------------------------

FOR MILLIONS OF SCHOOL-AGE American children, a typical weekday goes something like this.

For breakfast kids serve themselves chocolaty frosted cereal from a box that features a cartoon character. Often there's no time to eat breakfast at home, so they grab prepackaged snacks to eat in the car. One parent might get out sweetened juice drinks and "Lunchable" processed meals for them to eat at school or say, "Here's money for lunch—and snacks."

At school they shun the cafeteria's tasteless fare. Students flock to hallway vending machines, or to nearby fast-food outlets, and load up on "big grab" chips, "big gulp" sodas, "super-size" fries, and "grande" nachos. Their schedule blocks out time for computer lab, but not for recess or gym class. When school lets out they get rides home, since walking is considered unsafe, and they spend the remainder of the afternoon in front of the computer or television. Commercials whet their appetites for more sweet and salty snacks.

As night falls, one parent works late and the other turns to household chores. Neither has the time or energy to prepare a meal from scratch, and besides, a premade "value meal" is cheaper to buy. An extralarge "family-size" entrée—high in fat, salt, and calories—comes out of a box, goes into the microwave, and gets snatched up with fingers rather than forks. Between bites, family members alternately watch TV, talk on the phone, and wander off to do homework. Portions are so large that there's no need for second helpings. After supper the family regroups for "quality time"—to eat ice cream and watch a video.

What is missing almost entirely from this day? Fresh, wholesome food in reasonable portions; physical activity; and time to talk: "I wasn't chosen for the team; kids called me 'Fats' today."

What is the common characteristic of these children and their parents? They are fat—and getting fatter.

For myriad reasons, many involving the lifestyle and social environment sketched here, America faces a fast-growing epidemic of childhood obesity that threatens the long-term physical and psychological health of the nation's children. It is arguably the most pervasive and serious threat to children's health today and in the future. The rise in the number of cases of childhood obesity is entirely unprecedented and shows no sign of abating.[1]

The fact is that one out of three children in the United States is either overweight or at serious risk of becoming so. The number of overweight children ages six to nineteen has tripled within three decades; the rate of overweight *preschool* children is nearly as great. The accelerating rate indicates that the current generation of children will grow into the most obese generation of adults in history. Moreover, there is every expectation that the next generation of children will be even fatter and less fit. In 1995 researchers predicted that nearly all Americans would be overweight by the year 2030 if current trends continued.[2] That astonishing prediction—less than a decade old—is now in fast forward as greater numbers of very young overweight children give us an incredible head start.

While the public and media have begun to grasp the epidemic proportions of this problem, its causes, costs, and cures are far harder to untangle. This book aims to give other parents and all others who care about children—including educators, community leaders, health-care providers, and social workers—a clear understanding of the fatness epidemic, along with practical strategies to counter obesity. Any solution we apply must emerge from an awareness of its complex causes and consequences.

Some experts link the rise in childhood obesity to human biology and genetics. Others prefer to target fast food and soft drinks, which are nearly nutritionally empty but calorie-dense. Then there are those who focus on physical activity—or rather, the lack of it—and identify television and computers as the primary culprits. Still others say the fatness epidemic boils down to poor parenting. To varying degrees, these experts are correct. But the causes are even more numerous and interrelated; our whole society is complicit and therefore must be part of the solution. As one nurse at a national conference on childhood obesity put it, "It's bigger than all of us." Or as Oprah emphasized, on her show devoted to this topic, "no child is fat alone."

Understanding the interplay of these causes, and taking action to reverse the epidemic's rise, should be a priority for everyone at the start of this new millennium. Why? First and foremost, because many of our children are in pain, suffering from the merciless torment of a society that inflicts on its kids relentless discrimination as mindlessly as it inflicts on itself habits of overeating.[3] Second, overweight children do tend to become obese adults, putting themselves at a much greater risk, and at a much earlier age, for chronic illnesses such as diabetes and cardiovascular disease.[4] And while kids at all economic levels are getting fatter, the biggest burden is on those who can least afford it. Black, Hispanic, and Native American children, many of them from low-income families, have the highest incidence of obesity in America.

The point is this: with constant reminders—or more often teasing and bullying—about their weight, chubby kids easily become adults with disordered eating behaviors. Sooner or later, they may develop a long list of physical health problems, including diabetes, heart disease, sleep apnea, and premature death. Sooner, *not* later, the stigma of being fat shapes the way they view themselves and relate to others. These children suffer a devastating discrimination by adults and peers, resulting in a damaged sense of self-worth that exacerbates poor eating and exercise habits.

Growing up fat may seem far down on the list of woes that American children face in the twenty-first century. Educational achievement scores are flat or declining while rates of childhood poverty, suicide, and homicide are on the rise. America's national and international emergencies push these and other long-term health problems to the periphery. This book is a wake-up call, arguing that childhood obesity is, in fact, an urgent concern that demands and deserves the attention and resources necessary to combat it.

"This is an epidemic in the U.S. the likes of which we have not had before in chronic disease," noted Dr. William Dietz, director of the nutrition and physical activity division at the national Centers for Disease Control and Prevention (CDC). Obesity-related health costs to the general public are expected to run into the hundreds of billions by 2020, "making HIV look, economically, like a bad case of the flu."[5]

Dietz made his oft-quoted comments in 2001 during a conference on childhood obesity. Two years later at another national conference on the growing crisis of childhood obesity, the predictions were no less dire. U.S. Surgeon General Dr. Richard Carmona called the rise in childhood obesity a threat to national security: "Our preparedness as a nation depends on our health as individuals. . . . The military needs healthy recruits."[6] The conference had highlighted astonishing data to explain this concern: a statewide study of all California kids found not only high rates of overweight children but inadequate aerobic capacity as well in at least a quarter to half of the children (whether fat or not).[7] With similar weight statistics nationwide, there is little doubt that it's time to take action for all of our overweight *and* unfit children.

Why should any American *not* be concerned about our overweight children? My own concern comes from my personal role as a parent and grandparent, and from my professional training as a nutrition educator and registered dietitian. I am convinced that the scale and urgency of this problem pose a challenge to our national interest and certainly to everyone concerned with the health and well-being of our children.

For thirty-five years I have worked in the nutrition profession as an educator of consumers, teachers, and health-care providers, and of youth in classrooms, camps, and cooking workshops. My professional research and teaching have been international and cross-cultural, leading me to villages in South Asia to address diets that lack sufficient calories and vitamin A, then back to the markets and malls of America, where children consume foods that provide excess calories but insufficient nutrients. My purpose has always been to learn and to teach about food choices and food preparation in the interest of promoting health. Early on I believed that increased knowledge, positive attitudes, and practical skills led to a healthy diet. I came to realize that the process is more challenging and complex; nutrition education, a better attitude, and improved skills are not necessarily enough to counter the forces promoting obesity.

In the 1960s, during my early years of village development work in Asia, almost everyone there was underweight, especially women and children. In 1995, as a Fulbright scholar to Nepal, one of the world's poorest nations, I was struck by the number of overweight women among the relatively wealthy elite. Some showed off fat waistlines bulging from tight blouses while riding motor scooters—a sign of newly acquired wealth. Their children were fatter, too, and eager to eat and drink widely marketed processed products. The forces of globalization have put these relatively cheap foods and drinks—high in calories, low in nutrients—within reach of almost anyone, anywhere, giving childhood obesity a foothold in even the poorest countries. (See chapter 2's box on this topic, p. 32.)

Back in the United States in the 1970s and 1980s, my professional experience helped me develop therapeutic diets to manage diabetes and hypertension, diseases related to obesity. Nutritionists were just beginning to apply new knowledge about fat cells and energy regulation to curb obesity, and schools and government-funded programs were increasingly concerned with nutrition and health. I organized workshops to integrate physical education, school food programs, and classroom nutrition lessons. Students crowded the graduate courses I taught on weight management in the early 1990s to learn behavior modification and counseling techniques aimed at consumers concerned with fitness, athletic performance, and weight loss.

Meanwhile, in spite of society's preoccupation with losing weight to look fit and greater awareness about nutrition, both adults and children got fatter. I saw more and more overweight children in clinical practice, many depressed about their size and coping with adult diseases far too soon. "Now that Nina is taking medicine, she stays in her room and cries a lot. I just want her to get well." This and similar comments from mothers and relatives were all too common.

As the new century dawned, America showed signs of grasping the unprecedented scope of its weight problem. I began giving talks about childhood obesity to health professionals, school nurses, and day-care teachers, as well as to individuals involved with the federally funded Women, Infants, and Children program, which serves low-income mothers and their children who are nutritionally at risk. All were alarmed by the noticeable rise in obesity and obesity-related maladies among the very young. One doctor counseling young people in an obesity clinic described the situation well when he told a reporter: "It's like talking to someone who's eighty years old. Overweight kids have the same maladies [that seniors do]; they have trouble moving."[8]

Community and legislative leaders with a new sense of urgency have begun to act on the growing epidemic. In 2001 I testified before a group of New York City legislators intent on new initiatives to forestall obesity among minority children. I applauded their call for a variety of community programs that parents would consider safe alternatives to after-school television and video games. And colleagues familiar with my recently edited book for health professionals, *Overweight and Weight Management*, urged me to tackle the problem. The timing was right. This book—a scholarly yet practical diagnosis and prescription for our overweight children—grew from my desire to make a difference, so that toddlers I see as I enter Bellevue Hospital in New York City do not reach the unhealthy size of their siblings.

The first of the book's three parts, "How We Meet a Growing Epidemic," begins with an overview and then takes a closer look at the children most at risk in the epidemic, and the health and psychological consequences they may face. The second, "Why Kids Are Getting Fatter," untangles the multiple causes of the sharp rise in childhood obesity. A matter of both nature and nurture, obesity involves genetics, lifestyle, and many factors inside and outside the home. And part 3, "How We Can Fight the Epidemic," presents practical strategies and guidelines to help families, schools, and communities reverse the upward trend in weight gain. These chapters begin by teaching parents how to model and pass on healthy eating behavior to their children in order to prevent obesity. For children who already struggle with being overweight, part 3 critiques many popular weight-loss programs. I cull the best advice from them and draw on my own professional experience to put forth optimal guidelines for weight reduction and management. The final chapter then examines the critically important role the public and private sectors have to play in this fight.

Let's be clear about what this book does *not* include: quick fixes or easy answers or radical solutions. Simplistic and extreme remedies are the stock-in-trade of the $35 billion weight-loss product and service industry and scores of weight-loss gurus.[9] Their advice has fueled fads that increasingly pull America's diet out of whack while doing nothing to curb the rise in obesity.

During the past half century America's food choices, eating behavior, and activity levels have become seriously imbalanced. This book does not advocate a revolution in the American diet or even a departure from traditional American norms. It argues instead for a return to normalcy; the prescription comes from and develops the best of the diet and fitness of earlier generations. Not so long ago the average man, woman, and child actually engaged in moderate food consumption and sufficient physical activity.

I do not mean to glorify our past; we certainly do not want to turn the clock back to a time when infectious diseases were rampant. Yet for all our progress in health care, medical research, and technology, we as a society have fallen into an unhealthy pattern of overconsumption and underactivity that has no precedent in the country's history. Consider this: federal surveys that rate the quality of children's food consumption give the typical diets of today's children, ages two to eighteen, scores in the 60s (100 being the best possible). Fifty years ago, children's diet scores were in the 80s. Reporting a similar drop in the quality of children's diets in England, nutritionists noted, "Post-war rations gave toddlers and children a better start in life. They ate meat and two vegetables, filled up on bread and milk. Soft and fizzy drinks were scarce."[10]

Children can achieve and maintain a healthy weight through family strategies to regain a balance, or "normalcy," in nutrition and activity. To that end, I make a case—and a plea—for *moderation*. Moderation involves temperate, measured behavior in eating and physical activity patterns, rather than an overindulgence in serving sizes or an underestimation of the importance of daily physical activity. It involves reasonable expectations about body sizes and shapes, and tolerance toward less-than-perfect ones. It does not envisage a perfect diet, a perfect lifestyle, or a perfect body size. Rather, as we assess the amount of fatty foods to consume, hours of television to watch, or number of pounds to lose, Aristotle's ancient wisdom still prevails: "as a general principle, moderation is always best."

An approach to weight management through moderation has room for the reality of children's behavior as well as the reality of the time and financial pressures placed upon their parents. And parenting is complicated. Dozens of daily demands ramp up the challenges that families face. Because I am writing primarily for families, let's be clear about the family's role. Parents, siblings, and grandparents of overweight children create a home environment where risk factors for obesity, unintended and unknown, may flourish. But before we hold them responsible for causing and curing childhood obesity, we must recognize that overworked families cannot tackle this epidemic alone. Families need all the help they can get: from schools and communities to engage their children in physical activity during and after school; from the marketplace to gain better access to healthy food choices.

Coupled with this book's call for moderation is an appeal for *prevention,* a concept sorely lacking from the dialogue around obesity treatment. Here is the silver lining behind that cloud of bad news, for though obesity is the most prevalent health affliction in children, *it is also the most preventable.* A few years ago I was fielding questions from a group of medical residents who had gathered for a presentation on the nutritional management of children with "adult" type 2 diabetes. The majority of their questions centered on popular weight-loss diets and pharmaceutical treatments. Not one of these young doctors expressed an interest in preventing obesity. All asked the unrealistic and unanswerable question, which reflected the main concern of their patients: what is *the* magic bullet to lose weight?

There is no magic bullet for childhood obesity in the form of a pill. There are only pills to suppress appetite and potions to prevent fat absorption once the potato chips are in the stomach and on their way toward digestion. Likewise, there is no single social or governmental action that is a panacea for this overweight generation. Rather, there are many steps that we can take, individually and together as a community, to combat this epidemic.

Serving nutritious food in reasonable portions is an obvious first step; less obvious, but no less important, is learning how to listen for and respect internal cues of hunger and satiety. Raising kids to self-regulate their food choices in a healthy, balanced manner is one form of insurance against obesity in a society where the marketplace and media encourage extreme eating habits by pushing junk food and glorifying unrealistic body types.

Fighting the fatness epidemic will require a long-term commitment because it involves much more than going on a diet: it entails changing individuals' behavior and the choices available to them to sustain a healthy weight through balanced eating and physical activity, day in and day out. For individuals, it is a lifelong undertaking. If a significant number of overweight children are to reach and maintain a healthy weight, and if we hope to prevent widespread obesity in the next generation, then society as a whole must work to change the external factors that play such a large role in making people fatter. For these reasons, we need to take the long view in addressing childhood obesity and commit to a lasting campaign to deal with it. The British pediatrician Ronald J. Sokol has stated this point well:

> The sleeping giant has awakened. Our changing lifestyle, high-fat and fast foods, and developing computer-based technology with increased reliance on the Internet will most likely keep this childhood epidemic around for a long time, despite current efforts at improving nutritional health and raising the activity level of our youth. Hopefully, the obesity epidemic in children will not be akin to global warming, wherein engineers, architects, and others are planning new construction strategies, assuming that global warming is here to stay. Pediatric *obesitologists* will be faced with the challenge to develop methods for reversing the childhood obesity epidemic and dealing effectively with the complications of obesity. The challenge is there: who will take it?[11]

If the fatness epidemic's complexity and pervasiveness make it look insurmountable, we can gain inspiration and learn lessons from advocates who embarked on a campaign nearly forty years ago to tackle the smoking epidemic. In 1964 the U.S. surgeon general published a groundbreaking report that exposed evidence of smoking-related illness and early death. That public awareness led to a call for regulation of the tobacco industry. A grassroots movement gained momentum, supported by educators, legislators, and community activists, and their multifaceted, long-term campaign dramatically reduced smoking. In 1964 some 43 percent of Americans smoked; by 2000 the figure had dropped to 25 percent.[12] Such an all-out campaign is not too much to demand in the fight against childhood obesity. The long-term threat to the nation's health and security is not just comparable; it is much greater.

To make significant strides, community action is critical, because raising healthy kids "takes a village." We must reset personal and public priorities in a way that fosters healthy eating and activity. There are roles for everyone—families, health professionals, school leaders, the food industry, the media, and policy makers at all levels.

What are some of the potential outcomes if we opt to do nothing? More overweight children who face multimillion-dollar lifetime medical bills for diabetes treatment. More who never experience the joys and rewards of sports because they're too unfit or tormented by peers to participate, and because recreational opportunities are not available to them. More who grow up to produce another generation of obese youth who suffer because of their excessive weight. If we care about our children, then none of these outcomes is acceptable. The time for strong intervention—and even stronger prevention—is now.

# HOW WE MEET
# A GROWING EPIDEMIC

# 1

---

# COMING TO TERMS

---

HOW DO WE, as parents and as health professionals, decide if a child is seriously overweight? Children on the playground need only a couple of minutes to spot a fat kid. If everyone is a self-appointed expert when it comes to judging body size and shape, obesity should be easy to recognize and diagnose. It's simple, right?

In fact, diagnosing a child as clinically obese is quite complex. Children grow at very different rates, and growth is the priority. No doctor or parent wants the mention of a "weight problem" to backfire and lead to poor nutrition, which could hurt the child's long-term growth. Health professionals try to get the diagnosis right, because labeling a child "overweight" can risk not only his or her physical development but the child's social and emotional development as well. Obese children, especially girls, evidence significantly lower levels of self-esteem by early adolescence compared to non-obese children, according to several studies.[1]

Just talking about the problem is difficult because of confusion over proper terms and the shame associated with them. An expert committee studying obesity evaluation and treatment noted that owing to "the common belief that obesity results from laziness or lack of willpower, overweight children and their families often feel embarrassed and ashamed."[2] So clinicians as well as parents must be highly sensitive in their language and demeanor when broaching this subject with young people.

Perhaps not surprisingly, parents often react with defensiveness and denial when they first face the fact that they need to address their child's—and perhaps their own—excessive weight. As a dietitian in a metropolitan hospital clinic, I remember talking with a heavyset man, age twenty-five, who had seen his medical chart while waiting for the doctor to arrive. Obesity, his primary medical diagnosis, was written in large letters, and he was furious. "I am not obese! I'm a big man, and my whole family—kids, brothers, sisters—we're all large. The doctor is wrong; we're not obese." I asked, "What does obese mean to you?" He said, "A huge fatso who waddles . . . can't fit through the door . . . takes up two seats . . . looks gross." To explain the reasoning behind the diagnosis, I suggested comparing his height and weight to the recommended "healthy weight" chart. He looked at the chart and said "I don't believe it." Clearly, "obesity" is a term that's loaded with emotion and carries the potential for discrimination. Even preschool-age children notice obesity.[3]

This chapter sets out definitions and tools to help all of us determine whether children have a serious weight problem or are at risk for developing one. We'll consider how parents and peers view weight, since their *perception* of "overweight" often falls out of line with the medical reality. Finally, we'll look at the debate over whether obesity should rank as a disease.

## "OVERWEIGHT," "OBESE," OR JUST PLAIN "FAT"?

Health professionals and the media have been doing an interesting dance around the term "obesity." They use it freely in the abstract and in reference to the general population, but they apply it with caution when describing individuals, particularly children. When it comes to kids, "overweight" has developed into a more acceptable and sensitive synonym for "obese."

In this book I use the words "overweight" and "obese" interchangeably, as both scientific and popular literature do (though "overweight" can connote a milder degree of excess fat than "obese"). I personally prefer "overweight" as the general term and in my practice emphasize "healthy weight for *you*," an individual, positive way to talk about body size and health.

When we discuss growth and the body-mass index (BMI)—a relatively new method for measuring weight in relation to height—you'll see that growth charts approved by the government and medical establishment give doctors a reference point to gauge when individuals are truly "overweight." But the BMI is only one tool, and an imperfect one at that.

The medical community generally talks about an "obese child" and "the childhood obesity epidemic," yet these same health professionals are very cautious about labeling an individual child "obese." Instead, they classify a heavy or big child in one of two categories: *at risk of becoming overweight* or *overweight*. I keep these widely accepted categories to describe children whose BMI places them at or above the 85th percentile on BMI growth charts (explained below). Others, including British medical professionals, use "overweight" and "obese" to designate these two categories,[4] while some reports in scientific journals label children "obese" and "super-obese."

A 1998 report from the journal *Pediatrics* titled "Obesity Evaluation and Treatment" discussed obesity in children but then gave guidelines for classifying a child as "overweight" or "at risk of becoming overweight," not "obese." The report included a cautionary section on the appropriate language and demeanor for clinicians. Showing an evident concern about the label "obese," it admonished those who care for overweight children and their families to "treat them with sensitivity, compassion, and the conviction that obesity is an important, chronic medical problem that can be treated."[5] Apparently this new language protocol caught on, as evidenced by a July 2000 *Newsweek* cover story that pictured a big kid. The headline was "Fat for Life? Six Million Kids Are Seriously Overweight," and the article also ignored the term "obese."

Health professionals have yet another reason to sidestep the term: "obese" generally refers to an individual's amount, or percentage, of body fat, and kids' body fat levels rarely get measured. Ideally, the common classifications for children's body size would reflect both their weight-for-height *and* their percentage of body fat. But measuring body fat is often imprecise and rarely occurs for individual kids in health clinics.

Still others prefer "fat" because "overweight" means *over* some ideal weight, and there is no ideal weight for a given person. "Fat," they argue— and I agree in principle—is simply an adjective like "tall" or "thin" and should not be offensive. Kids are different from one another in many ways— short and tall, skinny and fat, dark skinned and light skinned. Ideally, we would all be as tolerant of different body types as we are of, say, different hair colors. But the reality is that fat is undesirable for any kid, and fatness can have serious health consequences.

Bottom line: the terminology may vary and evolve, but we can't redefine this problem out of existence. We face a real epidemic of childhood obesity, and the words we use to describe it carry equally real and formidable social discrimination.

## BEYOND THE SCALE: GROWTH CHARTS AND THE BMI

A scale reveals a child's weight, but that's all it reveals. Medical professionals also need to gather information about height, age, rate of growth, and fat-to-muscle ratio before they can begin to determine if that child is overweight.

Growth charts developed in the 1970s by the National Center for Health Statistics indicated height and weight percentile distributions in children of the same age. These charts were based predominantly on data about white children, an obvious shortcoming in today's increasingly diverse society. The federal Centers for Disease Control unveiled revised growth charts in 2000, based on data from several ethnic groups.[6] These charts incorporate the new body-mass index, which is a single number that evaluates an individual's weight in relation to height. Parents and pediatricians now have a more accurate tool for determining if a child's weight-for-height is appropriate for a given age, and for then classifying that child as underweight, at a healthy weight, or overweight.

Of interesting note—since it too shows that our society's weight gain outpaces medically accepted standards—is the new charts' purposely distorted view of the "average" for American children ages five to twenty. According to the charts, children in the 85th through the 94th percentile range are "at risk of becoming overweight," while children at or above the 95th percentile are "overweight." The charts imply that only 15 percent of American children are too heavy but, as we know, the incidence of overweight children in America is significantly higher—at 25 to 30 percent. For example, if the charts used current surveys of children's actual BMI, an eight-year-old whose BMI is at the 87th percentile (at risk) would fall near the 75th percentile (not at risk) because there are so many children (25 percent) who are heavier than she is. Yet her weight is a risk to her health. Hence the CDC used population surveys from before 1988 to establish the new growth chart percentiles for older children. The charts show recommended values for the healthy range of body-mass index, not actual values. But for recommended growth and BMI curves in children ages two to five they use recent actual values.

Walk through the following steps to determine your child's BMI and to assess his or her weight category according to the new growth charts.

## How to Calculate a Child's BMI and Gauge His or Her Size

1.  Measure your child's height and weight.

2.  Using the table in Appendix 1, find your child's height (in inches) on the left-hand column and corresponding weight (in pounds) across the row. Your child's BMI is at the top of the column where height and weight meet. For example, a child who is 36 inches tall and weighs 31 pounds has a BMI of 17. (Or you can calculate the BMI on your own: multiply weight [lb] by 703, then divide by height squared [ht × ht (in)].)

3.  To determine if your child's weight is healthy according to the governmental guidelines, choose the graph for girls or boys in Appendix 2. Find the point where BMI and age intersect. The dark gray section indicates overweight (95th percentile and above); the light gray section indicates at risk of becoming overweight (85th through 94th percentile).

4.  If your child's BMI is in these two ranges, further laboratory measures and medical assessment of diet and physical activity are recommended.

The 2000 pediatric growth charts, along with a BMI calculator, are available on the CDC Web site: www.cdc.gov/growthcharts/. See the box titled "Sensitivity Matters" for measuring techniques and ways to talk about the measurements.

If you carry out these calculations on yourself as well as on your child, be aware that the BMI for adults uses arbitrary cutoff points rather than percentiles. The National Institutes of Health established the following standards for adults: "overweight" is a BMI of 25 to 29.9; "obese" is a BMI of 30 and above. "Normal" healthy weight for adults is a BMI of 18.5 to 24.9. Governmental health agencies no longer use "ideal" to describe body weight of children or adults. I applaud their decision: it suggests that a variety of body sizes can be healthy and that weight management is realistic and attainable.

As we note in the Appendix 2 table, the body-mass index changes dramatically with age during childhood and adolescence. For example, the average BMI for age six or seven is about 16; at age seventeen, the average BMI is close to 22. Thus the BMI must always relate to age. Differences between boys and girls are most striking in the high percentiles.

## SENSITIVITY MATTERS
### HOW TO MEASURE KIDS AND TALK ABOUT THEIR SIZE

Children and adolescents who feel insecure about their size may experience a great deal of anxiety when asked to step on a scale, especially if the weight and height measurements are taken at school when peers are present. Adults can lessen that anxiety by following this list of "do's" and "don'ts."

- **Do** weigh and measure children in private, with no other children present. **Don't** have children weigh and measure each other and then compare their results.

- **Do** make neutral comments such as, "Thanks, you can get off the scale now." **Don't** make comments about any child's weight or height while he or she is being measured.

- If the child asks if he or she is too fat or too thin, **do** say, "Kids' bodies come in lots of different sizes and shapes" and "Children grow at different rates"; suggest that he or she ask a doctor that question. **Don't** make a medical diagnosis about the child's size or label the child "overweight."

Weighing kids at school is a hot topic, as is clear from the following comment reported in the *New York Times*. After one mother got a letter from the school nurse stating that her son was at risk of becoming overweight, she said, "I took offense to it; I really thought it was totally inappropriate for school to send a letter." She argued that her son wasn't overweight at all, "just a big, healthy kid who's tall for his age."

Others counter that, using this information, parents can encourage improved eating habits and more physical activity. "If we have information that may have some bearing on a child's future health, why just put it in a drawer? When an examination reveals a child has vision problems, hearing problems, we inform the family," says George Zolkowski, director of pupil personnel services, East Penn District, Philadelphia.

One study showed that sending a health report card to families about their child's health and weight had positive results, compared to sending general health information. The report should include weight and fitness information for each child and include follow-up for parents.

For methods for accurately weighing and measuring children in a private, respectful way, see *Guidelines for Collecting Heights and Weights on Children and Adolescents in School Settings* at http://nature.berkeley.edu/cwh/resources/childrenandweight.shtml.

*See p. 244 for source notes.*

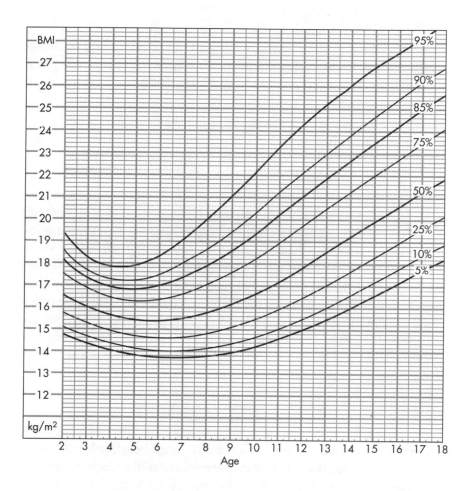

FIGURE 1. This part of the standard growth curve for boys shows the "adiposity rebound," a predictor of obesity later in life. A boy whose BMI reaches its lowest point and then begins swinging up around age four is more likely to become overweight than a boy whose BMI reaches its lowest point at age six. (Adapted from "Body Mass Index-for-Age Percentiles: Boys, Two to Twenty Years," Centers for Disease Control, National Center for Health Statistics, www.cdc.gov/growthcharts, 16 Oct 2000)

Also noteworthy is the dip in the growth curve that occurs in early childhood (Figure 1). Pediatricians often focus on this dip, as it can be a strong predictor of adult obesity. Healthy children normally drop in weight-for-height as they leave toddlerhood; they thin out after their second birthday. After the dip, their BMI holds steady for about a year, and then weight-for-height slowly increases at age seven or eight. This upswing from the dip is called the "adiposity rebound." If a child begins this fat-gain rebound earlier than age six or seven, the risk rises that obesity will persist, or "track," into adulthood. As we see in the figure, a boy in the 95th percentile reaches his lowest BMI at age four, whereas a boy in the 50th percentile reaches his lowest BMI at age six. The boy in the 95th percentile who begins regaining weight-for-height early may have a head start toward lifelong obesity.

Pediatricians and health-care providers in clinics should regularly measure children and calculate their BMI beginning at age two and continuing through age twenty in order to identify those who need further assessment and possible treatment.[7] A 2002 report of nearly 20,000 children studied from birth to age seven indicated a strong association between a high rate of weight gain during the first four months of life and the prevalence of being overweight at age seven.[8] Early screening for high weight gain as well as growth may be recommended in the future for children under two.

### A WORD OF CAUTION ABOUT THE BMI

On releasing the revised growth charts in 2000, Secretary of Health and Human Services Donna E. Shalala summed up their benefit when she noted that they give parents and health-care providers a tool to identify children who have the *potential* to become overweight years later. "The BMI is an early warning signal that is helpful as early as age two," she stated. "This means that parents have an opportunity to change their children's eating habits before a weight problem ever develops."[9]

Yet the BMI and corresponding growth charts don't show the whole picture, so use caution when studying where your child falls on the charts. First, they do not account for variation in the amount of body fat, and an individual child may have less fat and more lean or skeletal tissue compared to another with the same BMI.

Second, while the BMI provides a snapshot of a child's weight-for-height, it does not reveal the *rate* of growth: in particular, the rate of weight growth compared to the rate of height growth. Studying the rates of weight and height gain, and the relationship between them, is critical. Most experts

agree, and I concur, that if weight growth obviously outpaces height growth, steps should be taken to slow the rate of weight gain.

Ignoring body fat content and growth rate, as well as other factors in lifestyle and exercise habits, runs the risk of identifying a disproportionate number of tall, apparently overweight children while overlooking short overweight children who may be in greater need of help. Let's compare two girls to illustrate this point.

Karen's parents call her "Happy" because she has always been a bright, enthusiastic child. A school nurse refers Karen at age nine to her pediatrician because she is "big" for her age. Karen has a large bottom, emerging breast buds, and a BMI of 19 that is high for her age. Most nine-year-old girls as tall as Karen—5 feet 2 inches—weigh around 90 pounds, but Karen weighs 105 pounds.

Even so, Karen's amount of body fat compared to lean muscle is normal. Because she is tall for her age, her rate of weight gain does not outstrip her rate of growth in height. She also shows early signs of maturity, when fat accentuates gender-specific shape, especially breasts and hips. Karen is quite muscular, as she swims three to four times weekly. After considering these factors, Karen's pediatrician properly concludes that Karen's weight is healthy even though her BMI puts her slightly above the 85th percentile, "at risk for becoming overweight." The doctor praises Karen's passion for swimming and reassures her that her size is fine.

In contrast, Karen's nine-year-old friend Susan is short—4 feet 6 inches—and weighs 76 pounds. Her BMI of 18 places her near the 80th percentile on the chart, indicating she is within the healthy range. But her rate of growth in height is not keeping pace with her rate of weight gain. She has a double chin and an extra roll of fat at her waist. A measurement of her body fat indicates a high fat-to-muscle ratio. Though the risk is not immediately apparent, Susan could develop weight-related health problems. Because she is not very active, the doctor encourages her to get involved in recreational activities.

When assessing your child's body-mass index, remember:

· BMI is only a guideline. It does not measure bone, fat, or muscle.

· BMI values increase with age.

· There is no "right" BMI value for any single child at any age.

· Comparisons among children's BMI values are meaningless.

### HOW PARENTS VIEW THEIR CHILDREN'S WEIGHT

It's not uncommon to hear a parent say, "My son is just like his brothers—husky." Family members typically use comparisons to siblings and to other relatives to judge a child's body size. These comparisons strongly influence parents' opinion about proper weight and size—so much so that few seek and pay much attention to the textbook standards for growth and weight gain described above.[10]

A mother and father will develop firm ideas about the "right size" for their children but often disagree with extended family, friends, pediatricians, or even between themselves about what this right size is. Studies show that families' perception of an acceptable and physically attractive size differs from one racial or ethnic group to another. These cultural expectations, along with pride and protective instincts, all contribute to the parental definition of a "normal" size.

A child often gets caught between the family's definition of "normal" weight and society's definition, which is conveyed through the media and peers. This difference usually comes into focus during highly sensitive periods of development, such as early adolescence. Most parents naturally want their child to fit into his or her peer group. When the child experiences the pain of being stigmatized for being fat, this may trigger the parents to start worrying about their child's weight and to seek help for weight management.

My clients often come to me at this point. In one case, parents were seeking dietary help for their preteen, who was being teased for being fat. "They push leftovers toward me at school lunch and call me 'garbage truck.' I get so depressed after school that I go home where it's safe and I eat." He was eleven years old, 4 feet 10 inches, 170 pounds and tearful. His mother cried too. A ten-year-old girl, her large body covered in a giant T-shirt, told me with a wry smile, "I want to lose weight to get back at all those mean kids that make fun of me."

How well do parents guess and assess their child's weight? Not very. Studies show that parents—particularly those with low educational levels and low income—often mistake their child's weight. Mothers tend to underestimate, rather than overestimate, the size of overweight children.[11] One study asked low-income mothers whether they considered themselves and their preschool-age children overweight. Of those who actually were overweight and had overweight children, 95 percent of the mothers said they themselves were overweight, but only 21 percent believed their children

were.[12] So regardless of educational level, obese mothers' perception of their *own* weight was highly accurate.

What accounts for the misperception then? Researchers speculate that mothers may recognize their child's weight problem but choose not to acknowledge or address it. Or they may believe that young children will grow out of being overweight. Others may not think of being overweight as a problem and believe that having bigger children signifies good health and parental competence.[13] Some mothers say they don't worry about their child's weight if the child is active and has a healthy diet and a good appetite. Many of these mothers described their children as "thick" or "solid."[14]

Whatever the case, the mothers' view strongly influences their daughters. A nationwide study of more than 2,000 nine- and ten-year-old girls, black and white, found that 40 percent of those in all weight categories, and 75 percent of those who were in the heaviest category, were trying to lose weight. The main reason stated was "Mother telling me I am too fat." While equal numbers of daughters were trying to *lose* weight, significantly more black girls than white were trying to *gain* weight. Once again, the main reason was "Mother telling me I am too thin."[15] This suggests that mothers—and, we can assume, fathers too—can take a proactive approach and influence their children to manage their diet and lifestyle in a healthy fashion. Conversely, the parents' indifference can influence the children to be indifferent as well.

Surveys that try to gauge the level of parental concern about childhood obesity reveal a mixed picture about the degree to which parents care about their kids' weight. Concern certainly exists, but many parents simply do not consider weight among the top challenges facing kids. When asked, "How concerned are you about your child's weight?" 15 percent of the 1,500 parents in a nationwide survey in 2000 said "very," and 15 percent said "somewhat."[16] Because nearly 30 percent of children are overweight or at risk for it, the concern of these parents roughly matches the reported national prevalence of overweight children. What's more, those who answered "very" or "somewhat" spanned all income levels; nearly 40 percent earned less than $30,000 annually, 46 percent were middle-income earners, and 14 percent earned above $75,000.

Yet all parents—especially low-income—viewed other risks to their child's long-term health and quality of life as more pressing. Only 5 percent of the people in the same survey identified being overweight as the greatest risk to their child's health and quality of life. Parents were significantly more worried about illegal drugs, violence, smoking, alcohol, and sexually transmitted diseases.[17]

## HOW TEENS AND CHILDREN VIEW THEIR WEIGHT

Teenagers perceive their weight inaccurately as well—even more so than their parents do. A national study in 2000 involving more than 15,000 adolescents looked at the accuracy of teen and parental reports of obesity. It found that 44 percent of the overweight teenage children and their parents did *not* accurately report them to be overweight. Only 20 percent of both the teens and parents accurately reported that the teen was overweight; 30 percent of the parents, but not their teenage child, accurately recognized the teen as overweight. In the same study, among the adolescents with a *healthy* weight, 47 percent reported that they were overweight.[18] The problem is that, either way, perception does not represent reality; those who are overweight as well as those who are at a healthy weight have a distorted image of themselves.

As for younger children, plenty of evidence shows that they are aware of social standards for size and shape by age three or four. Many already judge body size as good or bad in kindergarten. Whether a child applies these notions of "good" and "bad" to his or her own body size that early is questionable. When friendships begin to form, body size may be a factor, like other characteristics that distinguish one child from another as reasons for friendship—or for discrimination.

Ethnicity and culture also shape a child's body image and influence young people's behavior in dealing with their body size. For example, while obesity rates are higher among black girls and adolescents, unhealthy dieting behaviors (such as using pills and vomiting) are more common among white adolescents. An overall cultural tolerance for large sizes in black women, and the stringent cultural standards for thinness in white women, are often cited for this discrepancy. Hispanic women are generally admired for larger hips and generous body size; Asian teens and independent young Asian women have a surprising incidence of eating disorders related to desire for thinness. We'll examine these differences in body image further in part 3.

## OBESITY: A DISEASE?

Given language, ethnicity, and varying perceptions of weight, we have to admit that recognizing or defining obesity is not nearly as simple as it may seem. The government and medical community have minimized these differences by establishing guidelines to indicate when a child is "overweight" and when an adult is "obese." Even so, they are nowhere close to reconciling different answers to a basic question: can we classify obesity as a disease among children in America?

If it were a disease, then almost everyone would agree that finding a cure for a disease affecting one out of three children should be a national priority. Yet there is heated controversy over its status. The positions of several key agencies and groups are summarized below.

National Institutes of Health: yes. Obesity is a disease with enormous negative effects on health and survival; also, health-care costs for treating diseases caused by obesity are estimated at $100 billion a year.

American Obesity Association: yes. Obesity is a disease; insurance plans should cover weight management services and tax deductions should be given for the costs of obesity treatments, as they are allowed for smoking cessation treatments.

American Dietetic Association: yes. Obesity should be classified as a disease; it is a significant risk factor for poor health. The goal of obesity interventions is health improvement that should be measured in terms of heart and lung performance, rates of admission to hospitals, and reduction in medication use.[19]

Internal Revenue Service: no. Until March 2002 obesity treatment did not qualify as a medical expense unless it was undertaken to treat another disease of the obese person, such as diabetes. Some treatments, but not diet foods, now qualify as deductions.[20]

Medicare and Medicaid: no. Obesity does not qualify as a disease; only related medical problems are covered by governmental health-financing programs.

National Association for Acceptance of Fat People: no. Fat people can be healthy and are therefore not suffering from a disease. It is not their weight that causes problems, but society's discrimination against fat people. They can do the same jobs and have the same abilities as thin people despite pervasive stereotypes to the contrary. The medical imperative to intervene in the lives of "disabled" people in order to "fix" them is repugnant to many fat people.[21]

The view I adopt is that obesity is *not* a disease, though it is clearly related to diseases such as diabetes and hypertension. My reasoning is that since obesity now characterizes the majority of the American population, we cannot reasonably diagnose most of the nation as "diseased." Applying a term like "sick society" to whole populations strips it of meaning. Most obese individuals suffer not from a physical or mental illness, but from *a condition of immoderation.* Overweight children and adults need a balanced lifestyle informed by healthy food and activity choices.

In the early twentieth century, obesity was described as a condition of patients who failed to lose weight during a period of low-calorie diet observation. These patients were thought to be unfortunate victims of disease, an abnormality of the thyroid or other gland that caused fat to be stored independent of physical activity or dietary habit. It remains true that, for a small minority of children (fewer than 1 percent), obesity is a disease with endocrine and genetic causes, as in Prader-Willi and Bardet-Biedl syndromes. But for the vast majority of obese children, their condition qualifies neither as disease nor as eating disorder. Obesity is a problem of energy balance: more calories consumed than those spent in physical activity.[22]

This debate over terminology has important consequences. If we label obesity a disease, then the implied remedy is medical treatment, pharmaceutical and/or surgical. These are not viable remedies for the majority of fat children, though these extreme interventions may be the last resort for some. Children require long-term preventive actions to establish healthy, moderate food and activity habits for life.

## SUMMARY

We've seen that diagnosing a child as overweight is a complex process since children grow at different rates and within a wide range of healthy sizes. The CDC's growth charts give parents and health professionals a tool for screening young people to determine if they are too heavy and at risk for weight-related health problems. These charts use the body-mass index, or BMI, which is calculated from weight and height measurements. A child whose BMI is at the 85th through 94th percentile ranks as "at risk of overweight," while one with a BMI at or above the 95th percentile is "overweight." These terms refer to any child whose excess body weight could pose medical, psychological, and social risks, whereas the term "obese" applies to adults whose BMI is over a certain level (30). "Overweight" and "obesity" often occur interchangeably in studies on the general problem of excess weight.

Recognizing a problem and raising the public's awareness of its threats and consequences are the first steps toward its resolution. In the case of a health crisis among children, we would expect parents to be especially alarmed by the early signals. Yet both because excessive weight gain is often imperceptible but steady, and because other, more immediate, challenges confront families today, these first public health steps are way behind schedule.

To sharpen our awareness of obesity's rapidly growing threat to children's health, in the next chapter we turn to its physical and psychological effects. Being overweight certainly puts children and adults at an increased risk for serious diseases. The treatment of their condition involves large doses of prevention and moderation.

# 2

---

# GAUGING OBESITY'S TOLL

---

EQUIPPED WITH A BETTER UNDERSTANDING of how to diagnose children as overweight, we can look more closely at who they are. This chapter explains which children are most overweight and consequently most at risk for obesity's physical and psychological consequences. It then focuses on the weight-related maladies that cause suffering.

A growing number of overweight youth experience health problems that are likely to carry over into adulthood. As this century progresses, that number is set to climb higher, for as the statistics that follow here show, kids are not only getting fatter; they are *getting fatter faster.* The number of overweight children and adolescents was relatively stable from the 1960s to 1980 but then nearly doubled by 1994. It has since continued to spike upward rather than plateau.

With the rapid climb in the incidence of overweight children comes an increase in diseases related to excessive weight and lack of physical fitness. Children who are as young as eight years old should not have "adult-onset" (type 2) diabetes, but they do.[1] Teenagers who are facing the ordinary stress of adolescence should not also have to cope with the physical discomfort of weight-related breathing problems along with the emotional pain of being ostracized for fatness. They do. And barring a significant reversal in the upward trend in obesity, these problems will only worsen over time.

American parents go to great lengths to ensure their children's health and safety. We buckle our babies into car seats, teach our kindergartners about traffic safety, and warn our preteens not to smoke. Yet by and large, we do not know—or choose to ignore—the very real health risks associated with overeating, poor food choices, and inactivity. Roughly one-quarter of America's children are too heavy and consequently are at an increased risk for illness and early death. Imagine the public outcry if unsafe drinking water or improperly installed seat belts put that many of the country's children at risk for illness or death. We can only hope that an increased awareness of obesity's physical and emotional toll propels a widespread effort to halt the epidemic.

## WHO'S FATTER NOW?

One out of three children and adolescents ages six to nineteen is overweight or at risk of becoming overweight. Their body-mass index places them in the 85th percentile or above on the growth charts published in 2000 by the Centers for Disease Control. Over half of these adolescents and six- to eleven-year-olds were in the fattest percentile (95th and above) in 2000.[2]

As we see in Figure 2, the younger age group has the same number of fat individuals as the adolescent age group—a clear sign of the epidemic's rise. The ratio holds even if the younger group expands to include children ages four and five. The number of overweight preschoolers and kindergartners is high and climbing, particularly among girls; the number of overweight girls in this young age group almost doubled from 5 percent in the early 1970s to 9 percent in 1994; by 2000, it had risen to over 11 percent. Altogether, the combined number of three- to five-year-old children at risk of overweight and those who are overweight comes to an astonishing 21 percent—one out of five.[3] And perhaps most troubling of all is that the prevalence of overweight babies and toddlers—newborn to two-year-old children—is over 11 percent. Younger children are fatter than ever.

Apparently children are following the lead of American adults, who are on record as the fattest, heaviest population group in the world. There is an adult obesity epidemic, too, and the rates are even more startling: 65 percent of adults in the United States are "overweight" (classified as a BMI ranging from 25 to 29.9) or "obese" (a BMI 30 or higher).[4] Two out of three Americans are overweight, and one of the two is also obese. As those formerly overweight became heavier and joined the ranks of the obese, the percentage of obese adults nearly doubled in the 1990s.[5]

For all age groups, as people grew heavier, those who had been at a healthy

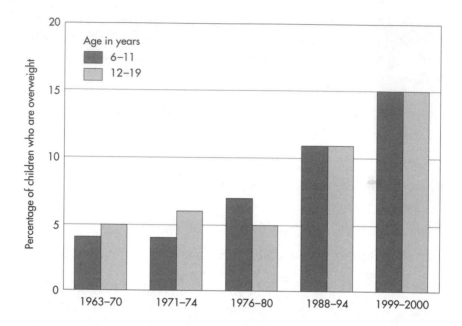

FIGURE 2. The number of overweight children—especially young children—has grown dramatically since 1963. Not shown on this graph, but of great concern, is the additional 15 percent of children and adolescents who were at risk of becoming overweight in 1999–2000. (Adapted from "Prevalence of Overweight among Children and Adolescents Ages 6–19 Years," Centers for Disease Control, National Center for Health Statistics, www.cdc.gov/nchs/products/pubs/pubd/hestats/over99fig1.htm, 12 Oct 2002)

weight grew overweight. And the BMI increased the most among children and adolescents in the top percentile. The heaviest kids in 1994 were markedly heavier than those in 1964. From 1994 to 2000 there was a 4 percent increase in the number of youth in the heaviest (top percentile) range.

For the growing number of heaviest kids, the chance of becoming obese adults is greater than ever before, especially in families where children learn behaviors that lead to adult obesity. Hence, with the increasing rate of adult obesity, the challenge is to slow and to stall, if not reverse, the weight gain of children *and* their families.

## RACE MATTERS

Of great concern is the fact that childhood obesity affects the government-designated "minority groups" at a significantly higher rate than the white population. The low socioeconomic status of these groups means that those children who are most likely to suffer health problems related to obesity are those who can least afford the high cost of treatment.

According to the National Health and Nutrition Examination Study (NHANES), which compared Mexican American childhood obesity rates with those of black and white children,[6] among boys ages six to eleven 43 percent of Mexican Americans and 36 percent of blacks are overweight or at risk of becoming overweight, compared with 29 percent of whites. Among girls in the six-to-eleven age group, 38 percent of blacks have a significantly higher rate of being or at risk of becoming overweight, compared to 35 percent of Mexican Americans and 23 percent of whites. If we look at younger children, ages two to five, we see that Mexican Americans have the highest prevalence of being at risk of becoming overweight—23 percent compared to 19 percent of blacks and 21 percent of whites. The number of overweight babies and toddlers, from birth to age two, is also increasing—again, black girls are ahead of the rest: 26 percent are already overweight before their second birthday![7] Of the cultural, socioeconomic, and other factors that underlie these differing rates of childhood obesity— especially for recent immigrants—a combination of unfamiliar (possibly unsafe) neighborhood environments, cultural notions that restrict active play among girls, and caretakers (often grandparents) easily seduced by high-calorie treats for children may drive the rapid weight gain of Mexican American and other Latino girls.[8] An overweight teenage mother who arrived in the United States when she was two described it well, "My grandmother wouldn't let me play outside because in Peru girls only played in their yard and here in the United States we didn't have a yard. My mother won't let my daughter out to play here either."

Another study, the National Longitudinal Survey of Youth, looked at more than 8,200 children ages four to twelve from 1986 to 1998 and found a significant increase in the number of black and Hispanic children in the "overweight" and "at risk" categories (85th percentile and above on growth charts) but not in the number of white children.[9] This suggests that the increase among white kids in these categories is leveling off. But wait; another federal study that follows the same girls by measuring them annually until age nineteen reported in 2002 that the rate of obesity during adolescence had doubled in both black and white girls. By age nineteen more than half of black girls and nearly half of white girls were overweight or obese. Of the heaviest, one in three black and one in five white girls was obese.[10] The striking increase among black and Mexican American adolescents

## CHILDHOOD OBESITY AROUND THE WORLD

While Americans hold the dubious distinction of being the world's fattest population, more and more young and older children around the globe are following their lead in becoming overweight. Globalization fuels the worldwide expansion of the behemoths of the American food industry, and as Whoppers and Frappuccinos spread to other lands, so do American-style food preferences and portion sizes. Relatively cheap food, high in nutritionally empty calories, is now within reach of families in developed and developing countries alike. In addition, more families in developing countries now have access to TVs, labor-saving devices, and, perhaps the most seductive of all gadgets for kids, video games. All contribute to a reduction in physical activity.

The problem of being underfed is still greater than the problem of being overfed; undernutrition, and the effects of malnutrition and starvation, remain of urgent concern everywhere. An estimated 28 percent of the world's two billion children are underweight, compared to 17 percent who are overweight. Overall, nearly half the world's children are soon to be either too thin or too fat. These two faces of malnutrition are two sides of one coin and carry the same message—children are not getting the food that supports healthy growth and development.

In strong support of this concern, the World Health Organization (WHO) calls overeating the world's "fastest growing form of malnourishment." "For the first time in history the number of people worldwide who are both overweight and malnourished, estimated at 1.1 billion, equals the number who are underweight and malnourished. Obesity rates in China have quadrupled in the past decade, and obesity in the urban middle class in India is epidemic. In Columbia 41 percent of adults are overweight. The global spread of diet-linked disease presents one of the greatest medical challenges of the twenty-first century."

Parts of Europe, Asia, and South America mirror the United States, with reports of childhood obesity doubling in both boys and girls between 1980 and 1996. The WHO cites rising obesity rates among urban Asian children in 2002: 16 percent in Thailand, 20 percent in China, 13 percent in Vietnam—all matched with rising incidence of diabetes.

Among preschool children, the global prevalence of being overweight was 3.3 percent, with considerably higher rates of overweight children in the Middle East, northern Africa, and Latin America. As in older children, the rates of wasting (undernutrition) in these very young children were generally higher than those of being overweight; Africa and Asia had wasting rates three to four times higher than overweight rates. A worsening problem is that, worldwide, impoverished urban children are likely to be the fattest future adult generation. A large study in Thailand illustrates this trend in developing countries affected by globalization: 23 percent of urban and 7 percent of rural children in the second and third grades are at or above the 95th percentile on growth charts. Thailand's poor, urban children are the fattest. Canada represents the same pattern occurring in developed countries. Among elementary school children in multiethnic, low-income, inner-city neighborhoods of Montreal, there was an 8 percent prevalence of being overweight in 1993 that increased 1 percent annually over the next five years.

A large study of schoolchildren in Belgium highlighted obesity-related social distinctions in Europe. In Belgium, the rate of obesity doubled, and severe obesity was greater in lower economic groups. The United Kingdom experienced a shocking 60 to 70 percent increase of obesity among three- and four-year-olds during the 1990s.

Report after report from countries rich and poor, more and less developed, document a "global epidemic of fat" and stress that—contrary to popular perception—children in developing nations are at a special risk of being overweight. Previously undernourished, they are vulnerable targets of global marketing of high-calorie, low-nutrient food and drink: an American lifestyle.

*See p. 246 for source notes.*

between the early 1990s and 2000 also showed up in the NHANES survey: the highest rate of obesity in these groups—44 percent—is among Mexican American boys and girls twelve to nineteen years old. Yet overall, 46 percent of black teens are the heaviest group in the United States.[11]

American Indian children compete for the worst obesity statistic: 39 percent are overweight, a fact that by itself demands immediate attention about ways to improve the health and living environment of this minority group.[12] In contrast, the six largest Asian American ethnic groups (Chinese, Filipino, Asian Indian, Japanese, Korean, Vietnamese) have a fairly low prevalence of being overweight. There is reason for caution here too, though, as that rate is increasing rapidly among those born in the United States, and the longer these families are in this country, the higher their risk of becoming overweight.[13] Children elsewhere are rapidly catching up— the obesity epidemic has "gone global." (For an overview of the ramifications, see the box "Childhood Obesity around the World.")

The socioeconomic and educational levels of these minority groups partly explain these differing rates, which we examine when we look at the causes of the childhood obesity epidemic. But culture plays a large role in shaping body image ideals and consequently factors into the differing obesity rates as well. In predominately black or Latino neighborhoods, obesity is becoming the norm rather than the exception because of the combined forces that promote fatness among people living there. For example, East Harlem has the highest obesity rate of adults and children in New York City. A health worker there commented to me, "When everyone in the neighborhood is big, big is normal! No one thinks there is an obesity epidemic."

## THREE CHILDREN, THREE LEVELS OF RISK

To put a face on these statistics, and give immediacy to the physical and psychological consequences of being overweight, I developed "snapshots" of three seven-year-old children. Eddie, Maria, and Dwayne represent dozens of firsthand observations, interviews, and studies, and we will come back to them in later chapters as we study the causes of and potential remedies for childhood obesity.

Eddie is an active child who likes a variety of food and is on his way to lifelong healthy weight. Maria loves food and daydreaming, spends little time outside in her urban neighborhood, and may be at risk for excessive weight gain. Dwayne eats super-size meals with gusto, loves video games, avoids physical activity because of asthma, and faces immediate and long-term health and social problems because of his heavy weight.

All three children are in a healthy height range of about 4 feet (the recommended 50th percentile for seven-year-old boys and girls). Eddie weighs 50 pounds and has a body-mass index of 15, which puts him near the 50th percentile on the CDC's pediatric growth charts—well within the healthy range. His risk of weight-related disease is low. Maria weighs 58 pounds and has a BMI of 18, which puts her at the 85th percentile for girls her age. She is considered at risk of becoming overweight, with a medium risk for disease. Dwayne, at 70 pounds, has a BMI of 21 and is "off the charts"—well above the 95th percentile. Dwayne definitely is overweight and at a high risk for disease.

The number of youngsters with a BMI like Eddie's is dropping; the number resembling Maria's and Dwayne's is rising. Maria typifies the 16 percent of U.S. children ages six to eleven who fall in the "at risk of becoming overweight" category (up from 11 percent in 1980). Dwayne is among the 15 percent of six- to eleven-year-olds who are "overweight" and thus in the heaviest category (up from 7 percent in 1980). Dwayne suffers from asthma, which contributes to his inactivity, and he also is the target of teasing. When he tries to join a basketball game at school, for example, other kids make fun of him for his slowness and breathing difficulties. His diet and lifestyle will put him on a fast track to early diabetes, sleep apnea, and other health problems.

Not all overweight children grow into overweight adults and not all overweight adults were overweight as children. But the odds are against Maria and even higher against Dwayne. The overarching risk of childhood obesity is that it will "track" into adulthood, thereby setting up lifelong weight problems. Tracking studies follow obese children for several years or review childhood records of obese adults to determine how many remain obese. The evidence shows a direct predictive relationship between the age when children became overweight and the rate at which they were overweight as adults: *the earlier a child becomes overweight, the greater the risk of becoming an overweight adult.* For example, 53 percent of obese children ages three to five become obese adults, compared to 12 percent of those with a normal weight. If teens are overweight, their chances of remaining so as adults are very high. An overweight adolescent has a 70 percent chance of becoming an obese adult.[14]

For some, knowing "it's only a risk" may make it easier to think "It won't happen to me" or "My kids won't develop those diseases." But the risk is real. Think of it this way: parents conscientiously apply sunscreen to their children and steer clear of secondhand smoke in an effort to reduce their children's risk of developing cancer. They would be wise to own up to the risk of obesity-related health problems as well and to try to minimize that risk by helping their children maintain a healthy weight and fitness.

## CHILDHOOD LOST
## TO ADULT DISEASES AND EARLY DEATH

Significant health problems can strike youth who are seriously overweight. The physical ailments that accompany childhood obesity persist and generally worsen in adulthood. Each year that a fat child gets fatter, the chances of developing the chronic diseases that are linked to adult obesity become greater. More shocking, an obese child can expect a shorter life. A boy who reaches a BMI of 45 in his twenties cuts thirteen or as many as twenty years from his expected life span.[15]

The list of chronic diseases related to being overweight and obese in adulthood is long and recited often by health professionals. Many of these now burden overweight children. The more widely known ailments related to adult obesity are diabetes, cardiovascular disease, high blood pressure, and breathing difficulties. Obesity also is associated with less common and lesser known medical consequences:

Orthopedic problems (including Blount's disease) from increased weight on the growth plate of the hip, which damages the cartilage and causes pain and limits movement. Worse still, studies that followed obese teenage girls for twenty-five years found that "weight wears out the hips"; they were three times likelier than healthy-weight women to need a hip replacement later.[16]

Headaches (pseudotumor cerebri and other forms), characterized by increased pressure within brain tissue. Nearly 50 percent of children with this problem are overweight.

Fatty liver disease (nonalcoholic steatohepatitis), caused by high concentrations of liver activity necessary to handle increased fats circulating in the body. Related problems like gallstones and inflammation of the gall bladder may occur, especially if people are trying to lose weight.

Menstrual irregularities related to obesity, such as ovarian cysts (polycystic ovary disease), with symptoms that are every young woman's nightmare: acne, mood swings, facial hair, and balding—even infertility.[17]

Thick, dark velvety skin growths (acanthosis nigricans) in folds and creases, especially around the neck, a common symptom among obese children.

All of these conditions require expensive medical treatment and have the potential to compromise the basic quality of life. If the fatness epidemic spreads unchecked, so too will the suffering and financial burden that these medical conditions cause.

### TYPE 2 DIABETES

Perhaps the most alarming obesity-related disease among children is type 2 diabetes—formerly known as "adult-onset diabetes," since it used to be rare in children. Type 2 diabetes develops when glucose—a simple form of sugar that supplies energy to body cells—cannot get into cells and builds up in the bloodstream. Glucose comes mainly from food, mostly in carbohydrates that break down to sugar in the intestine and cause blood glucose to rise. In response, the pancreas releases the hormone insulin, which directs glucose from the blood into the cells, either for immediate use or to be stored in fat and muscle.

Over 90 percent of people diagnosed with type 2 diabetes are overweight. Either their bodies don't make enough insulin, or their cells begin to resist it. One theory is that excess fat produces a hormone called resistin, which makes it harder for insulin to escort sugar into cells—possibly an energy conservation measure. The pancreas at first reacts by making extra insulin but over time gets exhausted. As the glucose and insulin levels swing up and down, blood vessels are damaged, causing harm to the heart, nerves, kidneys, eyes—and even early death. People with kidney failure spend many hours each week hooked to machines to clean their blood. Others suffer circulation problems and even amputation of a foot or leg. Diabetes accounts for about 20 percent of all deaths among people over age twenty-five in the United States.

In contrast, type 1 diabetes is generally not associated with obesity. It is an autoimmune disease, which means the body attacks itself. The defense cells that usually target germs and foreign invaders mistake insulin-making cells in the pancreas for toxins and destroy them. Insulin must then be provided through injections.

Though statistics are scarce, some estimates of case reports in health clinics are that one in every one hundred U.S. children has type 2 diabetes—five times more than have type 1. The incidence of type 2 diabetes is highest among Native Americans, with the rate among the Pima Indians of Arizona recorded as the highest in the world: 50 percent among adults and possibly 45 percent among children and adolescents. Typically, rates are also high among African American and Mexican American compared to white children. Diabetes disproportionately affects low-income populations: for example, the rate of adult type 2 diabetes is particularly high in New York City's poorest neighborhoods—14 to 15 percent; in San Antonio, the rate is 17 percent of those who are poor compared to 5 percent among high-wage earners.[18] Because the symptoms are often vague or "silent" in type 2 (frequent infections, fatigue) compared to type 1 (frequent urination, unusual thirst, weight loss), most experts suspect that the rate of undiagnosed type 2 diabetes is much higher than we know.

Diagnosed with type 1 diabetes when they are quite young, many children learn to manage their disease very well. They eat foods and meals in prescribed amounts, timed to match their daily insulin dose and spurts of physical activity. I've worked with some kids who knew exactly how much bread and butter they could trade for ice cream. They knew what to do when they got dizzy on the soccer field or when they got the flu. In contrast, kids with type 2 tend to be less well equipped to get their disease under control. When type 2 diabetes strikes children who have gained excessive weight, they have to deal with new patterns of eating and activity on top of coping with the health and social problems from the obesity itself. I remember holding back tears when a nine-year-old overweight girl and her mother were told by the doctor that she would have to take insulin shots twice a day, weigh her food, and plan to walk every day. Her mother sobbed, "I lost my sister and mother to diabetes, and now Rosa—she's so young! The trips to the clinic, the cost of the medicine, taking all those shots— it's terrible!"

If there is any good news among the swelling statistics about obesity and type 2 diabetes in kids, it is this: weight loss and increased physical activity can reverse many of the symptoms, especially for young children. Some successful programs target children ages eight to ten. But the direct medical cost of treatment and medication for diabetes in the United States is $44 billion dollars each year; much of it comes from public health funds, mainly Medicaid. The indirect annual cost is $54 billion (disability, work loss, years of life lost), and the total annual cost of diabetes is nearly a trillion dollars![19]

### HEART DISEASE AND HYPERTENSION

Over the past fifty years, the overall death rate from heart disease has gone down. But among young people, surprisingly, it has gone up. In 2002 federal health officials reported a 10 percent increase in the rate of sudden cardiac death among fifteen- to thirty-four-year-olds from 1989 to 1998. Obesity is a major risk factor responsible for this rising rate of early death among young people.[20]

Children who steadily gain weight but are not yet obese are also likely to have high blood pressure, with a diagnosis of hypertension.[21] High blood pressure forces the heart to work harder to pump blood through arteries inflamed and narrowed by high amounts of saturated fats and excessive body weight. Because an imbalance in body fluids that affects blood pressure relates to eating too many high-salt foods and too few fruits and vegetables, modifying food choices helps control hypertension. Childhood blood pressure and change in BMI are the two most powerful and consistent predictors of adult blood pressure.[22] Blood pressure screening is recommended at periodic physical examinations beginning at age three. Children who are physically fit have lower blood pressure than kids who are not physically active. Evidence points to greater mental fitness too.[23]

## BREATHING DIFFICULTIES

More young children who are overweight have trouble breathing. Pressure from excessive fat near the breathing passage restricts their airway, cutting down their oxygen supply. It results in drowsiness with a sudden arousal to gasp for air. Obstructive sleep apnea occurs frequently in obese children, causing them to wake up a dozen times a night, gasping for breath. Disturbed sleep and sleep deprivation in turn cause daytime sleepiness and decreased activity.

Asthma is on the rise among all children, fat and thin; inner-city children have more symptoms than others. But overweight children with asthma, compared to non-obese asthma sufferers, use more medicine, wheeze more, and have a greater proportion of unscheduled emergency hospital visits.[24] And evidence points toward the association of both asthma and obesity with lowered physical activity and unhealthy eating patterns. Most current treatment for asthma assumes that allergies cause it. Newer thinking suggests instead that a mechanical defect, possibly genetic, trips the hair-trigger alarm to set off the choking symptoms that afflict millions of kids. Whatever the cause, excess body weight worsens the condition. Dwayne eats too much, gets fat and unfit—factors that by themselves result in breathing difficulties. Because he takes medication, anti-inflammatory drugs such as steroids, he feels sluggish and is prone to obesity. He is among the group of inner-city children affected the most by both asthma and obesity.[25]

## EARLY MATURATION

An increase in body fatness is associated with early sexual maturation. Young children who reach sexual maturity earlier than others their age face more physical and psychological challenges than their peers. Obesity magnifies and complicates the inherent problems they must handle in this sensitive stage of development.

Maturing sexually at a younger than average age is not itself a health risk, but it exposes children to the risks that go with maturation before they may be prepared to manage them. For example, obesity often influences two fertility events for girls—menarche (initial menstruation) and pregnancy. Being overweight as a young child may lead to early menarche at eight or nine years old (among girls of healthy weight the average age of menarche is eleven). Scientists explain the link of puberty to body fat in what they call the "critical fat hypotheses": a girl must reach a certain weight before her brain sends a message that she is capable of sustaining a pregnancy; reaching that weight thus unleashes a cascade of biological events, including production of estrogen, that culminate in sexual maturity. The hormone leptin, produced in fat tissue, apparently triggers these events earlier in girls with more fat tissue.[26]

The series of events and risks may go as follows: increased leptin in obese girls sets off early menarche, which increases the risk of being more sexually precocious, resulting in teen pregnancy; early and frequent pregnancies increase the likelihood of obesity during adolescence and in adulthood.

Girls as well as boys who mature rapidly in adolescence are, in general, more overweight than slowly maturing adolescents.[27] In addition to being heavier, overweight girls and boys often are taller than their normal-weight peers. These physical differences affect the ways their peers and adults treat them, and the expectation that children can act or converse at a level above their age may lead to frustration or failure for big kids. They may then withdraw from outside relationships and grow more isolated and dependent on the family.

## OBESITY'S PSYCHOLOGICAL RISKS

Fat kids are at high risk of emotional pain from others' scorn and ridicule. For an untold number of kids, this psychological pain hurts as much as—if not more than—the pain associated with obesity-related physical health problems. "The most widespread consequences of childhood obesity are psychosocial," noted William Dietz, a pediatrician and youth obesity research expert. "Obese children become targets of early and systematic discrimination. As they mature, the effects of discrimination become more culture-bound and insidious."[28]

This discrimination will be examined in depth in chapter 8, but we must mention it here as well, because discrimination and the resulting loss of self-esteem pose substantial risks to the psychological health of overweight children.

The 2000 National Longitudinal Survey of Youth reported that self-esteem decreased significantly in obese, compared to normal-weight, white and Hispanic girls and boys nine to fourteen years old. It linked lower levels of self-esteem with increased rates of sadness, loneliness, and nervousness. Obese children with decreasing levels of self-esteem were also more likely than their normal-weight peers to smoke and drink alcohol.[29] Obese children ages five to eighteen rated their quality of life as low as that of children diagnosed with cancer in a 2003 study. A related news headline said, "Obese Children's Lives Found Full of Despair."[30]

Does weight loss help self-esteem? Some studies find that weight-loss treatment appears to improve self-esteem in adolescents but suggest that repeated weight loss and regain may have harmful psychological effects, especially if "weight cycling" or "yo-yo" weight changes begin in early childhood and continue into adulthood. Attempts to reshape body size through dieting reinforce feelings of failure and lack of control when they do not produce the expected result. Yet the pursuit of thinness drives the desire to try dieting again—and again.

Both Maria and Dwayne will likely experience lots of teasing and embarrassment, even as young children. Name calling—"fatso," "lard butt," "blubber"—will pick up as they enter their teens and could turn into threats. "Let's see if the air comes out when I poke the fat thing." Or "If I had those hips I'd cut 'em off with a butcher knife. Let's squeeze those hips behind the door." Small children's bruised feelings prickle and burn as they get older, dodge the daily insults, and muster the strength to face each day in our fat-prejudiced society. In addition, Maria and Dwayne will surely be targets and potential victims of the $6 billion diet industry, replete with seductive products for quick weight loss and perfect bodies.

## SUMMARY

This chapter took a close look at *who* is affected by the childhood obesity epidemic. It highlighted the fact that not only are children in all age groups getting fatter, they are getting *fatter faster* than ever before. Black, Hispanic, and Native American children have the highest rates of obesity in the United States. The global spread of obesity has reached children in both developed and developing countries, affecting children who are first undernourished and then become overnourished—both conditions are forms of malnutrition. We should not underestimate the danger of obesity's spread; the fatter these young people become, the more likely they are to experience a litany of costly physical and psychological problems that diminish their quality of life and in some cases lead to early death.

Part 1 laid a foundation for understanding this epidemic by presenting its definitions, scope, and costs. Now we can turn to part 2's essential question: *why* are kids getting fatter?

# PART TWO

# WHY KIDS
# ARE GETTING FATTER

# 3

---

# FAMILY MATTERS

---

"OBESE," FROM THE LATIN WORD "obesus," means "grown fat by eating." The term's origin clearly and correctly suggests that overeating is a major cause of the obesity epidemic. Teaching overweight children to eat less therefore is essential. But modifying behavior is no simple task, and eating too much is not the sole cause of obesity. Other factors play a role and must be well understood in order to reverse the epidemic and produce a healthier generation of children.

Comments I heard at a parent-teacher school board meeting in an inner-city New York district shed light on some of these less obvious contributing factors, such as limited access to healthy foods, unsafe settings for outdoor play, and a lack of parental awareness about what constitutes healthy eating. The meeting focused on students' health and the spike in obesity. "A trip to the farmer's market would be too dangerous in this neighborhood," a teacher said. "We usually call the kids in early from recess when they start fighting," noted a playground aide. One parent, herself obese, apparently believed that her children ate well and didn't need nutrition education: "When I was sick, my daughter set out the dips to go with the chicken nuggets—she knew what to do."

We have all observed that some individuals maintain a normal weight while others who eat the same amount grow fat. Some teenagers willingly eat a variety of vegetables and whole grains while others eat little from these food groups (other than fries and hamburger buns). And some kids regularly ride bikes and play soccer or pickup ball while others spend every afternoon glued to the television. What accounts for these differences? The answers—which begin to unlock the causes of the obesity epidemic—involve genetics, socioeconomic factors, culture, parenting styles, the marketplace, and public policy. "Nature" and "nurture" have conspired to produce an unprecedented number of overweight kids. This chapter focuses on *nature*—the hereditary factors that put children at a higher risk for becoming overweight—and then shifts to *nurture,* introducing the environmental factors that fatten the generations of today and tomorrow.

## NATURE'S PART IN THE EQUATION

Desperate for explanations, frustrated parents and sympathetic observers posit that genetics almost exclusively determines obesity. I often hear parents say that all their family members are big because "it runs in our genes." Echoing their parents, some fat children say they are "born that way." Their attitude shifts the blame away from personal behavior and social influences and toward human biology.

While those comments might sound to some like hackneyed excuses for being overweight, it is true that people with "fat genes" are "programmed" to gain more weight than others. But genetics alone cannot explain the obesity explosion, because the gene pool could not change as rapidly as the current rate of increased obesity has. Research suggests that inherited biological factors may affect body weight by as little as 20 percent or as much as 60 percent, which leaves a large margin for environmental factors to influence weight. Moreover, it is exceedingly difficult to quantify with any certainty the degree to which inherited factors cause obesity because, as we'll see below, biological and environmental factors are so tightly intertwined. (When I refer to "environmental factors," I'm using the term broadly to include behavior and lifestyle as well as the home and social setting.)

Nearly twenty-five hundred years ago, Plato gave us the concepts of *nature* and *nurture,* asserting that in the formation of any human behavior, both genetic endowment and cultural influences play essential roles.[1] Ever since then, scientists in various disciplines have sought to determine the degree to which genes or environment influence development, thus creating the ceaseless nature/nurture debate. Arguing for the primacy of one or the other sets up an unnecessary opposition. It is not a matter of genes *or* environment or of genes *versus* environment, but of genes *and* environment that act when a person becomes fat.

Think of it this way: just as undernourished children get sick first when a measles epidemic erupts, some kids are more vulnerable than others in the obesity epidemic. Genetics is one reason for this vulnerability. Certain genes increase a child's potential for becoming fat, and then other forces that fall under the nurture category trigger that genetic predisposition until he or she actually becomes overweight.

The human body has a marvelously complex system of regulating weight by controlling appetite and determining how much energy is burned or stored as excess fat. The brain and its chemical messengers, in the form of hormones and proteins, work to keep this system balanced and functioning. An individual's genetic makeup, or *genotype,* provides the blueprint for this system and thus affects its functioning in several ways. For example, genes are linked to *metabolism,* the way in which a body burns energy; to *set point,* the narrow range of weight a person gains or loses under normal conditions; and to *satiety,* the feeling of fullness. Genes determine whether a person is likely to store excess energy from food as fat or lean muscle or, regardless of diet, to burn more fat than carbohydrate.

Genes also determine where fat is stored, which in turn establishes a person's body shape. In lay terms, people generally inherit either an "apple-shape" body, which concentrates fat around the stomach, or a "pear-shape" body, which stores fat more on the lower body. A person with an apple shape may be a skinny apple if food is scarce and may become a fat apple if food is abundant, but no amount of dieting or overeating will change an "apple" body into a "pear." The traditional idea of the mesomorph (muscular, broad shoulders), endomorph (short, round shoulders, big bottom), and ectomorph (tall and skinny) classifications represents another way that different body shapes express our genetic blueprint (Figure 3). Genes therefore provide a primary (but not exclusive) explanation for why individuals who grow up in similar environments and eat similar diets—siblings, for instance—can have different body shapes and different rates for gaining or losing weight.

### SURVIVAL OF THE FATTEST

To protect against starvation, the evolutionary process promoted a genotype that encourages fatness and discourages thinness. It is a "thrifty" geno-

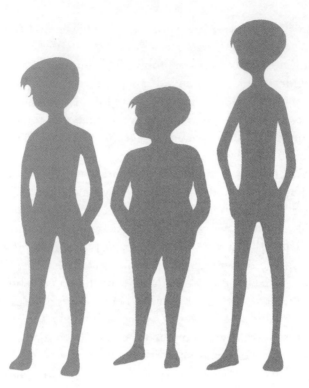

FIGURE 3. Children are genetically programmed to have different body types. (Adapted from "See How They Grow—Body Types Are Different," National Dairy Council, 1970)

type that puts on weight and keeps it on as a survival response to famine and other hardships that plagued earlier generations. People with a genetic predisposition to thinness—the ones we consider lucky these days—would not have survived the scarcity and harsh conditions that early humans faced, but the fittest *and fattest* thrived, passing on their genetic traits to future generations. In 1962 the geneticist J. V. Neel identified this thrifty genotype and proposed a fascinating hypothesis for obesity: that our genotype, essential to survival in the past, has instead become a detriment to good health in today's environment of excess food and easy living.[2] Our environment and lifestyle have changed quickly, in a matter of decades, but our biological systems have not caught up and adapted; they remain "pro-grammed" to pack on pounds rather than to resist excessive weight gain.

Neel's hypothesis has been supported by numerous studies of the Pima Indians in Arizona, a tribe that has been involved since the early 1960s in studies sponsored by the National Institutes of Health to understand the root causes of diabetes and obesity. The Pimas' genes, so protective of fat-ness during famine, became the enemy in the current environment, lead-ing to obesity and diabetes.[3]

Obesity runs in families because of these shared genes and because of shared environments as well. We know this from everyday observations and from research studies; children with two obese parents are more than six times as likely to become obese than children of non-obese parents. Ge-netic factors collaborate with behavioral and social factors to pass obesity from parents to kin. For example, infants with obese mothers suck more vigorously, which suggests a genetic basis to an infant's eating style.[4] Yet a mother of a vigorously sucking child is also likely to feed the child more milk than she would if the child showed less response. The mother's re-sponse can override the infant's internal cues of fullness and establish a feed-ing cycle that prompts overeating.

"Assortative mating," jargon for selecting a partner based on common char-acteristics, represents another way that genetic factors link with environ-mental ones to promote heavier kids. German researchers have found that assortative mating between obese adults is common among parents of seri-ously overweight children, and they propose that social stigmatization of fat people leads these overweight individuals to choose each other as partners.[5]

A complicated relationship between genetics and the environment also determines the body's ability to recognize fullness and regulate the amount of food consumed. Still, we (and mice) learn to override these signals. Stud-ies of obese mice suggest that the environment activates certain hormones, which cause them to eat past the point of fullness. A substance called melanin-concentrating hormone (MCH) is one of them, and this hor-mone's gene is two to three times more active in the brains of obese mice and possibly in ours. Seeing and smelling food may unleash MCH and cause a "pizza effect"; that is, if the smell of something tasty triggers the hormone's release, a subject will be inclined to eat again because "even though you are not hungry and you don't need the energy, you still eat the pizza because you know it will taste good."[6]

The manner and setting in which a child is fed and learns to eat often override that child's internal system for recognizing hunger and fullness.

While the body's chemistry sends out appetite signals in an effort to regulate the amount the child eats, environmental cues may blank out internal ones. The result—no surprise—is weight gain.

## RESETTING THE SYSTEM

Scientists studying the body's system for regulating weight have discovered that "yo-yo dieting" and overeating interfere with the body's finely tuned system in ways that ratchet up the difficulties for anyone who is obese and tries to reach and maintain a normal weight. People who repeatedly or drastically diet prompt their genetic protection against starvation to kick in; the body slows its metabolism and works to regain the lost weight. If the weight returns, the body clings to these fat stores defensively, making weight loss much harder the second or third time around. (Oprah's famous ups and downs in her battle of the bulge come to mind.) Extreme under- and overeating can also reset a person's "set point" and allow for greater range of weight gain than before. These findings support the commonsense wisdom that quickie weight-loss schemes ("Lose 30 pounds in 30 days on the ice cream diet!") generally do more harm than good. But moderate, long-term, and preventive strategies can work *with* rather than against the body's internal system to reach and keep a healthy weight.

Advances in the field of genetics have led to increased hope—and hype—that science will find a way to manipulate the body's chemistry, perhaps leading to clinical treatment or prevention applications. Pharmaceutical companies are racing to develop drugs they can market as a solution to obesity. But finding key molecules that are potential targets for manipulation is one step; "rewiring" the faulty circuits concerned with energy balance is another. Ongoing research involving the hormone leptin illustrates the complexities and challenges that face scientists in this field.

Leptin (from the Greek word for "thin" or "slender") regulates several functions involved in weight management, including appetite and food response in the brain and possibly physical activity and calorie burning in the body. When scientists discovered in 1994 that deficiencies in leptin caused mice to become grossly fat, the news brought hope to millions of obese people who thought that leptin supplements could be their ticket to thinness. It turns out, however, that fat people produce plenty of leptin, but they are resistant to it—possibly owing to consistent overeating.

On the whole, however, scientists are making rapid advances in understanding the genetic dimension of the obesity epidemic. Discoveries have been made of genetic disorders that result in severe obesity, such as Bardet-Biedl and Prader-Willi syndromes. These are rare disorders that are present at birth and result from genetic mutations. Bardet-Biedl, which is associated with mental retardation and impaired vision, affects one in a hundred thousand; Prader-Willi, caused by a missing gene on chromosome 15, is characterized by short stature, voracious appetite, and decreased mental capacity, and it affects one in twelve thousand children. We look to the genetic causes of these disorders with high hopes that they will reveal important clues for preventing and treating obesity in the general population.

A 1996 review identified several genes that contribute to the inheritance of body fat and its location in mice. And it linked at least eleven genes in humans to susceptibility to obesity.[7] The *Human Obesity Gene Map*, published in 2003, reported that twenty-five genetic disorders exhibiting obesity as a symptom have been mapped; there are now 250 genes, markers, and chromosomal regions linked with human obesity.[8] The authors note that the main tasks now are to identify how the genes and mutations combine to predispose a person to obesity and in what environmental circumstances they act. (See the box "A 'Fidget Factor'?")

Some researchers hope to establish that human obesity can result from a simple fault in the genetic regulation of energy balance "without the need to implicate complex social and environmental factors." "If this fact were known," they write, "obesity would be validated as a medical condition deserving of sympathetic handling and worthy of scientific study."[9] But there's no reason to wait for a scientific breakthrough to pursue and provide "sympathetic handling" of the social and environmental aspects of obesity. Its link to poverty, the marketplace, and discrimination makes those who struggle with their weight deserving of society's sympathetic concern, not scorn. Moreover, the goal of finding a purely genetic explanation for obesity seems far-fetched. A single genetic disorder leads to obesity only in very rare circumstances. (Thus when a child becomes seriously overweight, a specialist should screen for underlying conditions—like the genetic disorders Prader-Willi, Bardet-Biedl, and Cohen syndromes—that involve obesity as one of multiple symptoms.) In the vast majority of cases, a tangled and interdependent relation between nature and nurture causes an individual to become overweight. If only there were something beyond anyone's control—a genetic flaw, a malfunctioning gland, or even a virus—that caused obesity, it would be more likely to elicit sympathy than abhorrence and blame.

## A "FIDGET FACTOR"?

What about a genetic link to voluntary physical activity—do genes give some children a propensity to be spontaneously active and others to sit quietly? To some degree, yes. But, again, nature interacts with nurture. The body spends energy (measured as calories) in two ways: voluntary and involuntary activity. Voluntary activity is choosing to run or to sit. Involuntary activity is breathing, maintaining body temperature, digesting food, and moving nutrients and waste products throughout the body. Genes affect both types of activity.

Some people are more inclined to stand than to sit, to run than to walk—voluntary, but spontaneous, activities (as opposed to deliberate voluntary exercise, such as going to the gym). Family studies indicate that when both parents are spontaneously active, their children are more than five times as likely to be active as children with two inactive parents. And family and twins studies estimate the propensity to be spontaneously active as about 30 percent genetically based. One comparison of three- to five-year-old non-obese children with obese parents to children with lean parents shows that the former burn fewer calories during both rest and activity, suggesting that both involuntary and voluntary activity are partially genetically driven. Over time, burning less energy contributes to gaining weight, even if young children with obese parents seem as active as kids with lean parents.

From birth, some children spend more energy than others, even when participating in identical activities. Called the "fidget factor," energy spent in nonvoluntary physical activity—such as fidgeting or maintaining an erect posture and flexed muscles when sitting or standing—might explain why some children who spend long hours sitting at video games and television may not gain as much weight as others. The energy spent on these movements is called non-exercise activity thermogenesis (thermogenesis is the creation of heat or energy) and helps explain why some people are resistant to weight gain, even when they eat more or move less than others of the same body size.

Does a genetic bias toward inactivity show up in the cradle? A 1988 study using a sophisticated method to measure all the energy spent in voluntary and involuntary physical activity of three-month-old infants born to lean and overweight mothers suggested a genetic role in future activity level. But follow-up research made quite clear that excessive calories from food intake, not energy output, is the most significant factor in excessive body weight of one- and two-year-old infants.

For older children too, evidence of genetic bias is hard to pick up. Moving pictures taken of fat and lean girls playing tennis for identical time periods show that lean girls make significantly more body movements than fat girls. When Jean, whose BMI is 13, plays tennis with Sara, whose BMI is 16, Jean dances on her toes between shots, while Sara stands still. Perhaps

Sara is simply less fit than Jean and rests between shots, spending less energy. Even so, a genetic disposition toward less movement, even as a younger child, may partly explain Sara's current heavier weight and slower physical movement. But nothing shows which came first—Sara's slow movement, or her extra weight and low fitness.

Overall, maintaining energy balance—eating and spending the same number of calories—is the key to achieving a healthy body weight. An average five-year-old child consumes and spends (in both voluntary and involuntary activity) over half a million calories per year. Considering the large volume of calories a child's body must process, we marvel at the fine-tuning of energy balance healthy weight involves. Yet very small amounts of overeating and underactivity can lead to obesity. A startling fact is that over time, thirty calories of excess food a day—or fifteen minutes of daily television watching instead of play—can cause a child to become overweight! Genetics may tip the balance in favor of storing or spending energy, and less time spent in active play also matters, but the major reason for the current out-of-balance energy equation is overeating.

*See p. 250 for source notes.*

A fictional version of the wish for a physical cause plays out in a popular novel for teenagers, *Life in the Fat Lane,* by Cherie Bennett. Lara, the central character, first appears as a trim high school beauty pageant queen and then doubles her weight in a year. To explain this phenomenon, the author concocted a disease and added two scientists who discovered it among "teens who ate next to nothing, under strictly controlled circumstances, yet continued to gain weight." When Lara's shocked parents hear the diagnosis, they say, "At least you don't have cancer." Lara yells back, "I'd rather have cancer than this!" Her sole solace lies in the notion that her loathsome bulk is a physical illness—beyond her control.[10]

Unfortunately for overweight children outside her fictitious universe, research is far from finding a simple—or, for some, guilt-free—explanation for their condition.

## NURTURE WEIGHS IN

We cannot change nature (barring scientific breakthroughs), but to varying degrees we can control and modify the elements that constitute its co-conspirator—nurture. To a large extent, the environment in which we raise kids today drives the obesity epidemic. More than ever before, children are growing up in an environment, both inside and outside the home, that promotes excessive food intake and discourages physical activity. A review of the key factors that put some children at a higher risk for excessive weight gain shows that most relate to nurture, not nature.

What are these pivotal risk factors? Research and my own professional experience lead me to consider five elements when predicting whether children will become overweight:

Parental obesity: children with two obese parents are more than six times as likely to become obese than children with non-obese parents. Children with only one obese parent are twice as likely to become obese as adults.[11]

Unhealthful eating patterns and parenting styles: children raised in families who do not regularly prepare and eat family meals together are more likely to be overweight. Children whose parents exert an excessive degree of control over what and how much their children eat are more likely to be unable to regulate their food intake in a healthy manner.

Low physical activity: children are more likely to be overweight if they lack opportunities to participate in active recreation and sports and/or are not encouraged to engage in physical play.

Excessive "screen time": children who spend several hours daily watching television, playing video games, or working on the computer are at a greater risk for weight gain.

Low socioeconomic status: poverty and low education are predictors of obesity. The lower the family income, the greater the likelihood of being overweight.

## POVERTY AND OBESITY

In the following chapters I explore these risk factors. But perhaps the most intractable of them all, the one that shapes so many behaviors in the nurture category and poses perhaps the greatest challenge in the epidemic, is low socioeconomic status.

A large research literature analyzes how and why obesity relates to low social and economic status; the fields of history, sociology, nutrition, communications, psychology, and public health offer varying perspectives. Gender, culture, and discrimination all play a role. But however you approach it, the statistics are clear: children from low-income and less-educated families have a much greater risk for obesity. Federal statistics show that about 23 percent of whites and 34 percent of blacks who earn $15,000 or less annually are obese. Those obesity figures drop to about 16 percent of whites and 23 percent of blacks when they earn $50,000 or more. Children in families with parents who were educated beyond high school (thirteen or more years) are far less likely to be overweight than children from families whose parents are illiterate or poorly educated. The link between poverty and obesity isn't confined to America; developing countries view it as "a new public health challenge."[12]

Why are the poorest—those who presumably have the least amount of money to spend on food—the fattest? The answer, at once personal and political, has much to do with a "toxic environment" of unhealthy food choices, unsafe streets, and unavailable parents.

## A "TOXIC ENVIRONMENT"

The unfortunate truth is that today's environment puts *all* children, even those with few or no risk factors for obesity, at risk for excessive weight gain. "We live in a toxic environment, one that is almost supremely designed to cause us to gain weight," said David Ludwig, M.D., Ph.D., head of the Optimal Weight for Life program at Boston's Children's Hospital.[13] I agree—it is an environment that is slowly but surely sickening our population.

Kelly Brownell, Ph.D. and chair of the department of psychology at Yale University, coined the term "toxic environment" in a 1994 *New York Times* editorial. Looking for ways to reduce the availability of inexpensive, convenient foods high in both fat and calories, Brownell called for a tax on certain foods, including soda. During the controversy this acquired the label "Twinkie tax." Brownell and colleagues now argue, "As the environment worsens, so does obesity. Biology permits obesity to occur in the individual, but the environment causes obesity in the culture. We are preoccupied with why individuals are obese and how to help them, rather than with why society is obese and how to help it."[14]

In this environment, food high in calories and low in nutrients is available everywhere, and it's cheap; manufacturers push highly processed food products, loaded with excessive calories from added sugars and fats, for every age group; huge portion sizes are the norm at restaurants and, increasingly, at home. At school, soft drink industry giants compete for "pouring rights" while recess and physical education disappear from daily schedules. On television, in the grocery aisle, and at almost every turn, the marketplace hawks junk-food products and extols movement-saving devices. (Chapter 5 takes up these environmental factors outside the home.)

Crime—or the fear of it—also factors in and links obesity with low socioeconomic status. Kids who are not allowed to run outside and play are left with few alternatives but to sit around indoors. The *New York Times* profiled a family who keenly experienced these circumstances. An African American mother living on Chicago's South Side rarely allowed her two adolescent boys to venture outside because of the neighborhood's rampant crime. Robert, seventeen years old and 5 foot 9, ballooned to 415 pounds; Jeffrey, fifteen and 5 foot 8, grew to 280 pounds. Robert developed type 2 diabetes and spent several months in the hospital before dropping out of high school because he tired so quickly and got out of breath when he moved around.[15]

Fast-paced lives and tough economic times have made parents of all incomes and backgrounds busier than ever, constantly pressed for time and struggling to meet the demands of work and family life. Harried parents often are unavailable, too tired, or simply lacking in interest and know-how to prepare healthy meals and play actively with their kids. For them, fast-food takeout or "heat-'n'-eat" packaged meals are cheap and easy alternatives that prove irresistible. Parents grab food on the go and snack mindlessly while working or watching TV; their children follow suit.

## RECOMMENDATIONS VS. REALITY

The result of these environmental factors is a society in which fewer and fewer children and adults follow the most basic recommendations for healthy living. For eye-opening proof, consider the U.S. Department of Agriculture (USDA) dietary guidelines and the much-publicized Food Guide Pyramid. The guidelines synthesize reasonable recommendations that, if followed properly, would go a long way toward reducing obesity.[16]

Contrasting some of these government-endorsed recommendations with the reality proves what most of us already know from everyday observations: American families have a terribly unbalanced diet and inactive lifestyle. These facts alone speak volumes about the causes of the childhood obesity epidemic and serve as an informative backdrop to the chapters that follow.

| | |
|---|---|
| *Aim for a healthy weight.* | · 61 percent of American adults are overweight or obese. |
| | · 25 percent of youth ages twelve to nineteen and 33 percent of children six to eleven are overweight or at risk of becoming overweight. |
| *Be physically active each day.* | · Only 29 percent of high school students and 35 percent of middle school students participated in daily school physical education in 1999. Of those who did, only 38 percent were physically active in the class for more than twenty minutes. |
| | · At least 43 percent of adolescents watch television more than two hours every school day; children ages seven to eleven spend three hours playing video games or watching television daily. |
| | · 40 percent of adults engaged in no leisure-time physical activity in 1997.[17] |
| *Choose the recommended number of daily servings from the five major food groups; aim for variety and note serving size* (servings *are recommended amounts, whereas* portions *are amounts commonly offered*). | · Children typically eat less than the recommended number of servings from the vegetable, fruit, and dairy groups, and they eat an excessive number of servings from the meat and bread groups. Moreover, they tend to consume less-healthy alternatives from the meat and bread groups—in particular, red meat and white bread rather than lean poultry or fish and whole grains.[18] |
| | · The most commonly available food portions exceed standard serving sizes. The bagel as commonly offered, for example, is 5 inches in diameter, weighs 4 oz, and equals approximately *four* pyramid servings; 2 cups of spaghetti commonly offered as a single portion equal four of the ½ cup pyramid serving size; one medium order of fries (4 oz) equals four of the pyramid's portions (1 oz).[19] One McDonald's value meal, consisting of a 6 oz hamburger and large fries, includes three servings of meat, four servings of bread, and |

four servings of fried potatoes—enough for three children ages three to six or two older children.

*Eat at least two servings of fruits and at least three servings of vegetables each day.*

- Children eat only two to three servings of the five recommended vegetables and fruits daily, and one serving is likely to be fried potatoes or potato chips.[20]

- Many children, but especially children of overweight parents, have diets high in fat (high-calorie foods) and low in fruits and vegetables (low-calorie foods).[21]

*Choose beverages and foods to moderate your sugar consumption.*

- The American food supply provides 156 pounds of added sugars (mainly sucrose and corn syrup) per person per year. Children ages two to six consume about 13 teaspoons of added sugars a day (children ages one to three years should have no more than 6 teaspoons of added sugar a day; ages four to six, no more than 9 teaspoons). Adolescents and adults consume more than 33 teaspoons of added sugars a day. On a 2,000-calorie daily diet, no more than 10 teaspoons are recommended—the amount in one 12 oz soft drink.[22]

- About 35 percent of added sugars comes from soft drinks made with high-fructose corn syrup, about 15 percent from sweetened cereals and pastries, and 10 percent from fruit drinks. Sweetened cereals contain nearly 4 teaspoons of sugar per serving. A significant amount of added sugar is hidden in otherwise healthy food, such as spaghetti sauce, low-fat yogurt with added sweetened fruit, and even whole-wheat bread—sucrose and high-fructose corn syrup are often high up on the list of ingredients.[23]

- Annual sales of soda average 56 gallons per person in the United States. On any given day, 37 percent of children ages two to six consume an average of 10 oz of soda. Six-to eleven-year-olds drink an average of 15 oz a day; twelve- to nineteen-year-olds drink an average of 18 to 28 oz each day.[24] A 12 oz can of soda has the equivalent of 9 teaspoons of added sugar (usually corn syrup) and 150 calories.

· In 1978 children drank 4.0 times more milk than soft drinks; in 1998 they drank only 1.5 times more milk than soft drinks (soda), fruit drinks (5–10 percent fruit juice), and fruit-ades (fruit flavoring and sugar). Both the amount and the frequency of children's drinking these beverages were higher in 1998 than ever before.[25]

*Choose a diet that is low in saturated fat and cholesterol and moderate in total fat.*

· Girls and boys ages six to eleven consume at least 33 percent of all calories from fat (30 percent or less is recommended) and 12 percent from saturated fat (8–10 percent is recommended).[26]

· Between 1989 and 1996, adolescents ages eleven to eighteen increased total fat consumed by 4 percent, much of it from fried potatoes.[27]

· On a positive note, about 25 percent of whole milk consumed by six- to eleven-year-old children is now replaced by low-fat milk (which has less saturated fat). Elementary school meals dropped from 36 to 33 percent of calories from fat after implementation of revised USDA guidelines in 1998. Most restaurant meals contribute 36 percent from calories from fat (14 percent is saturated fat).[28]

Why are eating and activity patterns of American families so out of line with these recommendations? In the blame game of the childhood obesity epidemic, parents usually get tagged as the chief culprits. After all, parents are supposed to raise healthy children and steer them away from damaging influences. Many believe that having a fat child indicates some defect in the quality of parenting—and, regrettably, in some instances it does. But this blanket condemnation unfairly overlooks the genetic and environmental factors over which parents have little control.

## SUMMARY

We now know that nature and nurture have conspired to produce an unprecedented number of overweight children. Many genetic factors, often interrelated, predispose children to easy weight gain. Fat storage, appetite, body shape, and even activity level are to varying degrees genetically driven. Nurture's part of the obesity epidemic involves low socioeconomic status, unhealthful eating patterns and parenting styles, low physical activity, and excessive screen time (television, video games, computers). The marketplace and public policy allow an environment that some call "toxic," littered with highly advertised processed food products, loaded with excessive calories in huge portions available at school, at home, anytime. Comparison of the American family's unbalanced diet and inactive lifestyle to government-endorsed recommendations backs up that reality.

Just as children are born with certain hereditary factors that increase their risk for obesity, so too they inherit a demographic profile that can and often does put them at a higher risk for poor nutrition and excessive weight gain. The remainder of part 2 takes a closer look at the nurture factors that have cultural, economic, and political dimensions: chapter 4 explores ways in which parenting styles and the home setting influence a child's eating and activity patterns, while chapter 5 traces influences beyond the home that affect a child's weight. We often return to issues of class and culture, as they influence the parenting skills, lifestyles, and larger social context that encourage obesity.

# 4

--------------------------------------------------------

# AT HOME

--------------------------------------------------------

IN 1953 THE PSYCHIATRIST Hilde Bruch—the "mother" of our current understanding about overeating and eating disorders—said that to understand obese children, we need to remember that each of them accumulated their extra weight "while living in a family that, wittingly or unwittingly, encouraged overeating and inactivity."[1] A half century later, with obesity at epidemic levels, researchers are saying roughly the same thing: "Behaviors that contributed to the increase in overweight prevalence for adults may be transmitted within the family setting and affect the weight status of children."[2]

I agree that family behaviors and interactions undoubtedly contribute greatly to childhood obesity, but I caution against focusing so sharply on the family as to overlook factors outside the home that fuel the epidemic as well. Clearly we need to study the family at home to understand and curtail childhood obesity. Home is where the market's plentiful products show up, where children's habits form and flourish, and where fatness and fitness begin.

In attacking disease epidemics, public health workers look for three components: the host, the agent, and the environment. Any one is a potential point of intervention. In the fatness epidemic, the home harbors all three—the host is the child, the agent is excess calories from food and drink, and the environment encompasses the behavior, lifestyle, and surroundings that promote excess eating and insufficient activity. Home therefore is the logical—and potentially the most effective—starting point for intervention.

Home is not what it used to be. Traditional nuclear families dwindled to 23.5 percent of all households in 2000.[3] The balance may be single parents previously wed or never wed, some of their children living in shared-custody arrangements, "blended" families with children from other marriages, or unwed couples with children. The swiftly changing family unit is an easy target for assaults on the relentlessly fattening forces of the toxic environment. But whether kids are raised by a gay or unmarried couple, stepfamily, or single parent, what matters is that the parent(s) have the resources, interest, and know-how to raise children with healthy eating and activity habits. Even so, families who are struggling and in transition—among them many single-parent and blended-family households—often experience higher levels of stress and demands on their time, which in turn can foster overeating, excessive television watching, and little active playing.[4]

This chapter begins with glimpses of three children and their families as we try to trace the causes of childhood obesity that relate, directly or indirectly, to family dynamics and demographics. The remainder of this chapter elaborates on these causes, moving from prenatal care through early childhood and adolescence.

## INSIDE THE HOME

Studying a family's behavior is rather complicated. Short of using a "candid camera" to record what happens throughout the house, we can't observe and measure what actually takes place. Noted one researcher, "Even if we could accurately describe what occurs in a family, reality may not be as important as family members' perceptions of what occurs in explaining eating behaviors."[5] That said, research offers an overview of the ways in which family members and the home environment influence children's eating and activity.

We'll use that research, combined with my own personal and professional observations and interviews, as we turn to the three seven-year-old children—Eddie, Maria, and Dwayne—whom we met in chapter 2 and who represent the "normal," "at risk," and "overweight" categories for children their age and height.

### EDDIE

Eddie, a lanky redhead, is the youngest of three in a busy suburban family. His mother works as a fundraiser for a nonprofit organization, sometimes in the evening. Eddie's father is an architect. Eddie walks seven blocks to school with his older brother, who is ten. On two school days, he spends the afternoon at soccer or softball practice or swimming, coming home by carpool on those days. On other afternoons after school, Eddie and his brother participate in supervised after-school programs; when school is closed, they play in the yard or play video games indoors with their older sister in charge.

Dieting is not an issue in Eddie's home; it doesn't have to be, because the family's food and activities equal good weight management. On most nights their mom starts supper preparations around six o'clock, working from a menu planned by the whole family on Sunday evening. She calls the boys to help. Sometimes Eddie drags his feet and complains about turning off his Gameboy, but he is starting to enjoy his job of washing and cutting vegetables, sorting the pots and pans, setting the table, and an occasional juggling lesson using oranges with his brother. At least a couple of nights a week, his father returns from work early enough to prepare a favorite main course while his mother packs the next day's school lunches and helps Eddie's brother and sister with their homework.

Eddie's parents both work forty hours a week outside their home, so they divide up grocery shopping. One night when his father came home bearing grocery bags, Eddie demanded, "Did you get the cookie-crunch cereal I told you I liked at Roger's house?" His dad pulled out two cereal boxes— one the cookie-crunch kind, the other the whole-grain O's, saying, "You know the deal: the sweet stuff is for Saturdays or just for topping on the other one."

The kitchen is noisy—not from television, but from everyone talking. The one household TV set is in the family room. When Eddie and his father put the groceries away, the apples, tangerines, bags of baby carrots, cheese sticks, and applesauce go on the shelf labeled "snacks," along with a pitcher of water to remind refrigerator raiders what to drink. The wheat crackers and oatmeal cookies go on the cupboard shelf marked "packed lunches and snacks." Two small containers (not a huge tub) of ice cream favorites go into the freezer for family dessert a couple of nights a week. The weekly shopping includes fresh seasonal fruits, such as strawberries, mango, pineapple, or watermelon, for the family's twice-weekly dessert "fruit ceremony." This dessert event, begun when the children were first on solid foods, is a time to taste and talk about a new or different fruit.

Eddie likes cereal, milk, and fruit for breakfast and sometimes eats toast with peanut butter instead of cereal. His lunch usually consists of a piece of fruit, some veggies, a sandwich, pretzel, cookie, and milk. Ever since pre-school, his mother has packed cut-up veggies in his lunch. He has juice for a snack after school and drinks milk at meals and water when thirsty (soda is a treat reserved for going to the movies). At home, Eddie munches on red bell pepper or zucchini strips that his mom slices and puts on the counter for snacking or leaves on the refrigerator snack shelf. For dinner, everyone in the family likes baked sweet potatoes and baked fish or chicken. Eddie especially likes the crunchy type of chicken or fish "sticks" he makes with his mother and sister by dipping moist pieces in cornflakes he crushed with a bottle or rolling pin. The family has one pizza meal a week; they some-times order plain pizza and add their own veggie topping or make their own with a frozen pizza crust.

Eddie and his siblings sometimes say "yuck" over some vegetables, like dark orange squash, to which his dad replies, "It looks like sweet potatoes but feels different in your mouth, doesn't it?" Mom adds, "I didn't like squash when I was your age, but I really like it now. Try it if you want to, but you don't have to eat it." A few weeks later they again offer Eddie squash and enjoy eating it themselves but don't push it at him, knowing he is more likely to try new foods out of curiosity than coercion.

On weekends the family enjoys eating out and also likes to go hiking or bowling; sometimes they organize a volleyball game with the neighbors. Recently Eddie's dad helped the neighborhood kids build a fun house for Halloween.

Eddie is active, has friends to play with, eats a variety of foods, and takes part in individual, family, and community activities. In terms of healthy body weight, he represents about 80 percent of American children in 1980, but less than 70 percent of American children in 2000.


## MARIA

Maria, pudgy at 58 pounds, lives in a small city with parents who moved to the United States before she was born and who help support relatives in Mexico. Her mother works in a hotel housekeeping department, starting mornings early, and her father works the night shift in a local factory. Her seventeen-year-old sister cashiers at a convenience store after school until 8 or 9 most evenings. Maria's grandmother lives with the family and cooks traditional Mexican food, though the whole family seldom eats together.

Maria loves reading and helping her grandmother bake packaged cookie dough after school. "Eat more, you work so hard at school," her grandmother tells her, offering Maria unlimited soda with the cookies. At dinnertime Maria isn't very hungry but eats more because her mother chides her for picking at her meal. "To be strong you need to eat the rice, meat, and vegetables Gramma has cooked."

Maria eats breakfast with her grandmother—usually cooked cereal, milk, and doughnuts or pastry. She eats school lunch, which typically features chicken nuggets, canned corn, frozen and prefried reheated potatoes, sweetened applesauce, and milk. She sometimes eats second helpings and spends lots of time over her food as she watches other children talking with friends. Maria likes most foods and looks forward to all meals and snacks, especially pizza that her sister brings home after work in the late evening. Saturday afternoons Maria often goes to the movies with her sister, who Maria says looks "just like a movie star." Her sister's boyfriend buys large sodas, nachos with cheese, and candy bars; Maria looks forward to these treats and sometimes enjoys them more than the movie.

When she was preschool age, Maria loved the neighborhood playground, but now few children her age play there after school, and she prefers to be inside reading or watching television with her grandmother. Maria goes to one class each week at the Y called "Gym Magic" where fantasy, storytelling, and fitness activities teach a wide range of movement. She would like to keep going to the class, but no movement class like it is scheduled for seven-year-olds next year. "Total Jamming"—line dancing to the hottest new moves in rock and funk—is available, but it makes her fearful because she feels so awkward. Her mother and father don't encourage her to try the dance class or help her look for alternative recreational activities, because it is more affordable and convenient to have Maria spend each afternoon with her grandmother. Her grandmother, who never took part in organized fitness activities when she was a girl, thinks it's fine for Maria to spend the afternoons running errands or baking with her.

Maria likes a variety of food but eats and drinks too many high-calorie meals and snacks. She is sedentary and is becoming increasingly isolated from other children both during and after school. As a result, she is well above her recommended healthy weight range and is in the 13 percent of children in 2000 (up from 11 percent in 1980) within the 85th through 94th percentile range and considered *at risk* of becoming overweight. Maria represents the growing number of American children well on their way to lifelong physical and psychological body weight problems.

Dwayne, a well-established "husky" at nearly 70 pounds, gets laughs for winning the hotdog–eating contest at his table in the lunchroom at school. He lives with his parents and four siblings—three older, one younger—in a big, rundown house in a metropolitan neighborhood. He walks to school, three blocks away, but avoids playing on the street after school because his folks worry about "scary people" on the street corners. His dad works at a machine factory during the day and part-time as an evening security guard. His mom works long hours in a data-processing job.

For breakfast, Dwayne generally eats sugary cereals with whole milk or picks up sweet rolls or potato chips and soda on the way to school with his brother. Dwayne's favorite school lunch is chicken nuggets and fries with chocolate milk from the cafeteria. Two to three nights a week, the family eats super-size meals from a nearby McDonald's or brings home Chinese food. Dwayne gleefully looks forward to Kung Pau deep fried shrimp with fried rice. After school, the older children often bring home doughnuts from the nearby Krispy Kreme store, and Dwayne enjoys them too. There are always plenty of bargain-size soda bottles in the refrigerator or cupboard to go along with family-size bags of salty snacks. His mother rarely has time to cook but notices—and worries—that Dwayne eats a lot. "He will slim down during 'the big' growth spurt," say her friends at work. At home, she is too tired to talk with Dwayne; his older siblings call him "Fats." He likes their attention.

Dwayne especially likes family gatherings on weekends when aunts and uncles bring a lot of favorite foods and everyone has second and third helpings of everything. "Eat your greens" is easy for Dwayne because they taste so rich and salty with plenty of bacon. Someone always shows up with a delicious dish of macaroni and cheese on the side, and Dwayne takes some—even when he is too full for anything else.

When Dwayne tries to join a basketball game in the schoolyard at recess or after school, he is teased because of his slowness and heavy breathing from asthma. He prefers video games, especially the fast action ones that reward him for wiping out the enemy—he pretends they are the bullies on the playground, or the big kid who took the bike handed down to him from his brother. In spite of being overweight, he had nearly learned to balance the bike. Now he spends more time inside watching TV, even when his brothers and their friends are playing street hockey.

Overall Dwayne suffers from severe overweight, asthma, inactivity, and teasing. His high-calorie, high-fat diet will keep him on the fast track to early diabetes and other health problems. He may well be severely obese as a teenager and young adult because he is now in the 13 percent of heaviest American six- to eleven-year-olds. The incidence of obesity among this group has nearly doubled from 7 percent in 1980. When Dwayne is twelve, he may join the 15 percent of American children ages twelve to nineteen who make up the fattest category—a rate that has tripled since 1980.

Already at age seven Dwayne and, to a lesser extent, Maria face a lifelong struggle to manage their weight. Eddie, in contrast, has positive eating and activity habits that will help counterbalance the unhealthy food choices he encounters at school, at friends' houses, and practically everywhere else.

## NURTURE EVOLVES

There was no turning point in Dwayne's and Maria's young lives when they began to eat poorly and gain too much weight, just as there was no moment in Eddie's life when he suddenly got on the right track for a healthy weight. Rather, each one's health, size, and circumstances unfolded over time, starting in the womb. Let us turn now to the choices and actions that parents make—consciously or unconsciously, voluntarily or involuntarily—that influence a child's weight and risk for obesity.

### PRENATAL CARE AND NUTRITION

What a mother eats during pregnancy certainly matters to her unborn child's health. Proper nutrition is an essential component of prenatal care. But how much do a pregnant mother's food choices and lifestyle affect her child's birth weight and risk of obesity later in life?

Evidence showing a link between a mother's prenatal care and a child's later weight gain is limited, but we do know that a baby who has either a low birth weight or a high birth weight has an increased risk for becoming overweight later in life.

When a poorly nourished or underfed pregnant woman gains substantially less than the recommended weight-gain range, she risks having a low-birth-weight baby (under 5½ lb); conversely, if she herself is overweight or gains an excessive number of pounds during the pregnancy, then she is likely to have a big baby (10 lb or more). Pregnant women who follow guidelines for a healthy prenatal diet and stay within the recommended weight-gain range are more likely to have a normal-weight baby, and starting life

## EATING RIGHT FOR TWO

A mother who eats right during pregnancy and gains a proper amount of weight increases her chances for producing a healthy, normal-weight baby, which may help prevent obesity later in the child's life.

During pregnancy, the mother needs generous amounts of carbohydrate-rich foods (whole grains, legumes, starchy and other vegetables, and fruits) for energy; protein for tissue building and growth; and calcium for bone building. Food chosen wisely can provide all the nutrients needed to support healthy fetal development except iron and folic acid. For this reason, a prenatal vitamin is recommended. The goal is a diet based on the USDA Food Guide Pyramid guidelines (reviewed in chapter 7), plus about 300 additional daily calories (compared to the needs of a nonpregnant woman) during the last two trimesters. Pregnant teens, underweight women, and physically active women may need more calories for consistent, healthy weight gain. These extra calories should come from one extra serving from each of the five food groups. As with nonpregnant women, a pregnant woman's intake of highly processed foods with added sugars and fats should be sparing. Most American women do not need extra protein during pregnancy because they already exceed the recommendation.

What follows is a sample recommended daily menu for a pregnant woman:

BREAKFAST
¾ cup whole-grain cereal
1 cup low-fat milk
1 slice toast or ½ English muffin with 2 tablespoons peanut butter
½ to 1 cup fruit
1 cup 100% fruit juice

SNACK
1 cup 100% fruit juice
1 oz pretzels or whole-grain crackers
1 oz cheese

LUNCH
Sandwich (turkey and avocado on whole-wheat bread)
½ cup carrot sticks
1 cup low-fat milk

DINNER
Chicken Creole (4 oz chicken, ¾ cup stewed tomatoes)
1 cup rice
1 cup vegetables (zucchini, mushrooms, greens)
1 tablespoon olive oil

1 tablespoon Parmesan cheese
Sparkling water
½ cup ice cream

EVENING SNACK
1 cup low-fat milk
3 small oatmeal cookies

at a normal weight increases the baby's chances of maintaining a normal weight during childhood.[6]

How much a woman should gain during pregnancy depends on her pre-pregnancy weight. The American College of Obstetricians and Gynecologists recommends the following weight-gain ranges for pregnancy: underweight women should gain 28–40 lb; normal-weight women, 25–35 lb; overweight, 15–25 lb; obese, 15 lb; women carrying twins, 35–45 lb.[7] (See the box "Eating Right for Two.")

It might come as little surprise that large babies are more likely to grow into chubby children and fat adults. Higher-than-normal birth weight is consistently associated with an increased BMI in adulthood.[8] Children born large—10 lb and above—are likely to gain excess body fat in early childhood. According to research, these children may exceed the expected weight and height gain when three to six years old (during the "adiposity rebound" explained in chapter 1). Their size elevates their risk for later obesity. The risk for obesity is even greater for heavy infants born to overweight, compared to healthy-weight, mothers.[9] An added risk to consider: the infant of an obese mother may be large even if born prematurely, and the large pre-term baby may not be recognized as premature and thus not receive the special medical care it needs. Obese women should strive to attain healthy weights before pregnancy or between pregnancies—but not during, because dieting may interfere with meeting the nutritional needs of the growing fetus.

What is less well known and perhaps counterintuitive is the suggested link between *underweight* babies and obesity. Mothers undernourished during pregnancy often give birth to babies of low birth weight. Scientists are debating the connection between low-birth-weight babies and later development of obesity and diabetes. (Low birth weight, or LBW, is less than 5½ lb; very low birth weight, or VLBW, is less than 3½ lb.)

Low-birth-weight pre-term babies may first rapidly catch up, overcompensating for their scarcity of nutrients once out of the womb, and then follow a normal growth pattern. For instance, a "preemie" baby I know, born at 31 weeks and weighing 4 pounds, was extremely chubby by three months old—she had a triple chin and triple rolls on her thighs. By the time she reached toddlerhood, though, she had thinned out to a normal size. Other LBW babies, however, may continue to gain weight excessively.

We are still learning about the risk of obesity after catch-up growth of pre-term and full-term LBW babies.[10] The explanation may come from a basic condition of pregnancy—if nutrients are scarce, then the fetus conserves blood glucose and energy stores. The theory is that after birth, the child's body remains thrifty, hoards nutrients, and grows quickly to catch up to—and perhaps surpass—healthy size and weight. A thrifty fetus would have an advantage if born into a famine environment, but in our food-rich world, such a child faces a greater risk of obesity.[11] This theory might explain why undernourished fetuses who have a low birth weight become chubby and remain fat later in life, whereas preemies who gain weight rapidly after birth often settle into a normal weight range—the baby who was undernourished in utero developed "thrifty genes," but the infant who was born prematurely did not.

The suggestion that a mother who is underfed during pregnancy is likely to increase her child's risk of obesity came from follow-up studies of the children whose mothers were exposed to famine in 1944–45. Studies of these adults conceived during the Nazi occupation of Holland and the siege of Leningrad during World War II, whose mothers had barely enough food for survival, show that they had a higher rate of obesity at age fifty than the general population.[12] The findings support the theory that a mother's nutritional health during pregnancy affects the development and hormonal regulation of her child's fat tissue, and, if she is undernourished, that the child stores fat more readily in later life. Some evidence for this link also includes babies undernourished at birth from Brazil and other Latin American countries, where large numbers of children are obese.[13] Research also suggests a link among African Americans between high rates of low birth weight and obesity in their children.[14] African American women have a high rate of obesity, and their nutritional health may be compromised during pregnancy, resulting in a high rate of low-birth-weight babies, especially those born to very young mothers.

Do women who chronically diet before pregnancy increase the risk of future obesity in their unborn children? We do not know. We do know beyond question, however, that extreme dieting and poor nutrition compromise the health of both mother and fetus.

What about the link between prenatal nutrition and diabetes? Because type 2 (adult-onset) diabetes and obesity are closely linked, is a pregnant woman with type 2 diabetes putting her unborn child at a higher risk for obesity or diabetes, or both? The answer is maybe, but likely to be yes. A woman with type 2 diabetes is usually overweight, which in itself correlates to producing a child with high birth weight. Large babies have a good chance of becoming overweight children, adolescents, and adults. Paradoxically, a child born with low birth weight, as we saw earlier, has an increased risk of obesity and type 2 diabetes. In fact, in a study of over 70,000 female nurses, the women born with the lowest birth weights had twice the rate of type 2 diabetes as the women with the highest birth weights.[15] Either way, a mother with a healthy body weight who follows recommended nutrition guidelines during pregnancy is most likely to have a child with a healthy body weight and low risk of type 2 diabetes.

Children born to mothers with insulin-dependent diabetes (type 1) also have an increased risk of later obesity. During pregnancy a mother's glucose passes freely to the fetus, but her insulin does not. Since the fetus needs insulin to use the glucose for energy and growth, it produces insulin. When maternal glucose is too abundant (often the case in diabetes), fetal insulin may also be overabundant and act as a growth hormone, increasing the child's risk of a higher birth weight and continued excessive insulin production after birth.

Some pregnancies result in short-term gestational diabetes in mothers. Apparently, prenatal exposure to the effects of mild, diet-treated gestational diabetes does not increase the risk of childhood obesity.[16] Nonetheless, in gestational diabetes, attention to prenatal nutritional care is critical because fetal exposure to excessive insulin production may increase the vulnerability of a child to obesity and diabetes later in life—especially when the child is exposed to a plentiful food environment.

In sum, the evidence is strong that the nutritional environment of a mother's womb influences the lifelong health of her children.[17] And, beyond birth, the way children, and adults, continue to respond to their nutritional environment relates partly to "programming that occurs during fetal life." When exposed to a calorie-dense food environment, children whose energy regulation was disrupted in the womb are at an even greater risk of obesity or diabetes when growing up. This double exposure triggers a domino effect that in turn sensitizes their own children. Researchers call this a "feed forward" effect that makes the next generation even more susceptible to obesity.[18] To break this chain of events and stem the rapid rise of obesity, a scientific review of obesity's fetal origins concludes that measures to ward off obesity must start in childhood, and before. Otherwise, "Failure to address this epidemic could lead to a vicious cycle of obesity and its consequences because adolescent obesity among girls is likely to lead to [compromised] . . . pregnancies and, thus, increased obesity among their offspring."[19] Prenatal care and childhood feeding practices are obvious points at which to begin.

Before we move from prenatal care to infancy, consider an interesting hypothesis that relates weather-related environmental birth conditions to obesity: *where* a mother gives birth could make a difference in her child's susceptibility to unhealthy weight gain.

Could a child born in subfreezing climates have a greater chance of becoming overweight? Perhaps, according to an extensive analysis of body weight records of English men and women born between 1920 and 1930. Those born in the winter, particularly a very cold winter, had a greater risk of becoming overweight later in life, suggesting that early cold exposure is linked to obesity.[20] The biological mechanism is not clear but may involve the resting metabolic rate. The extreme temperature could cause the newborn's metabolism to slow down, as though hibernating, and signal the body to hold on to fat as a way to protect against the cold. While interesting, this possible link between cold weather and weight gain should not cause parents-to-be who live in areas with frigid winters to worry a great deal, since their bundled-up newborns are unlikely to be exposed at length to the cold outdoor temperatures. If, however, the cold climate leads the family to spend most of their time indoors and thus to be less active, then that is another matter—and could indeed speed up weight gain.[21]

### FIRST FEEDING: BREAST OR BOTTLE?

From day one in a newborn's life, parents have an opportunity to reduce their child's risk of later obesity by making every effort to breast-feed rather than to feed by bottle. For several reasons, involving both the method of bottle-feeding and the content of infant formula, breast-feeding reduces the risk of obesity later in life.

If we could offer a single solution, a "magic bullet" remedy for childhood obesity, would breast-feeding be it? Headline news on July 16, 1999, seemed to promise that solution: "Study: Breast-fed Kids Stay Slimmer." One authority, commenting on the largest study to date, involving nearly 10,000 German children, named breast-feeding a "powerful strategy for fighting the spiraling level of childhood obesity." Lawrence Gartner, chair of the American Academy of Pediatrics' group whose policy statement recommends breast-feeding for at least an infant's first six months, said of the German study that the link between breast-feeding and obesity "was something we all thought was likely to be true."[22]

In fact, what we have is not a magic bullet, but a trend—a very positive trend. Breast-fed children have a reduced risk of obesity. Among five- and six-year-old children who were breast-fed, the German study found, the rate of obesity was nearly half that of those who were not breast-fed.[23] In the nationwide American *Growing Up Today Study* and another study in the Czech Republic, the protective effect of breast-feeding against obesity was significant but smaller among older children, nine to fourteen years old, compared to younger children. Still, the longer the children were breast-fed, the lower their risk of being overweight during older childhood and adolescence.[24]

Breast-feeding is beneficial for many reasons; a lower rate of weight gain is one of them. Healthy overall eating behavior is another. Breast-feeding gives a baby the chance to learn self-regulation of food. A mother who breast-feeds offers her baby food and at the same time allows the baby to assume control over the amount of milk consumed.[25]

In bottle-feeding, the parent sets the pace. I often see well-intentioned parents or other caregivers encourage their baby to finish a bottle during a single feeding. It is understandable that they feel satisfied on seeing a whole bottle consumed; they can rest assured that they adequately nourished the baby, and they do not want to pour the contents—formula that was expensive to buy or breast milk that took effort to pump—down the drain. Yet the same precedent for feeding could inadvertently lead to overeating during childhood. Those who say while bottle-feeding, "Just one more ounce. There, good boy!" are more likely to say in later years, "Just one more bite. Good job!" In contrast, babies who breast-feed simply let go or fall asleep when full. The mother typically does not encourage the baby to latch on again and continue nursing. She respects the baby's signal of fullness, and the baby consequently is more likely to consume a proper amount. As the baby moves on to eating solid food, child and mother share the control over how much to eat; both have learned to respond to the child's hunger and fullness cues. Of course, self-regulation around food can be learned during bottle-feeding. It again requires attention to the infant's cues.

Breast-feeding also starts a child's taste training. It comes as a surprise to many mothers that a baby encounters a great variety of food flavors from breast milk. Because the taste and smell of foods eaten by the mother are passed on to the baby in breast milk, acceptance and appreciation of a variety of flavors start early for the breast-fed baby. They build a "flavor bridge" to a wide variety of solid foods and pave the way for a child's personal tastes to develop for a well-balanced diet.[26] The monotony and sweetness of infant formula feeding may set a lifelong affinity for sweet and monotonous foods.[27]

Overfeeding during early infancy—which is more likely to occur with babies who are bottle-fed—can lead to rapid weight gain and set the stage for later obesity.[28] If a child grows excessive fat cells at this stage, he or she has them for life. If the child's fat cells enlarge too much and divide into more fat cells through excessive eating, the extra cells speed the rate of obesity; the child gets fatter faster because excess fat cells secrete additional hormones, including estrogen and leptin, which affect metabolic rate and hunger. The prevalence of being overweight at age seven was found to be higher among babies for each *extra* 3.5 oz of weight gained per month. (A doubling of birth weight in the first four to six months is normal.)

There is some evidence that feeding solid foods before age three months— for instance, by adding cereal to the bottle—is associated with overweight beyond infancy.[29] Yet most studies do not support the idea that babies fed solid foods very early become overweight children.[30]

As babies and toddlers shift from breast or bottle to cup, and even before, juice drinking often takes a prominent role in their daily diets. Indeed, increased juice drinking, like soda consumption, has received a fair amount of blame for childhood obesity. I see many children drinking juice in baby bottles when they are only months old. In fact, I am often startled to see baby bottles filled with a fluid resembling blue window cleaner! Between 1990 and 2000, fruit juice consumed by young children increased significantly from an average of under 5 oz to over 7 oz daily, owing in part to ubiquitous juice boxes and other clever marketing. Since juice and juice drinks often replace nutrient-dense milk and lead to an early preference for sweetened fluid instead of water, the trend is of concern. And of greater concern is a link between excessive juice drinking and compromised growth and obesity. In particular, short stature has been tied to heavy use of apple and grape juice; obesity to excessive apple juice drinking.[31] The guideline is to limit juice to 6 oz or less a day for children ages one to six, and to limit it to 12 oz or less for kids ages seven to eighteen.[32]

In any case, juice drinking decreases as children get older—a trend in the wrong direction. Sadly, many children would prefer sipping soda if they weren't drinking juice, so at least juice is a preferable alternative. Since the average two-year-old drinks a cup of soda a day (and I see even young babies drinking soda from bottles), I suggest that 100 percent juice, preferably diluted with water, is acceptable for children and far preferable to carbonated beverages, tea, and juice drinks with added sugars. (The recommendation is that children ages two to six years drink two cups of low-fat milk daily, while younger children should have two to three cups of whole milk daily after the transition from breast milk or formula at twelve to fifteen months.)

Children of all ages should be encouraged to quench thirst by drinking water. Drinking water for thirst at an early age establishes an excellent lifetime habit. After living for several years in tropical countries with unsafe drinking water, my children remember dreaming of water from public fountains—which are still widely available but underused, though they provide an essential commodity, free and safe water, in America today.

## TASTE BUDS: HOW EATING HABITS
## AND TASTE PREFERENCES GROW

Once babies move from breast milk or formula to solids, eating patterns emerge and taste preferences kick into high gear. Food and learning to eat are central to children's development. Most aspects of social development and acculturation of children involve food. Still, the question remains: why do we, first as children and then as adults, eat what we eat? To learn how to reshape the way children eat in order to moderate body weight, we must be able to answer that question with some degree of certainty.

High on the list of reasons, after basic sustenance, is taste. Availability, accessibility, and convenience follow. In a situation where food is available and easily accessible, how can children develop taste preferences for foods that support a healthy weight? The answer lies primarily with the parents. Influences beyond the home—such as advertising, peers, and school lunches—will affect children, but usually not to a significant degree until they reach kindergarten age. For young children, parents are the decision makers, the gatekeepers.

What follows is a list that summarizes influences on children's food behaviors, all of which have direct or indirect connections to childhood obesity. These key facts and findings highlight the degree to which the eating routines and parenting styles that emerge during early childhood affect lifelong eating patterns and preferences.

By age three, children develop likes and dislikes for certain foods, notably vegetables.

Younger children are easier to induce to try novel foods and to change preferences for familiar foods than older children.

Children learn food preferences through repeated exposure to new food; a minimum of eight to ten times is required for children to accept and develop a preference for it.

Children consume a diet with less variety if variety is seldom available at home or dining out.

Children's, especially toddlers', acceptance of foods follows the example of parents and siblings.

Feeding tactics and behaviors—"clean your plate"; "eat your carrots so you can have dessert"—pass from one generation to the next.

Children who regularly eat a nutritious breakfast are likely to control body weight—overall, they eat less fat and fewer impulsive snacks.

Increased frequency of family dinners and companionship at meals relates to lower consumption of fried foods and higher consumption of vegetables—even at meals away from home.

Social atmosphere influences children's food habits: a positive meal experience increases preference for a food; a negative meal decreases it.

Just as educators and parents have come to appreciate the importance of early-childhood education for "wiring" young brains to learn, so must we recognize and respect the importance of early-childhood eating for establishing eating behavior. Studies show that before age three, neither the parents' genes nor the parents' personal food preferences strongly influence what children will like or not like to eat. Aside from an innate preference for sweetness, toddlers are open to trying anything and everything, free from preconceived notions of what's "yummy" or "yucky." We know that kids are willing to taste a great variety of food—especially vegetables and fruits—between twelve months and two years, *if offered.* We also know that most adults do not eat a variety of fruits and vegetables themselves and are unlikely to offer them to their children.

This is the window of opportunity to expose a child to a variety of tastes. It is the time to honor a child's rejection of big and frequent servings; young children know when they are full.

After age three, a child's obesity risk increases in some family environments, not only because of the unhealthy food choices available to the child, but also because of the example that parents set at mealtimes. Almost everyone remembers growing up with instructions to "do as I say, not as I do," but we soon learn that "actions speak louder than words." It is not rocket science to connect the way parents eat to the way their children do. There is plenty of evidence that role modeling matters.[33] Parents (and caretakers) of young children can seize this one opportunity to make a strike against obesity. Figuring out ways to cook, eat, and like foods with less fat and added sugar (and eat them with the kids) pays off for the whole family. For example, I worked with a father concerned with his own elevated blood sugar and triglycerides (fats in the blood often affected by high-sugar diets). It turned out that after substituting water for his favorite sweetened iced tea drink for a few weeks, his triglycerides dropped to a normal level. He also noted a change in his three-year-old: "Andy stopped demanding iced tea and now drinks water along with me." He said that Andy's one-and-a-half-year-old sister would likely do the same "because she tries to do everything Andy does."

## PARENTING STYLES THAT TRIGGER—OR INHIBIT—OBESITY

Eavesdrop on a family while they are eating together, and chances are you will hear a parent employ one of these timeworn tactics:

"You have to eat three bites of vegetables and finish your milk before you can be excused from the table."

"You may have dessert, but first you must pick up your toys."

"Fine, have a PopTart for dinner—just eat something!"

Comments such as these, if used regularly rather than as an occasional last resort, invariably do more harm than good. The first two show healthy food as something to rebel against (what *my folks* want) and unhealthy food as something to prize (what *I* want). The third sets no limits. Each comment points to a certain parenting style that influences children's eating behavior and obesity.

Parenting style about food choice ranges from *permissive* to *authoritarian*. Permissive style is "eat anything you want"; about one-third of parents (even parents of obese children) exercise little control over their children's eating. Authoritarian style is "do as I say or else" and involves using commands or coercion to get children to eat, or using food as a reward or punishment. About half of parents use food as a reward for good behavior or withhold favorite food as punishment for unwanted behavior.[34]

Permissive attitudes toward children's eating behavior often result in diets that are low in nutritional quality.[35] The authoritarian style backfires because restricting access to foods does not produce a dislike but rather may stimulate the children to eat the forbidden foods, even when full, especially if they are in an unrestricted setting away from parents.[36] Children whose parents order them to clean their plates are less responsive to fullness cues than are children taught to recognize hunger and fullness. Once again, we realize that parenting is a tricky business all around, but especially in guiding healthy eating behaviors. The permissive style can lead to overindulgence and become harmful, but the authoritarian style can lead to "pushing" and "restricting," both potentially harmful. I say, aim for the middle ground and strike a balance.

The middle ground is an *authoritative* style. It involves using dialogues such as, "I like crunchy broccoli and it makes me healthy; do you want some too?" It questions, negotiates, and reasons to guide the development of children's dietary self-control. Few parents find this middle ground, so there is little research on it. Authoritative parenting means giving small portions when introducing a new food and praising children for eating healthy foods. Its methods result in improved food selections among children. But do they prevent excess weight gain? Research on this fascinating issue is moving along quickly and with understandable urgency since we now recognize that untested recommendations may unnecessarily interfere with the parent-child feeding relationship, especially in diverse ethnic groups.[37] For example, the widespread recommendation, arising from research on white, middle-class children, *not* to impose too much control over children's eating is open to question. A study of parental control of diverse ethnic children found no evidence that control interfered with children's ability to regulate eating or led to their obesity.[38]

Culture and socioeconomic status undoubtedly affect parenting style. African American parents tend to role model both positive and negative food behaviors. They often sit with their children at mealtime and eat the food they would like their children to eat, yet they seldom eat the low-fat snacks, fruits, and vegetables their kids *ought* to eat. Thus unintended role modeling may encourage unbalanced eating habits.[39]

Hispanic American families appear to use bribes, threats, and other forms of punishment, especially among first-generation families trying to keep up traditional food patterns in a culture of seductive fast food. These parents are caught between using negative, authoritarian threats such as "You can't go with us if you don't eat your supper," and allowing "child-led" alternative choices of fast foods, thus losing their opportunity to preserve the children's preference for traditional healthy foods—and prevent obesity.[40] Both African American and Hispanic cultural food traditions include a variety of wholesome foods. These families need all the support they can get to preserve their traditions and serve these foods as nourishment for growing children. Because many Hispanic and African American families fall into the low-income bracket, some argue that they, and poor people in general, eat low-quality, high-calorie food because it is all they can afford and find available. Yes, fresh fruits are sometimes hard to find in Harlem, or South Chicago, or Watts, but beans, rice, vegetables, and chicken and fish are available, and relatively cheap. The tradition of planning meals, shopping, and cooking food "from scratch" is changing for numerous reasons (to be discussed in chapter 5).

Granted that healthy foods are available, does parenting style make kids fat? One intricate study carefully measured child-feeding practices, children's body fat, and the food children ate. Regarding children's body fat, the feeding behavior of parents was far more important than the amount of food (calories) the children ate. The conclusion was that "highly controlling feeding strategies may" interfere with children's ability to self-regulate their calorie consumption.[41] Other evidence that associates authoritarian or permissive feeding practices with higher child weight-for-height measurements comes from studies of mealtime practices in child-care programs and parents' small focus groups.[42]

One of the strongest studies to date of parental feeding style and obesity risk in children involved families with same-sex twins. It compared one hundred families in which both parents were overweight or obese with one hundred families in which both parents were at a normal weight or lean. Mothers in both groups were no different in offering food as comfort or as a reward, or in encouraging children to eat more or less than they wanted. Results suggest that the stereotype of the obese mother urging her children to eat more and more "is more likely to be myth than fact."[43] If anything, fatter mothers exerted less, not more, control in feeding their children. And a more permissive style may allow forces outside the home to have a larger impact in shaping children's eating behavior.

Given the several forces driving children to eat or not to eat, authoritative parenting—our middle ground—is an excellent tool for fostering lifelong healthy weight. Whether the power of parenting practices is large or small compared to forces beyond the home, authoritative guidance prepares children to make healthy food choices and manage their food environment—inside their home and beyond.

Parenting by example is understandably hard. Consistently eating balanced meals and drinking healthy fluids is hard. When describing to me what her children eat, a young single mother was at first defensive. Then, acknowledging the power of her role modeling, and the importance of vegetables in family meals, she sighed, "I would really like to have grilled fish or chicken and freshly cooked vegetables with my kids, but with my long working hours and my budget, I don't have money to shop for them or time to cook them, so we bring in fried chicken and pizza—a lot."

Chapter 6, which focuses on strategies to offset obesity, outlines an authoritative style that parents and caretakers can learn and adopt in order to give their children the best chance for developing a positive relationship with food.

## THE ENDANGERED FAMILY MEAL

It goes without saying that mealtimes are a vital time and place to develop kids' eating behaviors and food preferences. But mealtimes these days are more like flextime. Families who set a table and gather together for a home-cooked dinner are growing increasingly rare. Food surveys indicate that barely a majority of families still eat dinner together (or at least they say they do): half of the adults said the family sat down together for dinner four or more times a week. Less than a quarter of Americans eat three square meals—breakfast, lunch, and dinner—with few or no snacks in between.

Fewer families regularly eat meals together at home because family members eat throughout the day, and overloaded schedules leave little time for meal preparation.

"My kids end up eating in the car on the way to or from lessons, games, errands."

"I work evenings; it's hard to eat with the kids."

"We never cook. We just 'fix' food—from the freezer to the microwave—when we're hungry."

I hear it all the time. Marion Cunningham, a culinary icon and acclaimed cookbook author who strongly advocates the family meal, put it well: "Today, we are living motel lives where someone buys prepared food, and everyone eats whenever they like."[44] Portable foods and snacks have now become a main course. As the standard accompaniment to most activities—anywhere and anytime—eating has few off-limit locations. Sitting down to eat commonly pairs up with watching TV, playing video games, or riding in cars. Cup holders and insulated tote bags make it easier to eat in the car; refrigerated glove boxes and microwave ovens that plug into the cigarette lighter are coming soon.

As a result, fewer and fewer children sit down and eat in traditional ways, at a table with utensils and plates. A European visitor noted that few American children seem to eat with utensils. "They always eat with their hands, right out of bags or boxes or wrapped packages." A traditional method to modify eating behavior—slowing down—in order to recognize fullness signals is to "put your fork down between bites." When kids mostly eat from hand to mouth, while standing or walking, "put your fork down" is not an option.

Eating frequently with the family at home has a positive effect on overall diet quality, according to a study of nine- to fourteen-year-old children. The kids who ate dinner at home four or more times a week ate more fruits and vegetables and less fried foods, even on the occasions when they were eating away from home. But soda was the most frequent drink of choice—at home and away.[45] One lesson learned: families who drink soda at home as the regular source of fluid should take the obvious opportunity to make soda a "controlled substance."

Furthermore, overloaded schedules and eating on the go encourage fast eating, with little time to notice fullness signals. The average time spent at the dinner table at home is twenty-eight minutes, according to one family study. Children spend even less time eating school meals; an average eating time of twelve to fifteen minutes for middle and high school meals is common.[46] The speed of eating among children may be a factor in losing track of fullness and hunger cues. Teens, especially fast-growing boys, have traditionally been known to eat quickly—and to eat large amounts. Many mothers of active teenage boys describe their eating as "inhaling" food. But for many young children, eating too fast becomes a pattern that is difficult to change. Adults tell me how this pattern begins: "I started eating fast as a kid; otherwise the pizza would be all gone." "People always talked about eating too much and getting fat in my family, so I ate real fast hoping no one would notice how much I ate." "I sort of learned from my dad that eating goes with whatever I'm doing. Now when I eat while working at my desk, I quickly cram big bites into my mouth or eat the whole thing real fast in order to free up my hands for work." For families who think having a leisurely, pleasant meal together is an impossible dream, it can be a worthwhile goal—a few times a week.

## AT HOME WITH TAKE-OUT

Whereas meals together at home allow for healthier diets, they by no means stop excessive weight gain, because meals at home increasingly resemble restaurant take-out fare. Parents today are accustomed to bringing highly processed, high-fat fast food into the home for meals and snacks.

Popcorn, candy, and corn dogs, once reserved for baseball games and movies, are no longer special attractions away from home. Now children may heat up cheese-laden nachos and hot dogs at home, accompanied by 20 oz sodas from their own refrigerators. "Special treats" are so much the norm that breakfast and lunch food typically considered healthy—such as yogurt, cereal, or waffles—today feature chocolate chips and sugary sprinkles to entice children who will reject anything that seems too "boring" or plain.

Families are not only eating high-calorie food at home, they're eating huge helpings of it. Portion sizes have increased significantly at home and away from home for the most popular foods, including soft drinks, hamburgers, fries, and Mexican food—the largest increase being in hamburgers, cheeseburgers, and desserts eaten *at home*.[47] And worse, the more food that's in front of us, the more we eat. In an experiment with different portion sizes and instructions to eat as desired, individuals offered the largest size in one serving bowl ate an incredible 30 percent more than individuals offered the same amount but divided into small portions. The study participants all reported the same level of hunger and fullness regardless of how much they ate.

Related studies found that preschoolers ate an average of 25 percent more macaroni and cheese when given large portion sizes. When allowed to serve themselves, however, they ate "child-size" amounts. The kids who did overeat when serving themselves were also the ones who tended to eat the greatest amount of snack foods in the absence of hunger. These findings all suggest a link between increased susceptibility to the cue of super-size portions and decreased ability to recognize fullness.[48] The habits learned during childhood continue into adulthood.

For further evidence, consider the growth—in both size and popularity—of Kraft "Lunchables." In 1988 Lunchables were small, containing less than 300 calories. Each had a small piece of cheese, a small piece of ham, and a few crackers. The format allowed children to add a glass of milk and piece of fruit or raw vegetable to complete the meal. By 2003, the Lunchables "Mega Pack" contained 640 to 780 calories. Vitamins and minerals per calorie are low.

The 700 calorie "Deep Dish Pizza—Extra Cheesy—Mega Pack" (32 percent of calories from fat) holds half the calories small children require for the whole day. It includes a juice drink blend (10 percent juice; the rest is high-fructose corn syrup). The pizza sauce is laden with high-fructose corn syrup, and the crispy chocolate candies are high in sugar. The healthier choice offered is the "Fun Fuel" pack (440 calories; 27 percent of calories from fat), containing food from four of the food pyramid's groups: tortilla wraps, chicken, cheese, and fruit-flavored yogurt in a tube and 100 percent fruit juice punch. The "Cracker Low Fat Stackers" (400 calories; 25 percent fat), with lean ham and reduced-fat cheese, includes a 10 percent juice drink and low-fat pudding. The "Stackers" adds a very high-calorie, high-in-sugar snack when eaten with the other high-calorie "meals." On the plus side, all three packs supply, via the cheese, about the same amount of calcium as 1 cup of milk. On the minus side, all are high in sodium, low in fiber, and low in the vitamins and minerals a balanced lunch ought to include—for the calories they hold.

Why are Lunchables wildly popular? Parents say, "They're ready-to-go and cheap." "My kids say, '*Everyone* eats them,' and you know what that means—they want 'em too." How much does a Lunchable cost? The "mega" and the "fun" sizes cost the same—less than four dollars; the cracker stackers cost less than three dollars.

A homemade turkey and cheese sandwich on whole wheat or in a tortilla wrap with shredded carrots, tomato, and lettuce, a piece of fruit, and a carton of milk is cheaper and healthier, but it takes planning ahead. It is far easier for a parent to buy Lunchables than to prepare and pack a healthy, less calorie-laden lunch. Parents tell me that their ten- and eleven-year-olds eat two Lunchables a day: "Lunch and snack are so easy with school and soccer practice back to back, even if the grocery bill at my wholesale club is much more."

The "fun food" waffles, yogurts, and Lunchables are targeted to kids for breakfast, lunch, and snacks. A growing trend is marketing these highly processed meals to children as convenience dinners—the only meal where some kids still eat vegetables. Some parents and my nutritionist colleagues worry, "soon it will be fun fried food at every meal."

A *Wall Street Journal* headline sums it up: "Single-Serving Sales Increase as Snack Packs Get Bigger; Children Drive Demand. Result: People Eat More." The news story recounted the history of single-serve packaging from school-lunch milk cartons and candy bars to potato chips and juice boxes to repackaging "yummies so that they're easier to wolf down in the car." These single-food packs have become the major source of financial growth for the food industry. Parents stock their pantries with cartons of individual food packages: Oreo, Nutter Butter, and Chips Ahoy cookies wrapped several to a package; Gatorade in pull-up-top bottles; fruit roll-ups in packs of 80. One mother reports, "If you have them in the house, kids eat them." She finds food wrappers all over the house. The food executives talk about their packaging as "portion control," but Hot Pockets, the microwaveable sandwiches (a popular after-school treat), added 10 percent more filling, kept the price stable, and increased sales 32 percent. One executive admitted that the best-selling individual-serving foods come in larger than typical sizes. "That's kind of sad. You get used to it. Then it's a normal portion, and that's why everyone is so overweight."[49]

## AN ENVIRONMENT RIPE FOR "EMOTIONAL EATING"

As children get older and move into adolescence, they may begin turning to food for reasons having more to do with their psychological needs than with their appetite. The parent-child relationship and the home setting may work together to foster an environment that makes eating the best response to emotional distress.

Imagine a child arriving home to an empty house after school, with instructions to stay inside, away from potential stalkers, speeding cars, and unhelpful neighbors. This daily routine can lead to anxiety, anger, loneliness, and boredom. A television program, a full refrigerator, and a microwave oven may help cut anxiety, work off hostility (conscious or unconscious), counteract a feeling of being unloved, and offer pleasure—all responses to emotional distress. We hear a lot about "emotional eating" and "medicating with food" as factors in the rise of adult obesity. Whether or not the childhood situation described here leads to obesity in children (and there is very little information about what really happens at home after school and before adults arrive), one thing is clear: the "home alone" child is vulnerable to emotional distress. The idea, which is a pervasive if unproven theory, is that emotional distress leads to overeating.

The theory generally known as the psychosomatic model of obesity (PMO for short) applied to adults may or may not apply to children. The PMO supports a common cultural belief: overweight and obese adults eat in response to emotional distress and hence gain weight; food is their emotional defense against anxiety, depression, anger, boredom, and loneliness. While obese people overeat in response to emotional distress, people in a healthy weight range use other coping skills in similar situations. If this hypothesis is in fact true for adults, it may help explain the development of obesity begun in childhood.[50]

And when the model links emotional eating to a character flaw—a lack of self-control—it partially explains the ridicule and scorn directed at obese adults and children. Our culture values self-control and coping skills while imposing stresses at every turn. The widespread belief linking distress and overeating is evident in the vast literature that documents anti-fat attitudes in Western culture. Eating in response to stress is another adult behavior parents and caretakers frequently model for children. Among families followed for eleven years in a research study, children whose parents vacillated between severe dieting and episodes of bingeing were more likely to gain excessive weight throughout childhood than children with parents who were healthy eaters. These findings suggest that these behaviors pass on to children, affecting their ability to regulate their own food behavior.[51] There is no denying that both parents and children, fat or not, could benefit from learning healthy coping skills to handle the stresses and boredom in our living and working environments.

## TURN ON, SIT DOWN, GET FAT

Screen time is on the schedule of most family members each day. Video games offer an exciting activity in the "downtime" after a busy school day for many kids. A video serves as babysitter after Mom picks up the kids from day care and rushes to get dinner ready. The whole family gathers for their favorite TV series after an exhausting or boring work day. Overworked, sleep- and time-starved parents often have no time to play outside with their children. Or to walk or ride bikes and talk with their children about their needs, problems, and dreams. Many children are also time-starved—or at least think they are, with scheduled lessons, clubs, and homework—and parent-child communication suffers as a result. Exhausted parents and children both find television irresistible: "We'll talk about that later, after the program."

When all the pressures to eat—and overeat—collide with the relentless lure of sedentary activities, such as watching television, playing video games, and surfing the Internet, we have an answer to why children are getting fatter. Some facts speak for themselves:

- 99 percent of children live in a home with at least one TV set

- 32 percent of two- to seven-year-olds and 65 percent of eight- to twelve-year-olds have a TV set in their bedroom

- three to four hours a day is the average amount of time two- to five-year-old children spend watching TV

- five-and-a-half hours daily is the average time spent on combined media (TV/video, video games, computer) by children and adolescents

- the average child in the United States watches more than 1,250 hours of television and views over 38,000 commercials each year—the majority are for food products[52]

A classic 1985 study raised the question: do we fatten our children at the television set? By 1996 the answer was obvious: yes. Studies documented television viewing as a "cause of increasing obesity among children in the United States" between 1986 and 1990. In 2001, representative national data confirmed that the incidence of obesity is lowest among children watching one hour or less of TV daily, and highest among those who watch four or more hours a day.[53] As they go on connecting the dots, these and other studies consistently associate children's time spent viewing television with being overweight.

Screen time not only robs kids of more active entertainment but subverts healthy food choices as well. A study of ninety-one households found that when children are eating at home but families' television viewing is a normal part of meal routines, kids eat fewer fruits and vegetables and more pizzas, snack foods, and sodas than when families separate television viewing from eating. A project that helped kids learn to schedule and manage their screen time resulted in their eating healthier foods.[54]

It is clear that excessive TV watching is *likely to lead* to excessive weight gain. But for some children, we may have the cause and the effect backward. Watching excessive television may be the result and not the cause of being overweight. Overweight kids find it hard to move fast and keep up with others, so sedentary activity attracts them. Either way, excessive screen time and excessive weight are related.

It's not just the sitting; the "mind-bending" advertising, the "must-have" buying, and the eating exacerbate the problem. Watch a kids' TV channel such as *Nick Jr.* for an hour and count the food-related commercials. Take a minute to think about how the favorite characters on the channel's shows are exploited to sell certain food products. Marion Nestle, in her book *Food Politics: How the Food Industry Influences Nutrition and Health,* gives numerous examples of how this works. "Teletubbies, the public television program for toddlers, for example, was sponsored first by Burger King and later by McDonald's; McDonald's distributed toys representing the four characters."[55]

Preschool children see so many television commercials that they can sing advertising jingles and name product logos. In her vivid and closely documented investigation of creative food industry marketing, Nestle describes how kids are successfully exploited when advertisements aim at underage consumers. She reports studies that some children make requests for as many as twenty-five items a month that they have seen advertised.[56]

Another close analysis of the advertisement content on children's shows found that half of the nutrition-related information in commercials was misleading or inaccurate. Foods high in fat and sugar are among the most heavily advertised items.[57] Many young children cannot distinguish what they see from what is real; television messages influence their perceptions and behaviors. A 2001 study of television commercials' impact on food preferences of preschoolers confirmed what those planning ads know: to kids, commercials and programs are equally fascinating. Preschoolers exposed to embedded commercials were significantly more likely to choose the advertised items than those who saw the programs without commercials. Young children, in contrast to older children and adults, do not alter attention levels between commercials and programs.[58]

Commercial TV is not the only culprit. Computers and video games also monopolize kids' time. Between 1998 and 2003, both chat time with friends and electronic school work have doubled the amount of time kids spend sitting at the computer. When computer use is squeezed into a day already loaded with television watching and homework, it's no surprise to see that kids' physical activity is on the decline.

As kids get older, their amount of moderate or vigorous physical activity declines. Startling statistics for nine- to eighteen-year-old girls report a 35 percent decline in daily physical activity for white girls and an 83 percent decline for African American girls. Vigorous activity decreases among both girls and boys as they get older. Few children walk to school; less than 1 percent of children ride bicycles to school.[59]

Given less activity among kids and the low physical activity levels among adults, parents understandably spend little time in physical activities with their children. Once again, role modeling makes a difference. Parents who are physically active have kids who are more active, both on their own and together with their family.

Whether declining physical activity matches increasing food consumption in the rise of childhood obesity is of urgent interest to everyone involved: food and drink companies, media, technology makers, parents, communities, and health professionals—all who have a stake in the cause, the solution, or both. The next chapter investigates factors outside the home, particularly in schools, that have made today's generation the least fit ever.

## PARENTING: THE HARDEST JOB

Many parents and their children already have a fairly clear idea about the causes of childhood obesity, and they know that many of those causes involve their own behavior and their home environment. In one study, for example, parents of fourth-graders listed the following obstacles to eating healthy food and being physically active: lack of time or information, "bad" food preferences of other family members and caregivers, fatigue, expense, confusion about nutrition messages, feeling little influence over their kids, wanting to spend time in other ways, and stress.[60] Their children too partly blamed the family environment for poor eating and exercise habits. The kids' list mentioned barriers to healthy eating: fruit or juices are never available, no one says to drink water, so "we only drink soda." Or they felt little control over selection of diet—"Mom chooses what I eat." Some claim they didn't like lower-calorie foods—"Healthy food tastes bad." And they said parents hardly cared about their choice anyway: "I eat what I want." They acknowledged the connection between being overweight and lack of exercise but again blamed their situations: "My friends live far away," or "no kids like to play with me," or there is no place to get physical activity—"Mom says I can't play outside." Some held the media responsible for consumption of junk food: "They say it's good for you on TV."

If parents have at least a general understanding that their actions and home setting are unhealthy for their children, then why don't they do something to change—turn off the TV, prepare family meals, encourage active play? The answer lies in the fact that it's easier said than done. More than ever before, parenting is extremely challenging and undervalued. Parents—particularly working parents who are hard pressed financially—lack the time, energy, and support to carry out the positive changes that would help raise their kids to be healthy and fit.

In a lucid description of America's beleaguered moms and dads aptly entitled *The War Against Parents,* Sylvia Hewlett, president of the National Parenting Association, and Cornel West, university professor at Harvard, contend, "We live in a nation where market work, centered on competition and goods, crowds out caring, nurturing, cherishing—the essential components of good parenting; parenting is surely considered the ultimate non-market activity." If one institution after another makes parents responsible as both the culprits in and the cure for childhood obesity, then indeed parenting receives little support in America today. Parents get little assistance from the workplace: flexible work schedules are difficult to arrange, and adequate benefits often depend on double salaries or working overtime.

Hewlett and West do not mention obesity as a problem of the children they depict, yet the problems they describe contribute to the childhood obesity epidemic. They ask for help from all sectors of society to strengthen our families, communities, and chances for children, especially children in low-income homes and neighborhoods who have not had the luxury of material indulgence.

In contrast, in *Too Much of a Good Thing: Raising Children of Character in an Indulgent Age,* Daniel Kindlon describes parents who are comfortable financially but need other kinds of help—parents who are afraid to set limits, who want to be their children's friends rather than authority figures, and who also feel guilty about their work-obsessed lives. Whether poverty or luxury marks families, overworked and unavailable parents are more likely to alternate between being authoritarian and permissive—overcontrolling and overindulging their kids.

Effective child raising requires two special commodities (in addition to love, of course): energy and time. Both are usually in short supply to parents. It is worth considering why there is so little time available for raising children, when this is arguably among the most valuable investments parents, and society, can make. In *The Overworked American,* Juliet Schor describes how, in the 1990s, the average American worker put in about 164 extra hours of paid labor a year—the equivalent of an additional month of work—compared to twenty years earlier. This shift occurred just as the two-income household was becoming the middle-class norm. With greater time pressure at home as well as in the workplace, relaxation, civic participation, and caring for the young and the old compete for whatever energy is left.[61] Here, of course, in tracing the supply of time and energy we are particularly concerned with care of the young.

Long work hours may be a function of employers' hiring fewer workers to cut fringe costs or of employees' anxiously working more because of fears about unemployment—or both. Whatever the reason, Schor demonstrates that longer work hours create an "insidious cycle of work-and-spend." She cites several polls showing that Americans would prefer more leisure—like the 35-hour workweek in Germany and France—even at the price of reduced material living standards. Yet the American system rarely offers that explicit choice. Part-time work typically offers low pay and no fringe benefits.[62] There are likely other explanations for why Americans have less time and energy—less time for everyday family activities, talking, playing games, preparing and eating meals together; less energy for physical activities with children. But Schor's analysis in *The Overworked American* rings true when she argues that the quality of leisure activity has dropped as work hours have climbed. The main leisure activity of Americans is shopping; a close second is watching television, which conveys a relentless message to go out and shop some more. From the perspective of the family patterns that promote obesity, these leisure-time activities do matter. Both require minimal physical effort and go well with food. Shopping at the mall—and eating. Watching television—and eating.

Many parents say that working overtime or having two jobs is the only way they can afford to buy houses in safe neighborhoods with good schools—for their kids. Parents often feel as though they are expected to read from two or three scripts that tell them what is best for their kids. They become paralyzed by a host of contradictory demands. "I work two jobs to buy designer sneakers for my kids. Otherwise they wouldn't be seen on the playground. For them to play, I have to work more." For these reasons and more, many parents have become victims, rather than effective agents, in the struggle against childhood obesity.

## SUMMARY

To benefit overall health, but especially to guard against obesity, the degree to which families prepare meals together, eat together, and play together matters a lot. Families whose routines force them to be too busy and encourage kids and parents to eat away from home rather than together as a unit will be more likely to fall into a pattern of overeating, poor nutrition, and sedentary pastimes.

Looking at family dynamics and demographics, we examined the seeds of the blossoming epidemic of childhood obesity. From prenatal care to first feeding to children's food preferences, the indispensable, and often incredibly difficult, role of parenting helps trigger—or inhibit—the future fatness of our children. Two parenting styles regarding food choice—*authoritarian* (overcontrolling) and *permissive* (no limit setting)—contrast with *authoritative* parenting, which uses role modeling, negotiation, and reasoning to support healthy food behaviors. We learned about the importance of the endangered family meal and the difficulty of managing the super-size servings sold through the media, brought home in bulk, and available around the clock to even the youngest family members. From early childhood through adolescence, the decline in physical activity and the rise in screen time—video games and computers, and especially television, a focal point of so much family life—fatten our future.

The next chapter explores the growing trend of food-away-from-home and the degree to which children eat outside their parents' sphere of influence. It also assesses fast food, school food, and the many deterrents beyond the home to eating healthy food, staying active, and maintaining healthy weight.

# 5

---

# BEYOND THE HOME

---

WHEN SEVERAL OVERWEIGHT TEENAGERS from New York sued McDonald's, blaming the fast-food giant for their obesity and weight-related medical conditions, their case provided ample fodder in the debate over personal responsibility versus society's responsibility for causing and curbing fatness. The plaintiffs in the suit included a teenage girl—age nineteen, 5 feet 6 inches tall, 270 pounds—who said she ate a McMuffin for breakfast and a Big Mac meal with apple pie for dinner almost daily. Another plaintiff, a fifteen-year-old boy, said he grew to 400 pounds and developed diabetes because he had eaten McDonald's food every day since he was six. A U.S. district court judge dismissed the case in early 2003 but, in recognition of their compelling arguments, left the door open for the plaintiffs to amend and refile their complaints.[1]

The question on many people's minds was, what kind of parents would let their kids eat McDonald's food *every day?* Other questions that merit an equal level of concern and contempt come to mind: what forces are at work in the marketplace—not to mention schools and the media—to push aside healthier fare? Why are McDonald's and other fast-food outlets so available and attractive to so many Americans?

The judge—who famously described Chicken McNuggets as "a McFrankenstein creation of various elements not utilized by the home cook"—noted that kids are drawn to the restaurant chain not only for its food but also for its toy promotions and playground-like play areas. His remark raises two more questions. How do the food and restaurant industries target youth through clever marketing? And what opportunities for outdoor play and recreation are missing from these kids' lives that make them flock to a McDonald's PlayPlace?

As the questions above suggest, it is the interplay of societal and personal factors—not the parents' or children's behavior alone—that is responsible for young people such as these plaintiffs growing so fat.

After reviewing the McDonald's case with my teenage students, I polled them for an opinion. Of sixty students, fifty-seven agreed with the case dismissal, calling it "absurd" or "ridiculous," because "everyone knows that fast food is unhealthy." Most students held the parents responsible; the rest blamed the plaintiffs themselves for eating foods that made them fat. If pressed to choose, I would side with the judge's dismissal, and I am concerned that lawsuits may not achieve the desired results, but I would not characterize the case as "absurd." It is unreasonable to expect parents, already overburdened, to make a lone stand against fast foods touted to their kids (even as toddlers). And, as this chapter reveals, it is misguided to focus only on parents and the home when we study the causes and solutions for obesity.

When I observed my graduate students as they finished up a child nutrition field experience in a New York City Head Start program, they, too, held the parents responsible for promoting healthy weight in their children. Not yet parents themselves, they made comments such as "parents must set limits," "parents are supposed to be role models," and "parents are the problem and the solution." But the mothers of the Head Start children had a different perspective. They recognized that they were up against a society that does not support the family in making healthy choices and being physically active, and they appealed for outside help: "We need safe places for kids to play." "Healthy foods that kids like and don't make them fat would help." "Good child care while we work is hard to find." I agree with the viewpoints both groups expressed; my point is that they could learn from each other. We should likewise broaden our perspectives and acknowledge the complexity of this epidemic, rather than take sides and simplify it.

The previous chapter highlighted the benefits of families preparing and eating meals together at home. Family meals give parents the opportunity to serve nutritious food in appropriate portion sizes, to pass on healthy eating habits, and to strengthen family bonds through mealtime conversations.

But kids often eat away from home and apart from their parents: then who or what determines what they eat? This chapter goes beyond the home to finish answering the question of why children are getting fatter. We turn to the eating-away-from-home trend, driven in no small part by the popularity of fast food, and to the two main places kids spend their days—in school and around the neighborhood.

## EATING ANYWHERE, ANYTIME

More than ever before in American history, food is abundant and available around the clock. In fact, we have too much food: far more food is produced than is needed in the United States—about 3,800 calories per person per day in 2000, nearly twice as much as required by many adults and most children.[2] Our problem, then, in dealing with this enormous supply—cleverly marketed in many flavors and forms to create a demand—is with food choices.

Snacking is the standard accompaniment to activities throughout the day. For some, "an activity without food is like a day without sun," and there remain few off-limit locations for eating. To compete with bookstores, many libraries allow children to eat and read. Not long ago schools forbade chewing gum; students now bring doughnuts and candy to class. At most youth sports games, treats—generally candy, chips, and soda—are served at halftime and after the game. Kids come with extra soda and chips to fill in the downtime. This trend of eating-on-the-go and eating-as-entertainment is a big factor in increased obesity.[3]

Over the last three decades, calories from food prepared away from home increased from 18 percent to 32 percent of total calories. Americans now spend almost half of their food dollars on food away from home—47 percent, or $354.4 billion, in 1998. The majority was spent in commercial food service, including fast-food outlets, restaurants, lodging places, recreation and entertainment places, and "retail hosts" (who serve what is eaten at the mall and other public venues).[4] "Away-from-home" foods contain more total fat and saturated fat on a per-calorie basis than at-home food and—because restaurant meals contain large portions of highly palatable food—frequent restaurant patrons consume more high-fat, low-fiber foods than people who eat out less often.[5] Some families consider eating out to be a treat, a time to indulge, and the trouble is that American families eat dinner out at least two to three times weekly. When one study compared the frequency of eating restaurant meals to eating home-cooked ones, a high rate of away-from-home eating related to a higher rate of obesity.[6]

## FAST-FOOD FAMILIES

Americans forked over $110 billion to fast-food restaurants in 2002.[7] These restaurants report that half of their sales are now at the drive-by window—a high volume of backseat or dashboard dining that reflects the reality of today's hurried lifestyles and poses a threat to healthy eating.

Consider, for example, the difference between breakfast at home and breakfast from a drive-through. Breakfast, we're often told, is the most important meal of the day, which is especially true for school-age children. It is potentially their healthiest, most balanced meal and provides the energy they need to be mentally alert at school[8]—and eating breakfast helps control weight by keeping hunger in line. A breakfast of vitamin-fortified, lightly sweetened whole-grain cereal (such as Cheerios), fruit, and milk amounts to about 250–300 calories. But a child whose family swings by a McDonald's on the way to school might eat a 5.5 oz bacon, egg, and cheese biscuit (470 calories) or a 9 oz Spanish omelet bagel (680 calories). Add a couple of hash brown patties (300 calories) plus a 16 oz container of orange juice (220 calories), and the calorie total comes to around 1,000 calories. This is enough to feed four small children, two medium-size preteens, or one captain of a high school football team. The McDonald's meal, in addition to being excessively high-calorie, is a nutritional nightmare, containing high amounts of saturated fat and low amounts of the fiber, calcium, and vitamins that young (and older) bodies need. The "breakfast of champions" advertised on a Wheaties box—healthy cereal with milk and juice—is becoming a memory as high-calorie fast-food breakfasts become the norm.

In *Fast Food Nation,* Eric Schlosser uncovered the fast-food industry's efforts to reel in the youngest, most susceptible consumers. "Fast food," he claims, "has fueled an epidemic of obesity."[9] And how does the industry reel in the kids? Why do children and their parents eat so frequently at fast-food restaurants? "That's a 'no-brainer,'" I'm told when I ask families and kids what draws them to fast-food restaurants. "They're cheap, they're nearby, we love the food because you always know exactly what you're getting—and besides, everyone else goes and gets the toys."

Schlosser describes how McDonald's and Burger King operate over

10,000 playgrounds. He interviewed "Playlands" makers, who explained, "Playlands bring in children, who bring in parents, who bring in money." The seesaws and slides are effective lures but, Schlosser reports, "the key to attracting kids is toys, toys, toys."[10] A successful promotion easily doubles or triples the weekly volume of children's meals. Ronald McDonald is a "trusted friend" of most families, recognized by 96 percent of American children.

When I talked with people from the Bronx neighborhood who eat at the two McDonald's restaurants (only short blocks apart) sued by the teens for making them fat, it was easy to see how low-income minority neighborhoods are great "targets" for the promotions of fast-food chains. The food is cheap: "We use the coupons—buy one, get one free, like, 'Free Big Mac with purchase of a regular price Big Mac.'" "Extra Value meals give you a 32 oz soft drink [instead of 21 oz] and large fries too [instead of medium] for only 40 cents more." The place is familiar and comfortable: "My friends work here." "Cool place to hang out." The location is strategic: "McDonald's is right around the corner, open from 6 A.M. to midnight." And, above all, the food tastes good: "I love french fries—my favorite snack since I was a little kid." Yes indeed, McDonald's marketing formula reels in the young customers with taste, cost, and accessibility.

Two teens with both "size and style" told me, "Those girls who sued probably have families who work too much and don't have time to cook a well-balanced meal," and, "They do have a point about the McNuggets because the list of ingredients is so long and with things that only a nutritionist would know what it does to your body." One also noted that McDonald's has taken a few small steps toward a healthier menu: "McDonald's must be scared now because I just saw a commercial that said they have changed the McNuggets to all-white meat."

Consumers are demanding fresher ingredients and healthier choices in fast-food restaurants. As a nutritionist, I hope the move toward healthy fast food is real (all white meat and less grease), spurred by books like *Fast Food Nation* and eye-opening lawsuits. I was first delighted to see the "new all white meat chicken McNuggets" coupons appear shortly after the lawsuit hit the news—until I noticed the small print: "Only available in Manhattan south of 96th Street." Two plaintiffs in one suit live at least a forty-five-minute, two-dollar subway or bus ride away from the nearest McDonald's selling the new McNuggets, McVeggie Burgers, and the New Premium Salads with grilled chicken. Even if these healthier choices taste good and are priced right, they still are not accessible in the very neighborhood that ignited the movement toward healthier fast food. Nearly a year later, the customer representative said, "They are being test-marketed in selected stores."

## SUPER-SIZE PEOPLE

We also have the food industry to thank for the insidious super-sizing trend that has made this generation accustomed to portions that are larger and higher in calories than ever before. Consider that eating just one hundred calories more per day than needed adds about ten extra pounds in a year, and it is no wonder that super-size portions are leading to super-size people. In 1977, for example, the average cheeseburger weighed 5.8 oz and contained 397 calories; by 1996 it weighed 7.3 oz and provided 533 calories.[11]

"Meal deals" harness the desire of customers young and old to get the most for their money. For an extra 69 cents or so, they get extralarge portions of fries and sodas, which cost the restaurant only a few pennies more to produce. "It's a great sales technique," notes Nestle in the *Nutrition Action Healthletter*. "People buy larger sizes because they perceive them as good value. If they're going to spend all this money on food, especially in a restaurant, they figure they might as well get a lot to eat."[12]

Super-sizing spread from restaurants and convenience stores like 7-Eleven to the grocer's shelves; between the late 1970s and 1990s, the number of large-portion-size food products increased tenfold.[13] Old-fashioned "large" 16 oz bags of potato chips are now positively dwarfed by new "normal-size" 32 oz bags—get two for just a little more than the price of one, all in one bag! Coca Cola was sold in 6.5 oz bottles in the 1950s; single-serving 20 oz bottles are common in the new millennium. Family-size containers (64 oz) of cola are sometimes used as single servings, consumed in a few minutes by thirsty teens—and many preteens.

Super-sizing not only plays into the innate belief that bigger is better, it also manipulates the desire for food that people know is "bad" for them. Packaging unhealthy food in huge portions makes the consumer feel less guilty about eating large amounts. "People can often eat about 50 percent more of hedonistic foods like candy, chips, and popcorn when they come in bigger packs. With other foods, the increase is usually about 25 percent," reported Brian Wansink in the *Nutrition Action Healthletter*.[14] Value marketing is selling people "lots more" of something for "a little bit more" money (the profit is still considerable for the producer). It makes economic sense for the food industry.

Schools are partly responsible for the high fast-food consumption of youth. Schools sell junk food—through student stores, vending machines, and fund-raising drives—to students who rarely sit down to eat a balanced meal from the cafeteria or a nutritious brown-bag lunch from home. Why do schools compromise the health of youth this way? They argue that they need the money to make up gaps in their budgets and to support extracurricular activities.

We might hope that schools would provide a healthy oasis in an otherwise fattening environment, but quite the opposite is true: witness the remarks below.

"I pass six Pepsi machines on my way to lunch," reported a middle school student.

"We have to buy drinks, because the fountains are so gross," a high school student told me. Said others, "The lunch lines are so long, I just buy a big bag of chips and a candy bar from the school store. A girl asked if they could sell apples in the school store—they tried and the apples got rotten because nobody bought them."

"I usually eat school lunch because there are always fries, real cheap, on the line. One time the deep fryers broke down and we got up a student petition to have them fixed real soon. Ya just gotta have fries for lunch."

Elementary students tell me about Channel One, the televised newscast featured in many classrooms and supported by private advertising, "We have TV in our classroom with some interesting stuff about the world and how people live in other places, but I really think the funny little guy running to get Pepsi is the best."

Reported by a third-grade student: "My teacher is great! She teaches M&M math. If we get the problem she shows with the M&Ms right, we get to eat them! My sister gets a Milky Way if she reads another book in her class."

A 1996 nationwide study found that 68 percent of school foods were sold a la carte from school stores and the cafeteria's "trend" menu, which features less nutritious meals and snacks; 23 percent came from vending machines in the schools. Only 9 percent of food sold at schools came from the nutritionally well balanced Type A USDA-regulated lunch served in cafeterias and available to all, specifically to those eligible for reduced-price meals.[15]

Almost half of the student population reported shopping at student stores for lunch or snacks in a survey of twenty-four public middle schools in southern California.[16] Other studies report that 30 percent of high schools have student stores; most are open throughout the school day and 47 percent are open during lunch. The stores are meant to provide students with experience in planning and organization as well as provide a means to support special activities, speech debates, band trips, and the like. Yet the foods they sell—such as king-size candy bars, chips, cakes, cookies, and soft drinks—are generally high in fat, sugar, and calories, and low in nutrients.

We've reached a point where schools are compromising students' health in order to pay for educational opportunities—and where both parents and students help with fund-raising through candy sales. The 2002 national PTA president, Shirley Igo, told a *New York Times* reporter that when schools cannot pay for their instructional programs, PTAs help fill the gap, and that candy sales are one way to do so.[17] Athletic teams raise money the same way. Coaches have been known to tie grades to meeting candy sale quotas, or to threaten students with loss of participation in sports if sales fall short.

In moderation and offset with lots of physical activity, candy can be part of a balanced diet. But filling gaps in school budgets with candy sales discourages moderation, especially in children who are already gaining weight and don't get enough exercise. I believe schools can play a key role in slowing childhood obesity through comprehensive and coordinated nutrition services that provide nourishing and attractive foods kids like and encourage greater acceptance of less familiar foods, especially fruits and vegetables. Many kids tell me they would love freshly made salads and sandwiches in see-through containers, deli style, and fresh fruit salad or big pieces of melon. With appropriate financial support from parents, school boards, and all levels of government, along with strategic planning in schools that elevates nutritional health to a top priority, the cafeteria could provide taste, comfort, and easy access during lunch—just like McDonald's, but with healthier choices. The odds are that they could also win the competition with vending machines and school stores.

## VENDING MACHINES

Now a fixture in most schools, vending machines bring schools cash in return for a company's right to sell sodas and advertise. The commercial fight over exclusive "pouring rights" in schools is all about soft drink companies' competitive strategies to "put soft drinks within arm's reach of desire. . . .

Schools are one channel."[18] When schools sell more soda, companies reward them with more cash. Vending machines provide money for 98 percent of public high schools, 74 percent of middle schools, and 43 percent of elementary schools, according to the Centers for Disease Control. Some schools keep vending machines off-limits during the lunch hour, but more than half do not. Besides soft drinks, the foods in these machines are candy, potato chips, and other snack foods high in fat and sugar, low in vitamins and minerals—foods that displace the fruits, vegetables, and milk that are essential for children's health and that promote a healthy weight.

Efforts to ban vending machines have led to a brouhaha that divides educators, parents, and students as they debate whether to kick these machines off campus and suffer the loss of revenue. Several school districts have already made the leap; for example, San Francisco decided by early 2003 to ban junk-food sales on its campuses, even though it would mean a loss of approximately $546,000 from its annual school budget.[19] Several other districts in California have voted to take soft drinks off cafeteria menus and end the sale of soft drinks in vending machines by 2004—a loss of $4.5 million annually in Los Angeles alone.[20] Whether their action improves the health of kids remains to be seen. In some districts where vending machines are banned, such as Oakland, California, students can still get their soda and junk-food fix by shopping off campus.

One ambitious attempt to ban junk food in schools failed. In spite of voicing concern that childhood obesity is a serious problem, a state legislative committee in Maine unanimously rejected a bill to ban school candy and soda sales; the bill prohibited the sale in all schools of any food or beverage that has a high sugar or sweetener content, as well as any juice that is less than 100 percent "real fruit juice."[21] Other schools are leaving the machines on campus but offering healthier alternatives in them, such as milk and water, at a reduced price. The Haverford, Pennsylvania, school district sells milk and fruit juices in vending machines. Its food service director, Charles Damiani, told the *Philadelphia Inquirer,* "We couldn't keep them filled. It blew my mind. The milk machine outsells the soda machine two to one."[22]

I think offering healthy drinks (and foods) in vending machines makes sense. For schools that need the revenue, it is a healthier way to meet the bottom line. More important, this moderate move stands a good chance of improving food choices and stalling the rate of obesity. Another step is to improve water fountains so kids will use them—especially kids with less money in their pockets. California is legislating to raise bond funds that ensure modernization of fountains. Clean, cool water is not only calorie-free but supports healthy physical activity by replacing lost fluids.

Why do students spend so much of their lunch money on food and drinks with low nutritional value from student stores, vending machines, and nearby retail outlets? Besides school revenue, corporate marketing is certainly part of the reason. As one report noted, food manufacturers spent $7 billion in advertising in 1997. Most of this advertising focused on highly processed and highly packaged foods—which also tend to be the foods consumed in large quantities[23]—rather than foods that meet dietary recommendations. In fact, only $333 million was spent on nutrition education, about half the amount spent on advertising soda alone. Or beer, or candy, or breakfast cereals—each![24] For example, to increase teen sales and brand loyalty that continues into the school year, in the summer of 2003 PepsiCo planned to spend $100 million on hot-weather hoopla, including a television commercial showing a hip teen sitting in an exclusive club sipping Pepsi from a brandy snifter.[25]

Television commercials for food saturate the airwaves and target specific groups: four to five food commercials per thirty minutes on prime-time shows geared toward an African American audience compared to three food commercials per thirty minutes on general prime time. Candy is the feature in 30 percent of the food commercials, and soda in another 13 percent.[26]

But it is not just advertising that whets kids' appetites for unhealthy food; it also is the alternative—namely, the food prepared by school cafeterias—that makes the hallway vending machines and the food retailers even more tempting.

## SCHOOL LUNCHES

A big portion of noncommercial "food-away-from-home" food service includes schools and day-care centers. Almost all public schools participate in the National School Lunch Program, authorized in 1946 to be administered by the U.S. Department of Agriculture. The program served over 26 million children in 2000, while the companion School Breakfast Program served 17 million children. About 13 million children received free meals and 2 million children received reduced-price lunches, depending on their financial needs.[27] Many students these days participate in schools' extended-care and summer programs and therefore eat breakfast and after-school snacks as well as lunch at school.

The school lunch program can be a key player in the fight against childhood

## SAMPLE SCHOOL LUNCH MENUS

School cafeterias across the country dish up food from menus that vary widely in quality and popularity. Some school meals are subsidized and regulated by the government and are therefore relatively healthy, though generally less popular. Other meals come direct from fast-food vendors and are nutritionally inferior but typically more popular. The first menu lists several typical USDA Type A lunches at schools that participate in the national school lunch program; they are available to all students, including those eligible for reduced-price meals. They look fairly healthy and balanced but they are not very popular because the food is often frozen or canned. The nonsubsidized a la carte "trend menu" shown below is available in cafeterias as an alternative to the Type A lunch. The third menu lists food available in schools where Pizza Hut has a food contract.

USDA TYPE A
*Approximate calories: 600 (30% from fat)*

Teriyaki tenders
Rice pilaf
Peas (canned)
Mandarin orange segments
Milk

Chicken burger
Carrots (canned)
Chunky applesauce
Milk

Ricotta-stuffed shells in marinara sauce
Spinach (canned)
Peach crisp
Milk

A LA CARTE MENU
*Approximate calories: 600 (40% from fat)*

Grilled cheese sandwich
French fries
Carrot sticks
Brownie

Hot dog or hamburger
French fries
Baked beans
Peanut butter cookie

Fish nuggets
French fries
Coleslaw
Chocolate pudding

PIZZA HUT MENU
*Approximate calories: 800 (42% from fat)*

Pizza Hut Personal Pan cheese pizza
Iceburg lettuce salad with ranch dressing
Chocolate chip cookies

Pizza Hut Personal Pan pepperoni pizza
Potato wedges
Strawberry shortcake

Pizza Hut Personal Pan Hawaiian pizza (with pineapple and ham)
Spicy fries
Peach cup

obesity, since it reaches a growing number of children. Federal guidelines make these lunches relatively healthy. But the problem is that students do not want to eat them because the lunches do not taste very good (or kids think they don't), and because the students fill up on food from other sources.

When schools receive funds from the USDA for school food programs, certain guidelines about when and where to serve food apply, like not selling soft drinks in the cafeteria during lunch and serving the approved Type A balanced menu. Yet because USDA school food rules apply only to reimbursable meals based on a child's family income, various a la carte food options are allowed for students who pay full price. (See the box "Sample School Lunch Menus.") A la carte foods, such as a hot dog or hamburger with fries, or a grilled cheese sandwich, also with fries, do not meet the approved specifications—they are higher in fat, sugar, and calories—but students prefer them to the more nutritious federally subsidized meals. It is notable that some students who are eligible to take advantage of the subsidized menu do not do so, because of the real or imagined stigma attached to being in "that" cafeteria line.

Some schools have opted out of the USDA program altogether in order to take advantage of commercial cash revenue and other incentives (gigantic electronic football field scoreboards, school buses with billboard ads). As a result, chain restaurants have taken over many school cafeterias. Apparently, school principals like the revenue—and the students like the food. (One district food manager reports that participation in school lunch jumps 20 percent in his thirty schools every Wednesday, when pizza is served. He explains, "Pizza arrives on time, hot, freshly made, and evenly sliced.")[28]

It is worth noting that vegetables and fruits required by USDA school food guidelines are unlikely to be available for schools that opt out of governmental programs. But, unfortunately, they are unlikely to be missed. A study of fourth-graders found that half the children served vegetables did not eat them.[29] Veggies that come from a can and are overcooked aren't too appealing, but for many schools, serving fresh produce is difficult, if not impossible. Again, money is an issue. "I've been in school kitchens where they haven't the simplest tools like knives or equipment to store fresh fruits and vegetables, much less processors for shredding and chopping or containers and utensils for salad bars," Thomas Forster, of the nonprofit Community Food Security Coalition, told the *New York Times*.[30]

Many school districts with parent support are taking matters in hand and buying fresh foods, cooked by local people who know how to get kids to eat vegetables. "We figure you have to serve a new food item ten times before the kids actually eat it," said Melanie Payne, who oversees meals in an Alabama school district profiled in the *New York Times*. Compared to children in other schools, who usually choose fries as a vegetable, the children in this Alabama district choose (and eat) greens, peas, fresh sweet potatoes, and black-eyed peas.

New York City, with the largest school food service in the country, is beginning to make radical changes: to turn school cafeterias into attractive "dining destinations," to launch a "schools that cook" program, and to leverage its buying power for healthier food. Yet what threatens to stall these improvements is not the lack of equipment or even the desire of the food service staff to serve easy prepackaged foods, but rather administrative and political hurdles. I visited one of the newly constructed model high school buildings in New York City with an astonishing skyline view of New York harbor that fairly invites students to enjoy lunch at small tables. The food service manager was eager to provide attractive food, the cooks were happy to cook rather than open packages and reheat foods, and the students would enjoy freshly prepared salads and vegetables. What was the problem? Centralized buying contracts with corporate food companies and difficulties with food service unions were two barriers to on-site food preparation.

Congress is writing legislation to improve school food programs nationwide, which will require negotiating with the many competing interests that run counter to the aim of improving school food. Agribusiness has a big stake in the matter and undoubtedly wants the Department of Agriculture to continue buying surplus amounts of commodities from the nation's farmers (these are not small local farmers). The USDA uses the school lunch program to dispense these extra products, which accounts for the high-fat beef and dairy products on school menus.

Chapter 9 revisits the challenges and the possibilities of changing the nearly 5 billion school lunches produced every year into tasty, cheap, accessible, *and* healthy meals, served in attractive settings. Whether these changes earn money for the schools matters far less—we all agree—than children's health. Our urgent concern to improve food habits learned in school and reduce the number of obese children must drive the movement—a small tax increase would be money well spent.

## DAY-CARE DINING

Today's babies and toddlers eat away from home almost as much as their grade-school siblings do. For millions of children, responsibility to develop their eating behavior has shifted to child-care providers and preschools. Nearly 70 percent of children under five are cared for in another's home or in organized child-care facilities.[31] The majority of children in child-care centers eat one or two daily meals plus snacks there. Whether the food is prepared on site or sent from home, menu evaluations and my observations show that kids in child care typically consume excess fat and a limited amount of vegetables.

Many caregivers in private day-care programs fear children will overeat or waste food if left to choose their own portions. Few private child-care providers sit with children and consume the same foods during mealtime. Yet even trained caregivers who eat with the children often use authoritarian commands such as "You need to eat." Negative mealtime reprimands and verbal controls are common: "You need to clean your plate," "You have to taste each food at least once," "Hurry up and finish eating."

Governmental guidelines and resources, such as the USDA Child and Adult Care Food Program, are available for day-care providers at homes and in centers. Head Start, a federally funded preschool program for economically disadvantaged children, is the largest program in the U.S. providing food service to preschool children. It is regulated by the Administration for Children and Families, part of the U.S. Department of Health and Human Services. Head Start programs demonstrate positive mealtime routines that involve teachers eating the same food as children and children serving themselves and assisting with meal setup and cleanup. Still, a Head Start director told me recently that regulation reviews are "a headache because we have to meet guidelines from two agencies—one tells us we have too much fat in our menus, the other says we have to make sure the kids eat."

Head Start requires family-style meal service with small tables and utensils in order to teach serving and eating skills that allow children to recognize their hunger and fullness levels. In most cases in Head Start centers, according to one study, positive teacher attitudes and mealtime behaviors occurred more frequently than negative ones: naming food items, encouraging food tasting, general conversation.[32] Examples of positive interactions might be "This vegetable is called peas. Would you try some?" "When I was your age, my grandmother grew them in the garden. I would help pick them and take them out of their covers, called pea pods. I liked saying 'pea pod.'" There is no doubt about it: eating and enjoying vegetables and other healthy foods at this age are crucial steps toward weight management in the future.

It goes without saying that mealtimes and snacks at day care and school strongly influence children's weight gain. Another key determinant is physical activity at schools (or lack of it).

## SEE JANE (AND JASON) SIT

Today's students are less fit than ever before, in large part because school schedules often leave out physical activity. Ironically, educators' and administrators' well-meaning efforts to boost academic standards are partly to blame for the reduction in physical fitness, because students who are burdened with homework and busy at computer labs have less time and energy to run around for play or to take a gym class.

Recess has all but disappeared from the daily school schedule, often to make room for computer learning time. Headlines attest to this trend: "Is Recess on the Way Out?" and "Even for Sixth Graders, College Looms, the Academic Pressure Is On."[33] According to the American Association for a Child's Right to Play, an estimated 40 percent of all elementary schools have dropped or are in the process of dropping recess.[34]

Even in schools that have recess breaks, the amount of energetic "running around" has declined. I watched a bunch of fourth-grade students in an inner-city school (with a paucity of play equipment) start to "fool around" by chasing one classmate and then another; the aide blew the whistle to go in early so the "kids wouldn't fight and get hurt." Principals complain that they don't have money to hire aides to supervise children in playgrounds, yet at the same time school grounds need more supervision than in the past because parents demand increased assurance of safety. The rules are so rigid in one suburban school playground that seventh-grade girls started playing cards during their recess breaks. Another reason for less running around on school grounds is that kids are simply more sedentary and less fit and don't want to be active at recess or in physical education class.

The facts speak for themselves: in 1991, 46 percent of high school students and 57 percent of middle school students took a daily PE class. By 1999, those figures had dropped to 29 percent of high school students and 35 percent of middle school students. Of those participating, only 38 percent were physically active in the class for more than twenty minutes. If not daily, we might expect participation in physical activity at school a minimum of two to three days a week. But 2000 statistics show that only 40 percent of high school students *enrolled* in physical education; by twelfth grade, the number dipped to 37 percent. Girls have lower rates of physical activity than boys; starting in adolescence, girls' physical activity declines at least 7 percent per year, while boys' activity decreases nearly 3 percent per year.[35]

Perhaps more startling than the drop in physical education participation is the worsening level of physical fitness among children of all ages. Only 3 percent of children surveyed by the CDC in 2001 met the standard for thirty minutes of continuous vigorous physical activity (aerobic capacity measured by heart rate).[36] One PE teacher for grades K–8 noted that her twice-weekly class is the only strenuous exercise most children at her school get. "In any given class, there's close to 50 percent of the kids who are overweight," the teacher told a reporter for a parenting magazine. "It's scary when you look at some of these kids, they get tired doing thirty seconds of exercise—I mean, really, *really* tired. They just quit."[37]

In a study of overweight African American eight- to ten-year-old girls in Texas, some voiced typical complaints about physical education class: "I hate running laps in the hot sun. Some of my friends are always ahead of us. The rest of us feel tired and exhausted."[38] Running laps at school is one thing, but plain old walking is another. A volunteer teen leader working with sixth- and seventh-grade African American girls in a HeartSmart school project in Harlem told me the girls on a walking field trip begged to sit down because, they said, "our legs hurt."

The overall decline in school physical activity translates into lower participation in team sports too. Working part-time jobs after school affects participation by both low- and middle-income students. City kids working at McDonald's earn money for CD players and clothes. Suburban kids cashiering at the supermarket say, "I have to work to run my car."

Even as the rate of physical activity falls and obesity rises, both parents and kids still pay lip service to the importance of physical education at school. Over 80 percent of adults and 70 percent of teens believe that daily PE should be mandatory in schools. One way to get attention and respect for physical activity is to revamp the old "PE for athletes" into "PE for fitness." This New PE philosophy encourages gym teachers to focus at least as much on poorly conditioned kids as they do on the students with more athletic abilities. As reported in *Newsweek,* "Instead of helping the natural athletes refine the perfect jump shot, proponents of the New PE say their goal is to get 'mouse potatoes' moving again."[39]

Thankfully, momentum seems to be building among educators and legislators to salvage PE and make it a priority. But let us not overlook the importance of getting kids to move more throughout the day, during and after school. Experts find that children are likely to get fat not only because they spend less energy in physical activity, but because they are simply less fit aerobically. Inactivity has a far stronger effect on obesity than lack of vigorous activity.[40] *Any* activity is better than none, to stall the increasing rate of obesity among all children.

### UNSAFE STREETS, UNFIT KIDS

Earlier generations did not need school recesses and PE classes as much as today's children do. For them, exercise was as much a spontaneous activity as a scheduled one. Kids rode their bikes or walked to and from school, then played freely with friends around the neighborhood in the hours between school and dinner. Hopscotch on the sidewalk or ball games in the park happened whenever kids took the initiative to play them. A young father lamented to me, "It's hard to find any kids who know how to play kick-the-can anymore."

Today, less than 1 percent of children ride bicycles to school. Walking and bicycling, even short distances, by children ages five to fifteen dropped 40 percent between 1977 and 1997.[41] Enjoyable outdoor activities and trips to the playground usually take place during scheduled play dates and involve adult supervision and transportation. Children learn early on that

"Go play outside" means go to the enclosed backyard, *not* out the front door.

Where do kids play after school when they return to a home without a backyard, without a parent present? For millions of children, the answer is that they play inside. Limited to indoors, "play" is likely to involve sitting rather than movement. Working parents whose children have few recreational opportunities are left with little choice but to tell their kids to return home from school by bus or carpool (rather than on foot), and then to remain indoors with the door locked.

Between 5 million and 7 million latchkey children go home to an empty house after school, and fully one-third of all twelve-year-olds regularly fend for themselves while their parents are at work. For them, playing video games and eating snacks are the only choices they are allowed for fun. "These children are at higher risk of truancy, school failure, substance abuse, violent or unhealthy behavior. Preteens and especially adolescents who crave excitement, are, if unsupervised, likely to become involved in something dangerous to themselves or others. Eating and watching TV are often considered safe and even healthy activities in comparison."[42]

Beyond discouraging recreation, unsafe neighborhoods and poverty foster childhood obesity for other reasons. In particular, these conditions lead to a fear of crime and a preoccupation with subsistence that push health and nutrition lower on everyone's list of concerns. A conversation I had with a group of overweight teenage single mothers, black and white, some as young as fourteen, made this abundantly clear. A few hoped to get their bodies "in shape," but neither their weight nor their ruptured education matched their worries of being physically abused and the fear of violence in their home and neighborhood. They told me, "My Mama always said stay away from the streets and the park—they're bad." "I went to the park with my baby—a gang of real big guys followed me saying bad stuff." "There are so many bullies and bad people watching, I get scared."

The safety, quality, and availability of a community's parks factor into the fatness epidemic. Unsafe or nonexistent parks and broken-down playground equipment can't compete with the cleaner, safer, and "climate-controlled" environment of food-rich shopping malls where parents and their youth spend leisure time.

A community's food choices also serve as a predictor of obesity. Fast food is everywhere, especially in low-income neighborhoods, but not the high-quality supermarkets with premium produce that suburbanites enjoy. Grocery stores that serve lower-income populations and rural communities are less likely to sell attractive fruits and vegetables and more likely to stock the budget-oriented food products that are higher in calories and lower in nutritional value.

The surgeon general's call to action in 2001 promoted the joint/shared use of facilities among parks, libraries, and community-based organizations for physical activity and urged communities to advocate for grocery stores carrying high-quality and affordable fresh produce.[43] Some communities have taken these steps, as we will see in chapter 9.

## REPORT CARD ON KIDS' EATING

Having considered the environmental factors that affect children's eating—in home, at school, and throughout the community—we can take stock of children's diets and look more specifically at what and how much they eat. Food intake surveys show that children's diets are overindulgent in certain areas and seriously deficient in others, earning close to a failing grade.

### SO MUCH SODA

Soda consumption weighs in as a major factor in the declining quality of children's diets. Carbonated drinks (sodas) are the single biggest source of refined sugars in the American diet, as high as 30 percent of total calories for some children and adolescents. From 1965 to 1996 boys raised their soda intake by 287 percent, and girls by 224 percent.[44]

Nearly half of all children six to eleven years old drink an average of 15 oz daily. Many have been drinking 8 to 10 oz a day since age two. One-fourth of thirteen- to eighteen-year-old soda drinkers consume two or more cans a day, some as many as five 12 oz cans daily. Because they drink it constantly, on average American children get 11 percent of their calories from soda; "heavy drinkers" get over 18 percent of their calories from it (that is, 35 oz per day, about 350 calories).[45] Twenty years ago the typical consumer of soft drinks drank about half this amount. Vending machines that dispense sodas are present not only on campuses but nearly everywhere kids go; in 1997, 2.8 million soft drink vending machines dispensed 27 billion drinks to Americans, particularly American youth.[46]

Harvard researchers noted children's soda consumption and weight change for two years and concluded that for each additional serving of sugar-sweetened drink consumed per day by a child, the chance of developing obesity increases. That holds true regardless of initial body mass, diet, television-viewing habits, and physical activity.[47] The lead researcher, the pediatrician David Ludwig, told *Eating Well* magazine, "When a heavy child eats the equivalent of 20 teaspoons of added sugar a day, 320 calories go straight into additional weight gain. Once a child has established this pattern of eating, it's a very difficult rhythm to break."[48]

Soda is sweetened, as are most fruit drinks, with high-fructose corn syrup and some sucrose (both are forms of sugar). Like sucrose, corn syrup is a good source of energy. But because corn syrup and sucrose are completely devoid of any other nutrients, when soda crowds out milk as a main beverage, it compromises bone building, especially in teenage girls.[49] Of equal concern for all children who eat and drink high amounts of corn syrup and sucrose is their susceptibility to coronary heart disease (especially elevated blood fats called triglycerides) and type 2 diabetes—made worse with obesity.

Scientists debate whether corn syrup is a major villain in the rise of obesity, but as Dr. George Bray, a leading obesity researcher and professor of medicine at Louisiana State University Medical Center observed about the meteoric rise in consumption of corn syrup and the jump in obesity rates, "Nothing else in the food supply [correlates like] this. It's a very, very striking relationship."[50]

### FAR FROM FIVE A DAY

Federal data from the most recent *Continuing Survey of Food Intakes by Individuals,* a nationally representative survey containing information on the diets of about 5,000 children, show the average six- to eleven-year-old consumed just over three servings of fruits and vegetables a day of the "five a day" recommended. Here are the top fifteen sources of energy (calories) for children ages two to eighteen, in order of popularity.

milk

bread

cakes/cookies/doughnuts

beef (ground)

ready-to-eat cereal (sweetened)

soft drinks

cheese

potato and corn chips

sugars/syrups/jams

poultry

ice cream/frozen yogurt

pasta

margarine

fruit drinks

white potatoes (fries)

As sources for bread, beef, and cheese, read big burgers and pizza. Poultry is a code for fried chicken nuggets and buckets of fried chicken parts. And milk means shakes and chocolate milk.[51]

Because vegetables and fruits are naturally low in calories, we might not expect to find them on this list of top calorie-contributing foods. Yet fruit drinks and potatoes do show up. Fruit drinks get a calorie boost from added sugar. The potatoes, generally consumed as chips or fries, are packed with fat. An astonishing 27 percent of vegetable servings for white children were fried potatoes and potato chips; 37 percent for black children. In contrast, fries and potato chips make up about 17 percent of vegetable consumption for the American population as a whole.

A daily diet of high-calorie fries, chips, burgers, and pizza together with high-calorie soft drinks equals a high-calorie diet (no surprise here). Though the surveys do not rate sufficiency or excess of total calories for individual children, we do know that excess food energy is available in the food supply. We also know that nearly two-thirds of children eat more than the recommended amount of fat for health. All things considered, we have some pretty sound evidence that excessive calorie consumption relates strongly to the childhood obesity epidemic.

The Healthy Eating Index, compiled by the USDA, gives us another overall picture of the type and quantity of foods kids eat. It rates the quality of children's diets—giving us a "report card" based on adequacy, moderation, and variety. This index has ten components, each representing one aspect of a healthy diet. The first five measure the degree the diet conforms to the recommended portions from five major food groups (grain, vegetable, fruit, dairy, and high-protein). The other five evaluate total fat, saturated fat, dietary cholesterol, sodium, and the degree of variety in the child's diet. Each component of the index has a maximum score of 10, so the maximum combined score for the ten components is 100. Thus any Healthy Eating Index score above 80 indicates "a good diet"; between 51 and 80 indicates a diet that "needs improvement"; 51 and below indicates "a poor diet."

So how do American children score? Nearly all are stuck in the "needs improvement" category, and their diets get worse as they get older.

Children ages two to three earn the best score—73.8. It falls steadily to 60.7 for boys ages fifteen to eighteen. As children get older, the percentage having a diet that needs improvement increases. Much of the decline in diet quality for children occurs between the age groups two to three and four to six—from 35 to 16 percent. Not surprisingly, the decline begins when children come into contact with multiple forces outside the home: fast-food restaurants, ubiquitous soda machines, mega single-size lunches, and the increasing lure of sitting in front of electronic screens. It picks up speed for the seven-to-ten and eleven-to-fourteen age groups—from 14 to 7 percent. The decline relates to a low fruit and milk score as children get older. Though children two to three have the best total fat score, only 40 percent meet the dietary recommendation of 30 percent or less total calories from fat. Boys eleven to eighteen have the worst fat score, which means they eat the highest percent of fat beyond the recommendation of any age group.[52]

As a professor of nutrition concerned with childhood obesity, how would I grade children's diet? C+ for two- to three-year olds; D for middle school kids; and for most teenagers, an F.

## SUMMARY

We now know why children are getting fatter. They eat excess high-sucrose/corn syrup foods (everyone is born with the liking for sweet). They learn early on to like what is offered (high-calorie foods and few low-calorie vegetables and fruits). They quickly respond to seductive cues in their environment (advertising, availability, and accessibility of food and drink an arm's reach away). They sit more than they move.

Though as a species we have evolved excellent physiological mechanisms to defend against body weight loss, we have only weak defenses against weight gain when food is abundant. Control of portion size, consumption of a diet high in fruits and vegetables and low in fat, and regular physical activity are behaviors that protect against obesity. Nothing in the current environment, however, encourages children to adopt and maintain these behaviors.

As this chapter confirms, kids have more homework after school and, in unsafe neighborhoods, fewer opportunities to play outdoors. At school they encounter increased academic requirements and reduced PE requirements. Dispensed by vending machines and sold in school stores, fast food is ubiquitous. School lunch (often from fast-food franchised restaurants on campus) is available in large portions, with few vegetables and fruits.

On a scale of 1 to 100, the quality of children's diets rates only in the 60s and low 70s. Are those passing grades? Most would agree that, at a minimum, the scores betray a vast need for improvement. In the final part of this book, we will study ways to improve those scores and get children on the move again. The following chapter focuses on *slowing* obesity, a task which everyone agrees is essential for turning the tide in this epidemic, but which few are able (or willing) to tackle.

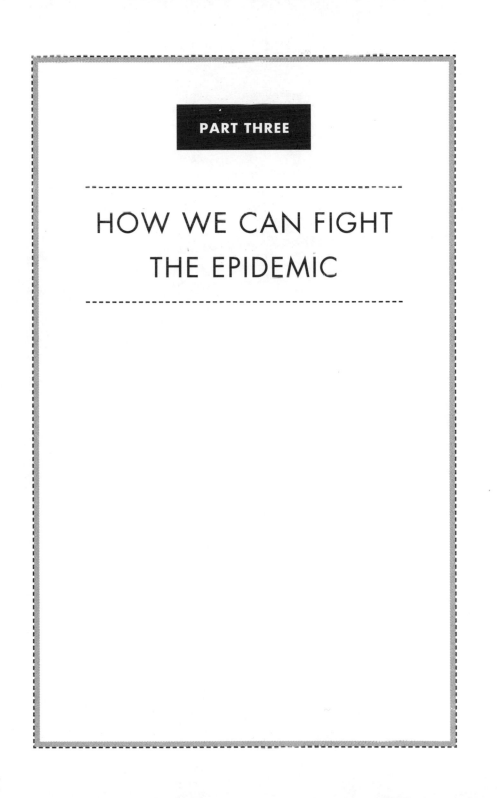

**PART THREE**

# HOW WE CAN FIGHT
# THE EPIDEMIC

# 6

----

# NURTURING HEALTHY
# AND ACTIVE LIFESTYLES

----

ONE QUESTION FROM TWENTY YEARS AGO haunts my memory. I was leading a workshop with health professionals representing a variety of agencies that served parents and children. The topic was childhood obesity. Most of the participants were mothers and grandmothers; about half were African American and Hispanic; the majority worked in government and health-care programs, as administrators or directly with patients; many were in minority or low-income communities. The objectives of the workshop were ones this book shares: to understand obesity's causes and to explore and suggest appropriate, effective remedies.

I showed a video clip from a documentary dramatization of four- and five-year-old children being asked to look at drawings of children and pick one they would like to have as a friend. The drawings showed children with various physical difficulties; one was obese. Invariably the obese child came last. Most participants nodded in recognition, and some told of similar experiences among children they knew. Two or three spoke passionately about the injustice of fat discrimination.

I had just summarized prevalence data and was about to discuss the health risks of childhood obesity when an impatient voice demanded, "I want to hear something new." An articulate Hispanic director of a small center for immigrant children from the Dominican Republic worked with children she described as chronically overweight. She began by stressing the severity of the problem and said she felt frustrated and burned-out. She knew what caused the problem—"They eat big fast-food meals every day and drink lots of whole milk as they're glued to TV"—but she had no remedies, no way to help these families stop or treat the children's unhealthy weight gain. Then she spoke the challenge that could only come from intense experience and rings in my ears as I recall it now:

> Professor, I know how to identify fat children, to talk to them so they don't feel miserable. I know why these kids are fat and getting fatter. What I don't know and am increasingly impatient to hear is what the experts claim is most likely to work when we try to help parents with fat kids. I've read the literature that says families should eat together. But after telling people that for seven years, I have no idea of how they can do it. The same is true for exercise; parents are rarely good role models for this, and even if they are themselves slim and active, that can't compete with a peer group watching some wild video together and munching chips. Parental role modeling? Health workers like us handing out advice? Please, Professor Dalton, tell us something that actually brings results!

Shouts of "Amen!" and loud applause rang out when she finished.

The response I gave at that workshop at least began well. I agreed with the group that as health professionals we needed to find ways to help and also encourage people to help themselves. I listed the kinds of support experts propose to prevent and treat childhood obesity. I pointed out that some of the advice draws on research data but has very little evidence about what is effective, especially in the long term, and that there are many more questions about what works than there are answers. We then pooled ideas and experiences of how to treat childhood obesity.

Yet my response was surely inadequate. The problem *is* challenging and her question stands: what really works to motivate and help children who are at risk or already struggling with obesity?

This book's final part takes up and tries to answer her question. The general approaches and practical advice I advocate on the following pages may appear relatively simple and basic. They are, because they must be. Imagine asking parents, many of whom have struggled with being overweight their entire lives, to do all of the following: decipher nutritional labels, count their children's calories, measure their portion sizes, and keep track of their protein-carbohydrate-fat ratio at every meal—and while they do so, to avoid sugar, soda, fried foods, and certain kinds of fats but not others; to exercise daily, cook healthy meals from scratch, and fix family members' schedules so everyone can eat dinner together; *and* to banish the TV. Many parents would throw up their hands in frustration and give up trying to lead healthier lives. In fact many do give up, and thus the epidemic grows. Therefore, to help the families hardest hit by this epidemic—those on the lower end of the socioeconomic scale, who face multiple challenges in their lives that compete for their resources and attention—we must deemphasize the complexity of the issue and put forth feasible and realistic remedies everyone can adopt for the long term.

Hence we focus on understandable, general guidelines with practical strategies to implement them, and then leverage a handful of manageable and moderate steps to make a significant impact on children's health.

For example, we know that children need to become more physically active. Parents on a budget and pressed for time may think they cannot get their children to exercise more because of the cost and time needed for organized recreational classes such as gymnastics or karate. My message to everyone is that physical activity does not have to be complicated, costly, or very time consuming. Parents should try instead to turn off the television an extra hour each day and use the time to encourage their children to engage in more active pastimes, which can be as simple as playing tag or dancing to pop music. As one report noted, "Opportunities for spontaneous play may be the only requirement that young children need to increase their physical activity. Reducing the amount of time that children are allowed to watch television is one strategy that offers children opportunities for activity, and it is likely to alter requests for advertised foods as well."[1]

Similarly, we know that many children eat too much and therefore need to reduce their calorie intake. Parents need to know that this does *not* have to involve embarking on a strict or trendy diet. Moderate steps to change eating behavior—such as sharing family meals, offering children a variety of healthy foods, and respecting children's choices not to eat a specified amount—will go a long way toward reducing young children's access to and consumption of foods that are fattening.[2]

These are not novel approaches. In fact, they were the norm a generation ago, when there were fewer alternatives. Now a return to basics seems essential. Why? Because we have few other strategies, because none of these interventions is likely to have adverse effects, and because all of these actions will improve the quality of family life. But the basics are simpler in theory than in practice, because they require that parents and children manage their many choices for eating food and spending time. It is not enough to educate ourselves on what we should do; we need strategies for how to do it.

To that end, this chapter offers strategies to help lay a foundation for healthy eating and activity in practice, not just in theory. The focus here is on the *prevention* of excessive weight gain. We examine ways that all parents can exert the appropriate degree of control in feeding and raising children so children are more likely to self-regulate their eating and spend their time in a healthy manner. Building on that foundation, I present my top recommendations for lifelong healthy weight management and discuss ways to raise resilient children equipped to withstand the fattening forces beyond their home. Chapter 7 targets treatment, conveying specific nutritional guidance and evaluating popular weight-loss programs, as well as examining the risks, among children, associated with weight loss (namely, disordered eating and unhealthy body image). Because the line between "prevention" and "treatment" is fuzzy, strategies for prevention are also sound suggestions for children who already are too heavy and need to slow their rate of weight gain.

## PREVENTION: THE FIRST—AND BEST— COURSE OF TREATMENT

Obesity is the most prevalent but also the most preventable health affliction of children today. If prevention were easy, we would not need treatment for childhood obesity. With one out of four children already overweight or at risk of becoming overweight, we clearly need both prevention and treatment strategies, now, at all levels—for individual children, families, communities, and schools, as well as in health care and other social and institutional networks.

So often, the predictable response to obesity is to put resources toward treatment, with little attention to prevention. Consider, for instance, a recent addition to the already frighteningly long list of medical complications obese children often experience, a liver disease called NASH, for *nonalcoholic steatohepatitis*.[3] How dreadful: obese fourteen-year-olds are getting a liver disease similar to one induced by excess alcohol in adults! One of the first questions that spring to mind is, which medication will treat the malfunctioning liver that results from obesity? The drug industry is working to develop a medication to improve liver function in obese children with NASH. Of course, we all worry about serious afflictions like this among children and hope a medical remedy can be found. But developing medical treatments for obesity is a Band-Aid solution. Prevention, not medicine, represents the best hope for protecting our children from potentially life-threatening afflictions related to obesity and a lifetime of clinical treatment that may have side effects—at overwhelming cost to families and our health-care system.

Parents hold the keys to prevention; they determine what young children eat and their choice of physical activities. Choices of older children and adolescents, including what they eat and how they spend time, involve a larger group of their parents, teachers, and peers. And to some degree, all age groups respond to the lure of products on TV, at the supermarket, and at the mall. Nonetheless, given the importance of early childhood in patterns for eating habits and the primary influence that parents exert, we must look to parents as the starting point for any strategies against childhood obesity. Recall the key risk factors for obesity, outlined in chapter 3: parental obesity; unhealthful eating patterns and eating styles; low physical activity; excessive television and computer time; low socioeconomic status. Individual parents may not be able to curb their own obesity and raise their socioeconomic status, but they can take steps to minimize the other risk factors on that list.

Obesity is not a disease that eludes prevention or recovery. Scientists know that mice, caged in an experimental laboratory, can be made fat on a typical American diet. They can be made thin if food is reduced and made thin much faster if placed on a treadmill. But we are dealing with children, not mice. We cannot force them onto a treadmill and feed them a carefully controlled diet day in and day out, because their finicky nature and their yearning for autonomy will lead them to rebel against such heavy-handed measures to control their activity and eating. Moreover, we raise them in an environment full of choices—a fully stocked refrigerator, a multichannel television set—and those choices multiply once they reach school age, gain independence, and venture out on their own. We believe in choice and want plenty of food easily available, but how can we help our children learn to choose food in moderation and participate in adequate physical activity? Becoming an authoritative parent is one path toward this goal—a path any parent can and should take.

## BECOME AN AUTHORITATIVE PARENT

Authoritative parenting, as outlined in chapter 4, is the middle ground between permissive and authoritarian styles. Whereas permissive parents might have abundant high-calorie snacks always and easily available or authoritarian parents might strictly forbid eating them at all, authoritative parents have a firm but flexible structure for when and how to enjoy a variety of foods as snacks. Authoritative parents neither give their children free rein nor hold them in too tightly; rather, they set parameters for their children that help them learn how to set limits on their own and how to exercise self-control. Parents who set limits to keep their children's world a manageable size are doing the right thing, because they are showing them how to structure the many choices available for eating and spending time. Raising children to manage their lifestyle choices is one form of insurance against obesity in an environment that can be so contrary to a healthy lifestyle.

Limit setting becomes an obstacle course for some children if caregivers first encourage them to eat more than they want or need during early childhood (ages one to three) and then restrict foods later (ages three to five). For example, a parent might serve second helpings to a two-year-old—even though the child did not indicate she wanted more—and then tell her, "You have to make all that chicken and rice disappear from your plate before you can leave the table." Later, when the child reaches age four, the same parent might say, "No more second helpings or dessert for you after all the snacking you did this afternoon." In one study, overweight and normal-weight eight- to twelve-year-old children ate at significantly different paces only when the mother was in the room too. In her presence, overweight children ate faster and with larger bites than the normal-weight children and speeded up eating near the end of the meal. One interpretation is that as toddlers, they learned this response to reinforcement to "clean the plate." Or it could be a learned coping response to stress among older overweight children.[4] "If I hurry, no one will notice how much I ate." Either way, the study shows that parental presence and practices affect overweight children's eating behavior more than that of children with normal weight. If parents are too pushy and then too restrictive, children get mixed messages.

Key to being an authoritative parent is finding an appropriate level of control and structure in feeding a child, with the goal being to nurture the child's self-control as well as a liking for a variety of foods. Children need limits and guidance, but the evidence is quite strong that strictly prohibiting foods usually backfires when kids later on have a free choice of foods, and restricting their food likely leads to overeating.[5] Even so, being overly permissive and serving unlimited portions of whatever older children desire leads to overeating too. Young children generally stop eating when they feel full, while older children—above age six or so—will eat beyond fullness when consistently exposed to large portions. Their bodies will expand by getting fatter and so will their stomach capacity as they override their satiety signals, until eating too much becomes habitual.

Because parents' own eating behavior is as important as their style of parenting regarding food, children often get confusing messages. For example, a mother who is "always on a diet" and tells her child to "clean your plate" demonstrates food restriction while simultaneously sending the message to "eat more." Modifying parent behavior is a good place to begin in preventing a child from experiencing difficulty in noticing fullness or from overeating "forbidden foods" when he or she gets a chance.[6]

Rather than force a child to eat specified amounts of certain foods or, at the other extreme, adopt a laissez-faire approach at mealtimes, parents should aim for moderation. To find that golden mean, I strongly recommend a method developed by Ellyn Satter and described in her book *Child of Mine: Feeding with Love and Good Sense*. Out of all the alternatives, her research and its application are outstanding and remain valid today. Satter encourages parents to observe what she calls "the division of responsibility" in child feeding:

· Parents are responsible for the *what, when,* and *where* of feeding.

· Children are responsible for *how much* they eat and *if* they eat some foods.

For parents, Satter stresses "the importance of providing the food and feeding environment and then letting go. This means controlling what food comes into the house, the making and presenting of meals, and regulating the timing and content of snacks. However, children are responsible for how much they eat. They also determine, based on the food provided, whether they will eat it or not. The idea is that if each party sticks to its division of responsibility, a child will grow according to his genetic blueprint— maybe fatter or thinner, shorter or taller than expected, but the right size and shape for him."[7]

Thus parents and caretakers divide up the shopping and cooking tasks among family members and are responsible for what foods are available, and when. For example, parents stick to their shopping list at the grocery store, responding to children's requests consistently rather than caving in to multiple demands; preparing and deciding when food is served to younger children; and choosing what foods are eaten in restaurants (older children, who can read the menu, should have some latitude to order for themselves when dining out, but guidelines are still in place; for example, if milk or water is usually served at home during family meals, an older child might have one soda at the restaurant, but refills will be water). Parents plan menus and shopping strategies; decide the number and type of meals together/away/brought in; designate who shops/cooks/cleans up; and set meal and snacking guidelines—for instance, the availability of "anytime, sometimes, seldom" foods—and so determine the *what, when,* and *where* of feeding.

Once the food is served, children take over. Within meal and snacking guidelines, they are responsible for deciding if they eat a food and how much they eat. It's their prerogative to be picky. At home or eating out, an un-eaten meal can be wrapped up and made available later. The parents might comment on the tastiness of the food and why they like it, but in general they should try to seem unconcerned whether and how much children eat. (When kids reject a new food, however, parents should not give up but offer it at a later date; sometimes it takes ten to fifteen "exposures" for children to try and to like a new food.) Bribes or threats that aim to get children to eat their meal—"You can have ice cream for dessert if you eat all your peas," "You cannot watch television unless you finish your milk"—should always be avoided, as should excessive praise when kids eat everything on the plate.

What about dessert? Dessert can be a part of the meal, but in a child-size portion. If the main meal was not eaten, extra dessert should not be what kids fill up on. In sum, parents choose and serve a variety of foods that they enjoy eating with their children; children eat (or do not eat) the amount they decide from the choices available.

Satter's division of responsibility sets the authoritative approach apart not only from a highly controlling one with strict rules and forbidden foods, but also from a more permissive "self-demand" approach. One "self-demand" method, especially recommended for adults and children who already have trouble eating in a balanced manner—possibly because of previous excessive parental control—involves "legalizing" all food. The authors of *Preventing Childhood Eating Problems,* Jane Hirschmann and Carol Munter, recommend having all foods available: fresh fruits and vegetables, meats, whole grains, and dairy products, as well as candy and ice cream.[8] Nothing is forbidden. But such a permissive approach has risks. I believe children need to learn how to control their eating behavior, and learning how to respect boundaries as well as how to be in charge requires guidance and support. Dividing responsibility and exhibiting moderation from the start avoid the need to deal with the notion of "illegal" foods later.

With so much advice available, it's no wonder that parents, trying to do their best, either control too much or too little. The underlying principle is that it's critically important to trust kids to know if they are hungry and how much to eat. This trust applies to all kinds of foods. In order to develop a sensible relationship to high-fat and high-sugar foods, parents and caregivers should offer children foods and snacks that vary in sugar, fat, and calories. This means some ice cream and cake as well as a wide variety of fruits and vegetables—all in moderation. Children learn to like what they are offered.

A man who had struggled with his weight since childhood once told me, "If only I had learned to eat as a kid." He recalled a moment when he was back with his family during a reunion and, trying to be healthy, came down to eat his cereal before anyone else got up: "I opened the fridge, and there were three banana cream pies. And the pie was right in front of the milk—just like when I was a kid. It was there, so I ate it. All of it. I felt awful all day." It is difficult, if not impossible, to learn to trust and "to listen to your body" after ignoring fullness signals for years. If we can help children learn to enjoy a variety of food, in moderation, they will find eating to be one of life's great pleasures—not a dieting land mine.

There is wide agreement on the importance of rediscovering the pleasure and ritual of family mealtimes, the theme of another Satter book, *Secrets of Feeding a Healthy Family.*[9] The pleasure comes not from overindulgent eating, but from making room for mealtimes. It comes from slowing down and taking the time to notice and enjoy the food being served. And— I believe—it helps kids and their parents develop lifelong balanced eating patterns that will curb obesity. Learning to eat for enjoyment and taste, and noticing fullness, are the basics. Some of what we nutritionists teach—about sufficient vitamins and minerals and too much fat—are not the reasons kids (or grown-ups) eat what they eat. In fact, "new" advice that conflicts with "old" advice blurs both. Concern with news about cholesterol and trans-fats causes some parents to forbid certain foods and overuse others. The basics of moderation and balance get lost in the terminology and news-breaks. The essential take-away lesson is this: kids eat foods that taste good and are available. So parents need to make healthy foods that taste good available—and enjoy eating them with their children.

## MAKE IT WORK: MY TOP RECOMMENDATIONS TO PARENTS

How can parents carry out the fundamental approach outlined above— not just for a month, or for a year, but for life? What follow are five key recommendations to help them—to help all of us—become authoritative parents who teach by example and exercise an appropriate level of control in feeding and raising children. These recommendations are simple to understand but may seem hard to carry out, which is why I add tips for implementing each one. They stem from my professional experience as well as from other expert guidelines. With time and a reasonable degree of effort, these recommendations become part of a family's everyday life.[10]

1.  Eat moderately, parents—kids will copy.

2.  Plan and eat meals and snacks together, emphasizing variety.

3.  Foster a preference for healthier alternatives—in particular, fruits, vegetables and whole grains—by repeated tasting and enjoying by the whole family.

4.  Talk, walk, and play together indoors and outdoors as an alternative to watching television.

5.  Get enough sleep (children need at least nine hours).

The method I use here—analyzing the recommendations first in theory and then in practice—is the same method I use in workshops with health advocates; I work with participants to examine the theories from reported studies on weight management, and together we try to apply them to the reality of our collective group experience. Under each "practice" discussion are tips on how to make it work.

### **1** *Eat moderately, parents—kids will copy.*
*The theory.* Children stand a greater chance of learning to eat in a healthy manner and to manage weight when using a family-based approach rather than going it on their own. Children are better copycats than listeners: they are more likely to do what their parents do, rather than what their parents say. Parents who themselves alternate between control (restrictive dieting) and loss of control (binge eating) are likely to pass on these eating habits to children.[11] Children do not naturally restrict food and then overeat later—unless they learn this behavior from an adult. Parents themselves should seize the opportunity to become agents of change by eating moderately and aiming for a healthy weight themselves. Several studies confirm that when an outside health professional *and* parents coach obese children,

they are more likely to change eating habits and show greater weight loss than with the conventional approach of diet advice without parental support.[12] In fact, when parents improve their own eating behaviors without actively including children, the impact of their role modeling alone positively affects children's eating behavior.

An important element of role modeling is wise social and emotional use of food, to help kids learn not to use food when they need love or other support. Comfort means a hug and attention—not M&M's. Ditto for grown-ups. Eating after stress, or erratic eating between meals, can contribute to becoming overweight.

*The practice.* The demands of our lifestyle and the lure of enticing food products in the marketplace make it hard for parents to be healthy and eat moderately, especially when food comes in "mega" sizes and, even at home, in restaurant-size portions (see the box "Common Portions vs. Recommended Servings"). Children try junk food at friends' houses and at school, which makes them desire it at home, too.

The practice of eating moderately means cutting down exposure to unhealthy food. How? Just as we learned to limit sun exposure because of the perils of skin cancer, so we must limit exposure to high-calorie "super-size" food or drink because of their excess calories from fat and sugar. Parents can show their children that it is okay to savor high-calorie foods, but in small amounts and only occasionally. Potato chips or Oreo cookies? If they are always available, they will replace meals. If they are forbidden, they become more desirable. Better to buy them only from time to time—for the occasional snacks or dessert—rather than keep them in the house and limit children's access to them. Bottom line: offer and also eat mainly healthy foods.

How to eat moderately?

**Instead of** serving overly large portions to adults at meals and equally large portions for children, **try** following suggested serving sizes and eating slowly so the body can recognize fullness, then serve second helpings only if family members are still hungry. Offer children small servings and allow them to ask for more if they finish and are still hungry.

**Instead of** reaching for a high-calorie snack when bored or upset from stress, **try** a planned distraction. Have a list ready to go with doable suggestions: take a five-minute walk around the block, make a phone call to a friend, or do a few stretches to favorite music.

## COMMON PORTIONS VS. RECOMMENDED SERVINGS

Eating moderately involves following suggested serving sizes and offering more only if hunger truly persists after the first serving is finished. Here are some sample food portions commonly served compared to the Food Guide Pyramid's recommended servings for these foods. First, consider the difference between the two terms:

· A *portion* is the amount of food you choose to eat. There is no standard portion size and no single right or wrong portion size.

· A *serving* is a standard amount and a guide on how much to eat.

| Food | Typical portion size | Food Guide Pyramid's recommended serving size | Number of servings in a typical portion |
| --- | --- | --- | --- |
| Bagel | 1 bagel (5" dia, 4 oz) | ½ bagel (3" dia, 1 oz) | 4 |
| English muffin | 1 muffin | ½ muffin | 2 |
| Sweet roll | 1 large (6 oz) | 1 small (1.5 oz) | 4 |
| Pasta | 2 cups (cooked) | ½ cup (cooked) | 4 |
| Rice | 1 cup (cooked) | ½ cup (cooked) | 2 |
| Popcorn | 16 cups (= medium, at movie theater) | 2 cups | 8 |
| Fries | 1 medium order (4 oz) | ½ cup (1 oz) | 4 |
| Fried chicken | 3 pieces (7–8 oz) | 2–3 oz | 3 |
| Broiled fish | 6–9 oz | 2–3 oz | 3 |
| Sirloin steak | 8 oz (cooked, trimmed) | 2–3 oz | 3 |
| Tuna salad sandwich | 6 oz | 2–3 oz | 2 |

**Instead of** drinking soda and juice several times a day, **try** quenching thirst with water. Parents should try to drink water or milk at mealtimes rather than soda. Let kids shop for a special water bottle; fill it with water, and pack it for school in lieu of a can of soda or fruit punch.

**Instead of** ordering a super-size value meal for each family member at restaurants, **try** ordering smaller portions, or ordering one super-size meal for a parent and child to share.

**Instead of** rewarding yourself or your child with an indulgent treat after accomplishing something challenging, **try** buying a nonedible special item—such as clothing, books, or toys—as a reward.

**2** *Plan and eat meals and snacks together, emphasizing variety.*

*The theory.* Children ages nine to fourteen who frequently eat with their parents are likely to have healthier eating habits than those who rarely eat with parents. One study compared the diet quality of children who never or seldom ate a family dinner with the diet of children who ate with their family most days or every day. Family meals were associated with healthful foods: more fruits and vegetables, less fried food and soda, and more fiber, vitamins, minerals from foods. Other studies have likewise established that eating a family sit-down meal together rather than eating while standing or while doing other activities (such as watching TV, reading, doing homework) reduces the risk of uncontrolled overeating in both parents and children.[13]

Variety also is a hallmark of better diets. The traditional wisdom, backed by scientific research, is that offering children a variety of food provides the basic nutrients for health. And indeed, variety increases the chances of their eating sufficient vitamins and minerals. Variety stimulates the taste buds, whereas eating a single, specific food may dampen them. Of course, the greater the variety of food offered, the more people eat. Hence the popularity—and overconsumption—of food served in "all you can eat" buffet-style restaurants. This means that while variety is good for getting sufficient nutrients, it is not so good for weight management. In fact, to reduce the amount of food people eat, diets for weight loss often rely on a very few foods. Laboratory studies that measure how much people eat when offered single foods versus a variety of foods show that older children and adults eat more food when there are more choices, less when choices are few.[14] Yet, given people's set choices of the same foods at fast-food restaurants (remember that the McDonald's lawsuit involved daily Quarter-Pounders), perhaps kids who did not have a varied diet never developed the "taste" for variety and can overindulge on monotonous diets.

If we adapt this research for young children, a good approach would be to offer them *more* variety of vegetables and fruits and thus increase consumption—which would be a positive change, since most kids' diets are deficient in fruits and vegetables, and these lower-calorie fruits and vegetables can take the place of higher-calorie, less nutritious snacks.

Yet because children are exposed to hundreds of choices in the supermarket and at the mall, and because families frequently dine at restaurants, children have opportunities to eat more, often too much. Managing these choices is a major skill that helps them resist the overwhelming presence of food and drink in their environment. What and how much people eat in restaurants really matter. A high rate of away-from-home eating relates directly to a higher rate of obesity because the variety of foods available in restaurants, combined with oversize servings, usually proves irresistible.[15] Food fixed and eaten at home does provide the opportunity to reduce the portions in size and number, as well as to add vegetables to the pizza, to use whole-wheat buns for the burgers, and to have fruit for dessert.

*The practice.* Most parents think family meals are important, but long commutes from work, varying work shifts, and the children's after-school and homework commitments obviously make eating together difficult. Moreover, children often eat most of their snacks and meals at child care or school rather than at home. Family meals have become exceedingly hard to organize. One answer may be to aim for at least four out of seven dinners during the week as family meals. Dividing responsibility for preparing dinners among all family members also improves the chance of having time for family meals. Children as young as two can get involved by helping the parents wipe tabletops, tear lettuce, and bring ingredients or utensils from one place to another; kindergarten-age children can help make a shopping list, measure ingredients, set the table, and cut with a dull knife.

Breakfast is a good place to start. As emphasized earlier, breakfast improves school (and job) performance and reduces inappropriate snacking (and weight gain). As with all meals, getting kids to eat a nutritious breakfast works better if they eat at home with a parent—and whole fruit is far too messy to eat in the car on the way to school or work. But even eaten at home, breakfast is a meal with a lot of nutritional land mines, owing to the rise in popularity of sugary cereals (Oreo and S'more cereals seem to be big these days), so parents have to be more proactive to plan and serve a low-sugar balanced breakfast.

Family mealtimes will be more successful and pleasant if parents stick to a routine and have a consistent policy for responding to requests to leave the table or refusals to try new food. In *Feeding Your Child for Lifelong Health,* the authors Susan Roberts and Melvin Heyman recommend the following: make it a rule that everyone stay at the table through the main course; leave refused foods within reach so your child can try them later in the meal; offer one plain alternative such as cereal and milk or bread, cheese, and fruit with little or no comment; let your child see you enjoy some of the food she refused.[16] This is appropriate limit setting that follows the division of responsibility and curbs overly controlled parenting.

How to plan and eat meals and snacks together and incorporate variety into the family's diet?

**Instead of** arguing with your child over what can or cannot be purchased at the supermarket, **try** working together to make a shopping list for the week's meals and snacks; have the child write down the ingredients on the list and help find the products in the store. If he or she begs for a junk-food item not on the list, then review the list and the basic menu and snack plan. Decide if and where the coveted item fits in—maybe a trade with another "seldom" item on the list.

**Instead of** eating doughnuts in the car on the way to school and work because parents are too rushed getting to work to prepare breakfast, **try** getting kids involved in planning and making their own healthy breakfasts—slicing fresh fruit, toasting whole-wheat bread, serving low-sugar cereal.

**Instead of** piling a cupboard with bulk-size packages of salty and sweet snacks (which are often high in fat and sugar and low in nutrients), **try** labeling a shelf in the fridge and another in the cupboard as "snacks"; stock the fridge shelf with packages of fruit, sliced carrots and bell pepper strips, cheese, and yogurt, and stock the snack cupboard with low-sugar cereal, graham crackers, dried fruit, and a few salty and sweet snacks—purchased in small sizes, not bulk.

**Instead of** preparing the same tried-and-true meals over and over again, **try** branching out by cooking with unfamiliar ingredients and experimenting with ethnic cuisines. Once a month, have kids help plan and prepare an "international" dish from a country or region of their choice. Use this as an opportunity to learn about that part of the world.

**3** *Foster a preference for healthier alternatives—in particular, fruits, vegetables and whole grains—by repeated tasting and enjoying by the whole family.*
*The theory.* The scientific evidence that fruits and vegetables are critically important to health is piling up so rapidly that there are many proposals to make them the foundation of the new Food Guide Pyramid, pushing grains and cereals (preferably whole) onto the second level. Besides their obvious role in weight management as low-cal/nutrient-dense foods, there is growing evidence that fruit and vegetables are linked to cancer prevention and blood pressure reduction. The five daily recommended servings

of fruits and vegetables will soon be "five to nine a day." The gap between recommendations and reality will widen further. Few children meet the minimal "five a day" recommendation of three vegetable servings and two fruit servings; few children get the health benefits of whole grains since they eat refined flour products. Both you and your children can grow healthier by eating more dark green vegetables (asparagus, broccoli, collards), deep yellow or orange vegetables (yellow squash, carrots), fruits (oranges, kiwis), and whole-grain products (graham crackers, oatmeal, whole-wheat bread and pasta).

The best way to foster a preference for fruits and vegetables is to offer a new item from time to time for tasting and enjoying at family mealtimes—*not* to withhold preferred foods until kids eat the new one. Not only do children learn to dislike a food, such as vegetables, that they eat only to obtain a reward (dessert), but they develop an exaggerated preference for high-fat, energy-dense foods; they limit their acceptance of a variety of foods; and they alter internal signals of hunger and satiety. A new food, especially vegetables and fruits, sometimes requires up to twenty low-key taste opportunities for a child to eat it. Some evidence suggests that early introduction of a variety of these foods acts as some sort of "buffer" against a strong dislike or "neophobia" of new foods.[17] As discussed earlier, a family should divide responsibility at mealtimes: parents decide what and when; children determine if they will eat the food that is given and how much.

*The practice.* Parents are not always convinced that their baby has eaten enough when the baby pushes it away, so they force more food. As the child grows they worry about his or her eating right and not eating "junk food," so they restrict the unhealthier food. Then parents tire of offering a new food when a kid refuses it a couple of times. Two strategies usually work: offer a wide variety of healthy foods during the twelve- to twenty-month "window" during toddlerhood when children explore everything with their mouth; and eat with your kids most of the time, so they see what you do. Eat and enjoy your vegetables and fruits so your kids will too.

That said, in practice it can be hard for parents to buy and prepare tasty vegetable dishes. The produce in markets in poorer neighborhoods is often not very fresh or appealing; parents accustomed to eating fried and prepackaged food often don't know how to cook appetizing vegetable dishes for their kids.

How to foster a preference for healthier fare?

**Instead of** using dessert as an incentive or reward for eating vegetables at dinnertime, **try** making dessert a part of the meal, most frequently fruit or low-sugar pudding; serve high-sugar, high-fat pastries as "seldom" foods. Serve vegetables in small portions that the child can try, then serve more if child asks for more.

**Instead of** repeatedly buying and serving the same vegetables and fruits, **try** buying and tasting one new fruit or vegetable every week. Have a weekly fruit/vegetable ceremony to taste the new produce item—take a bite, then discuss the color and texture and where the item comes from. Or the family can hold a fruit- and vegetable-tasting event where kids vote on the favorite color, texture, taste, shape, and "It looks just like . . ."

**Instead of** assuming a toddler doesn't like a fruit or vegetable because he or she refused to eat it the first couple of times it was offered, **try** waiting a few months and then reintroduce it in a slightly different way. For example, a two-year-old who doesn't like cooked and mashed peas might like to munch on a crunchy pea pod.

**Instead of** salty, high-fat crackers and dips to tide hungry kids over during the time it takes to cook, **try** offering them vegetables and salsa or bean dip—some kids will eat almost any new food as long as they can dip it.

**4** *Talk, walk, and play together indoors and outdoors as an alternative to watching television.*

*The theory.* Physical activity behaviors among children and adolescents are determined by a number of factors: the children's stage of growth and fitness; access to safe facilities for sports and play; opportunities for sedentary activities such as television watching or computer games; confidence in their own physical capability; and parental role modeling or support. As with eating, the parents' role is key. Actively playing and enjoying a physical activity with kids is a major way parents can help children develop and continue it (see Figure 4). A parent-child walk together to school, in the park, to the store, across the field, or to piano lessons pays big dividends for the time investment in setting physical activity patterns early and in bringing about an interval together without interruptions from television and phone calls (if the cell phone is turned off!).

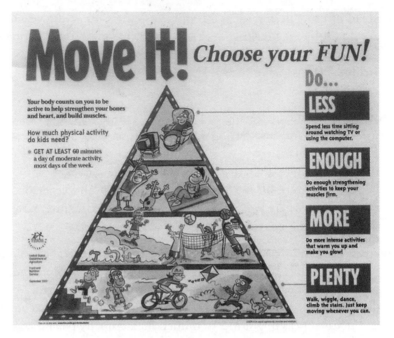

FIGURE 4. At each level of activity, kids can choose ways to reach and keep a healthy weight. (U.S. Department of Agriculture, Food and Nutrition Service, www.fns.usda.gov/tn/)

Reducing sedentary activity is itself likely to increase physical movement. Not only does turning off the TV encourage young people to be more active; it also reduces their exposure to commercials that whet their appetite for junk food. Studies have shown that children who learned to manage their TV time (and spent more time playing creative games) decreased overall sedentary activity and ate fewer high-calorie snacks and had lower body fat than children who watched more TV.[18]

In addition, mealtimes are more relaxed if the television is off. Many kitchens and dining rooms now have TVs; a family's mealtime focus should be on talking among themselves and on noticing food, not eating mindlessly while watching the evening news. This is a tough rule to follow. A report on "TV-dinner kids" found that 42 percent of dinners eaten at home are consumed in front of the TV but that the percentage for overweight children is 50, compared to 35 percent for normal-weight kids.[19]

Parents who strive to make physical activity—not food or television—the focal point during parties and family gatherings will send a message to their children that physical activity can be fun and sociable. When food is a side attraction—not the main event—at gatherings, kids (and adults) are less likely to overeat.

*The practice.* If kids aren't watching television or playing video games, they have to fill the void. What can compete with TV and the computer? Kids don't like to be the only ones in the park, and if they are, parents understandably worry about their safety. Children today may know how to play freeze tag or kick the can, but who are they going to play with if their friends are still watching the tube?

One answer is to get kids into after-school programs with activities like dancing and creative games where they have fun, instead of being at home with nothing to do but sit and snack. Many parents want schools to provide these opportunities, but schools are often overburdened too. (Chapter 9 discusses how schools and communities can be a part of the solution in this epidemic.) For the safety of small children, and to make efficient use of parents' time, some neighborhoods have a rotation system for supervising four or five children, so that each parent joins in or supervises an hour of vigorous play once a week. Parents and caregivers can become proactive with imaginative ideas for promoting physical activity. For instance, some parents in Harlem took to the sidewalks, chalk in hand, and after a brief demonstration got hopscotch going in the neighborhood. Others organized a jump rope contest and held workshops for two weeks in advance to teach kids how to do it and to practice. More adults, even grandparents, who are bored with treadmills are returning to children's games like kickball; kids are watching, and some will emulate these enjoyable and vigorous activities. Research from programs to promote healthy weight among children clearly shows that when kids choose a physical activity and parents reinforce it by joining in, it becomes increasingly enjoyable.[20] The point is to offer a wide range of choices and to cultivate the pleasure of participating in games, dancing, and just running around.

What exactly can parents do to limit excess television time? Americans know well how very seductive and mesmerizing television can be. Here too research evidence is clear: if you monitor the amount of watching time, make program choices, and come up with alternatives for the "freed-up" time, everyone ends up at a healthier body weight.

Most parents need guidance on how to tear kids (and themselves) away from the TV and computers. Parents and caregivers need not banish TV but can reduce a negative action by replacing it with a positive one. For example, make a goal to reduce TV watching by half an hour (the length of one show) every weekend day and every weekday afternoon, then make a parent-child play date for this time. Turning off the TV for thirty minutes a day for an activity together is a win-win. It's not enough to *tell* kids to turn off the TV; parents or caregivers must help plan and join in a casual, active alternative. Be creative; for instance, parents can make taking walks—an alternative to TV—more enticing if they make it an "adventure walk" that involves searching for fallen leaves of different colors or for tracks in the dirt or snow. This keeps interest high and allows for differences in age and ability, as do skipping, walking backward, or hopping.

How to talk, walk, and play together indoors and outdoors?

**Instead of** always suggesting "a walk," **try** going on a scavenger hunt around the neighborhood, using certain landmarks, trees, or plants as "findings" (evidence could be leaves, word pictures, photos with instant cameras); or walking to a specific destination (movie, mall, or local event).

**Instead of** watching cartoons for two to three hours on Saturday mornings, **try** limiting Saturday-morning television to one hour and planning an hour-long family outing or game to follow it.

**Instead of** letting friends watch television together at each other's houses during play dates, **try** making a pact with the friend's parents that the TV will be off-limits during play dates; help children get started with alternative activities such as putting on a mock dance contest or building a fort.

**Instead of** holding kids' birthday parties at pizza parlors or fast-food restaurants, where food is the focus, **try** having kids' parties and family gatherings at a park. Rather than ask other adults to bring potluck dishes and desserts, ask them to be in charge of planning an activity.

**5** *Get enough sleep (children need at least nine hours).*

*The theory.* Some may be surprised to see "sleep" on this list of recommendations. But time for sleep has a role in eating well and being active. Children ages seven to eighteen need at least nine hours of sleep a night.[21] Younger children need more. Research has demonstrated that tired children are much more likely to eat excess foods in search of more energy to keep going. They are also much less likely to engage in the recommended one hour of vigorous physical daily activity when they are tired. In at least two studies, a strong inverse association was observed between sleeping hours and childhood obesity: less sleep, more body fat.[22]

*The practice.* Many children get only seven or eight hours of sleep; adolescents get even less. With homework assignments expanding in tandem with competition for college admission, and the lure of television and video games as distractions from the stress of the overscheduled kids' and parents' daily lives, cutting down on sleep is the only way to get everything done. Erratic work and household activities interfere with regular sleep schedules. The imperative is to define goals for the family's and each child's health and success. Learning time-management skills will help both children and their parents.

How to get enough sleep?

**Instead of** letting children stay up late watching television, working on the computer, or talking on the phone, **try** having a consistent bedtime policy—for parents as well as for children. If this means cutting corners on housework or homework in order to make time for sleep, so be it; let your children know that getting enough sleep and being healthy is a top priority.

**Instead of** saving child's homework for after dinner, which can push back bedtime, **try** setting a goal of finishing an hour of homework before dinner. Have children work on homework at the kitchen table during dinner preparation so parents and children can interact during both homework and meal preparation.

**Instead of** overscheduling and overcommitting to extracurricular activities, which spread the family thin and interfere with sleep and family mealtimes, **try** being realistic and curbing expectations of what kids—and parents—can accomplish in twenty-four hours.

## RAISE RESILIENT CHILDREN

A complementary approach in authoritative parenting is to encourage resilience in both young and older children, an idea set forth by Robert Brooks and Sam Goldstein in *Raising Resilient Children*.[23] The following discussion is especially indebted to that book's inspiring conceptual analysis. The authors ask what most parents want for their children and conclude that whether it is happiness, success in school, satisfaction with their lives, or solid friendships, "realization of these goals requires that children have the inner strength to deal competently and successfully, day after day, with the challenges and demands they encounter." They call that capacity to cope and feel competent *resilience.*

If kids in general need to learn resilience to deal more effectively with stress and pressure, fat children need double doses of resilience to cope better with everyday challenges; to bounce back from disappointments, adversity, and trauma; to solve problems; and to treat themselves with respect. These skills, if learned early, may go a long way toward preventing the behaviors and series of events that lead to obesity.

Brooks and Goldstein speak to parents who increasingly view the world as a hostile place in which to raise children and who think that the solution is to construct taller walls around families and double-lock front doors to keep out a seemingly toxic culture. This solution, these psychologists believe and I concur, is unrealistic. But we can shield children by helping them build resilience to thrive in our culture.

To remain healthy and to achieve the expectations we place on them, children need all the help available. Parents who have an explicit or intuitive understanding of resilience can cultivate a similar mindset and behaviors in their children. If children learn self-nurturing (taking care of their needs in healthy ways, such as playing a game with a friend when bored) and limit setting (controlling urges for still more food or TV), they are more likely to avoid "emotional eating." Children who are resilient and self-nurturing will likely find comfort and pleasure from sources other than food—friends, physical activities, games, and the like. Children who have learned limit setting feel safe and successful and have reasonable expectations of themselves.

## GUIDELINES FOR RESILIENCE

One barrier to raising resilient children is the lack of know-how. Some parents are better than others at being empathic, communicative, positive rather than negative, and realistic about strengths and weaknesses—characteristics that help build resilience in their children. Even so, these abilities can be learned. And in many cases, parents have these abilities but feel too burdened with the pressures of work and worry to use them with their children.

To ask any parents to invest energy and effort in learning how to nurture resilience in their children by first learning and applying a resilient personal mindset is a tall order. To ask parents of overweight children in minority, low-income, or low-education groups to do so may seem totally unreasonable. Yet many of these parents already have resilient mindsets. With basic support from safer environments for play and better child care, increased supervised after-school activities and encouragement from healthcare providers and others in the community, a family is more likely to follow guidelines that foster resilience. In looking to reverse the childhood obesity epidemic, our first step is to develop resilient children.

The guidelines Brooks and Goldstein present use violence as an example of the toxic culture. But instead we turn back to Eddie, Maria, and Dwayne and apply each guideline to the toxic forces that make children fat. Can Eddie, currently at a healthy weight, keep his resilience? Can Maria, at risk of becoming overweight, learn more resilience? And can Dwayne, already overweight, learn to become a resilient child? Let's look at ways these three may respond to parents and caretakers who follow the guidelines for raising resilient children.

**1** *Be empathic; accept children for who they are and help them set realistic expectations and goals.*
Parents eager for their children's success may urge overweight or clumsy children to "try harder." Rather than assume a child must have a certain body size and shape to gain popularity with friends, or expect a child to excel in sports or school achievement, parents need to reevaluate whether these goals are realistic and reasonable and remember how they responded to similar pressure from their own parents.

Empathic parents put themselves inside the shoes of their children to appreciate their point of view. Being empathic is easy when our children are warm and responsive, but it is hard when we are upset or disappointed with our children.

Eddie at first enjoyed soccer but then began finding excuses for not going to practice. "I don't like everyone shouting at me during games," he said. His parents responded, "Just don't pay attention to them," but when he claimed he had a stomachache just before game time they got upset and accused him of faking it. When they put themselves in his shoes, they asked themselves, "Would I want my folks to believe me when I say shouting makes me upset and I have a stomachache?" Then, instead of lecturing him, "Ignore the shouting; your stomachache will go away," they helped Eddie take a leave from the soccer team. By encouraging him to work on a special project—putting together a Halloween fun house—they supported an alternative activity that validated his self-worth. Parents who are empathic toward the problem of childhood obesity and see a fat boy as a "good helper with little Sam" or "best finder of lost items"—any label but "fat kid"—are encouraging him (and other overweight children) to identify themselves as valuable, resilient.

Overweight kids often are better at empathy than their parents and other adults. A new parent recently e-mailed me for information about childhood obesity. He explained, "I was obese as a child and lost about 100 pounds when I was twenty-four. I don't want my son to grow up obese. On the other hand, I don't want him to grow up an entitled, spoiled punk, as he might if he is too good-looking. Kids who are constantly deferred to because they are good-looking tend to be spoiled. I think maybe I'm a nicer, better person for having grown up a fatso." Daniel Goleman's concept of *emotional intelligence* can be construed as another name for empathy; he describes empathy as the fundamental "people skill," one that builds on emotional self-awareness.[24] Fat kids are likely to have high levels of emotional intelligence because they have developed a keen sense of "what it feels like to be different," and they often display empathy toward other children who are different from mainstream kids in a variety of ways.

Child psychologists usually ask parents what they did to handle a difficult child, and if it worked. Oddly enough, they seldom ask parents what they believe the difficult child thought or felt. Questions parents could ask themselves might be: "How does my child feel when I tell him to eat his vegetables or to stop watching TV and do homework?" "What words would my child use to describe me as a parent?" A cornerstone of raising resilient children is conveying empathy as a way of fostering strength, hope, and optimism.

## 2 *Communicate effectively and listen actively.*

By validating what children are attempting to say, and by not telling them how they should feel, parents can effectively communicate and develop resilience in children. For example, Maria's grandmother worried that Maria rarely played with other children or talked about school friends. Without asking Maria, her mother arranged a play date with Jenny, who lived on their street. Maria was so anxious that she tried to get Jenny to play with all of her games at once and gave her loads of candy she thought Jenny would like. Jenny never asked Maria to play at her house and on several occasions refused to come back to Maria's house again. Later, Maria did not want to have a birthday party. After listening carefully, her grandmother and mother realized Maria was afraid no one would come. Her mother said she understood Maria's concern and then searched for a recreation class

Maria could attend two days a week after school. Maria's older sister persuaded her to start swimming classes on Saturdays and took her to them. (Perhaps another time her mother will ask Maria first if she wants to play with a friend.)

**3** *Change "negative scripts."*

Parents often nag their kids the same way, using the same words for years, "Eat your vegetables or . . . ." When nagging doesn't work, it's time to change the script.

Dwayne's weight became a family issue when the school nurse informed his parents that he was seriously overweight and ought to have a restricted diet. His parents then told him, no more trips to McDonald's with his siblings. When he went anyway, they said, "You always show disrespect." One brother tattled, "Dwayne's eating another doughnut," and his sisters teased him about his extra servings of macaroni and cheese. Each negative script fed the power struggle over his diet. Had his parents stopped all negative comments on Dwayne's eating behavior or encouraged his efforts to ride a bike or be successful at one activity, they could have showed him other ways to solve problems. Rethinking and rewording *any* issue is very hard—it takes attention and practice.

**4** *Help children experience success by identifying and reinforcing their "islands of competence."*

When some children feel hopeless about their abilities, it is hard for them to "hear" (or believe) any positive feedback. It's better to guide them to something they can do to build competence.

Dwayne's dad and older brother often told him to fight back when bullies taunted him at school. After an especially humiliating experience when five kids ganged up on him and tried to force a whole doughnut into his mouth at once—shouting, "He'll eat anything"—Dwayne's brother threatened to find the gang and beat them up. Had the family switched from "fight back" to help Dwayne learn a new skill such as karate or swimming, he could have built an "island of competence" to emphasize his strengths rather than his weakness.

**5** *Help children recognize that mistakes are experiences from which to learn.*

Nobody intuitively views mistakes as opportunities for learning. More often children experience mistakes as failures. They may retreat from challenges, feel inadequate, and blame others for their problems. If Eddie makes mistake after mistake on the soccer field without encouragement to find alternative physical activities, he may dive into video games, where no one notices mistakes. If Maria continues to overmanage her playmates without an opportunity to learn interpersonal skills in a group with guidance, she may more often turn to food for comfort. If Dwayne just blames others for bullying him without finding an island of competence in physical activity, he may remain a victim and learn to bully others when he grows up.

**6** *Love children in ways that help them feel special and appreciated.*
A basic ingredient for building resilience is the presence of at least one adult who believes in the worth of each child. Such belief helps redirect a child toward a more productive, satisfying life. Brooks and Goldstein call such adults "charismatic" because their personal appeal and engagement give them a compelling quality, and they become stakeholders in the children's future development. Helping children feel special without indulging them requires giving love unconditionally. It does not mean an absence of discipline but rather acceptance and love, whatever the children's shortcomings and mistakes.

Maria's mother tried to schedule "special times" each evening with Maria to read aloud or just talk. Maria looked forward to this time. Nonetheless, when the phone rang, her mother would interrupt their special time to answer. Maria soon chose to watch television rather than feel unimportant. Parental behavior sends a strong message about the value of family activities; for example, answering the phone during meals is often a signal to children that mealtime is worthless.

### MORE IDEAS FOR ADOLESCENTS

For the purposes of this discussion, let's fast-forward these three children's lives and imagine they are now thirteen years old. Additional guidelines for raising resilient children are apropos as these children enter adolescence.

**1** *Develop responsibility, compassion, and a social conscience by providing children with opportunities to contribute.*
Parents often teach kids to learn responsibility by giving them chores. It's hard to stay motivated to do chores but often much easier with the chance to help others.

Maria, at thirteen, has held her own in terms of weight. She is still at risk of becoming overweight, but she has not crossed into the overweight category. She remains an avid reader and now feels rewarded by reading aloud to her grandmother and to several other elderly people she visits three days a week. She even walks several blocks and up several flights of stairs to their apartments. Her growing competence provided encouragement to try out for drama club. She is now rehearsing for her first play and likes all aspects of participating in the group. She has less time alone to turn to food for comfort.

### 2 *Teach children to solve problems and make decisions.*
Instead of telling children what to do, parents teach problem solving best by engaging kids in brainstorming solutions. A regular family meeting time to discuss problems and solutions is a good place to do this.

Eddie has lots of friends and is quite popular. Many of his friends are now dropping out of sports and spending more time hanging around the house after school, playing video games, swallowing lots of soda and snacks. Eddie prefers to go down to a nearby stream and paddle his kayak but couldn't get any friends to go along. During the weekly family meeting, everyone joined in to make a list of ways he could solve the problem. One way was to organize a kayak club. He asked the athletic director at school for help; a twelfth-grader volunteered to provide supervision for a kayak club after school. Eddie has learned to negotiate choices and looks to a charismatic adult for help.

### 3 *Discipline in a way that promotes self-discipline and self-worth.*
Brooks and Goldstein point out that the word *discipline* relates to *disciple* and thus is a teaching process. Discipline can reinforce or weaken self-esteem, self-control, and resilience. Well-meaning parents often impose rules and consequences that provoke resentment, rather than learning. One alternative that worked for Maria when her mother kept after her to do a fitness workout every day was to work together in setting the rules (Mom: "I will stop nagging") as well as the consequences (Maria: "I will not get to talk on the computer chat room tonight if I skip my workout").

Whatever you do, parents be warned: pick each "self-discipline learning" project carefully, and keep the list short. A cartoon I saw illustrated the importance of choosing battles rather than expecting a child to do everything right all at once. The cartoon showed the table of contents for a book called *The Big Book of Parent-Child Fights*. The topic of chapter one, "Food Arguments," ran from page 1 to 832. "Bedtime Feuds" ran from page 833 to

1247, where "Personal-Hygiene Tiffs" picked up. "Messy-Room Run-Ins" and "Sibling Skirmishes" went on into the thousands. If you start early as a parental role model in how to eat moderately, exercise self-discipline, and lead a healthy life, you can go a long way toward reducing the volume of parent-child fights as children get older.

## SUMMARY

The final part of this book focuses on ways to reverse the fatness epidemic. We started in this chapter by focusing on prevention—specifically, what parents can do, from early childhood through adolescence and to adulthood, to raise children who have a lifelong balanced, healthy approach to eating and who lead active lives. (The next chapter examines treatment options, looking first at the diet culture in America and then reviewing some popular weight-loss programs for children.) I presented my top recommendations here, with tips for implementing them, along with a complementary approach for raising resilient children. Much of this advice parents and caregivers already know. Many, however, do not follow it because it is hard—and it requires support and practice. Parents, just like their children, are lifelong learners. Even small adjustments in parenting style often yield large benefits in children's behavior. An example of one recommendation to forestall and curb childhood obesity is to set bedtime limits so children get enough sleep as a step toward improving eating and physical activity behavior. To observe bedtime limits themselves as parents is a second step. The goal of this chapter is to encourage parents to take at least one or more similar steps toward slowing the obesity epidemic affecting all of our children. As parents, our best precept is our example. Mahatma Gandhi's words are apt: "You must be the change you wish to see in the world." And the poem "You Can Only Demonstrate" echoes the advice.

If you carry great expectations
for your children,
they will carry great burdens.
If you try to make them good,
you will create instead their vices.

Let your teaching be subtle.
Let your strength reside
in your flexibility.
Let your virtues be natural
and not affected.

If your children are treated
with modesty,
grace,
forgiveness,
and joy,
what are they likely to learn?

There is nothing more important
than the integrity of your life.
You cannot teach,
impose,
control,
coerce,
or force
any virtue.
You can only demonstrate.
Put your best effort forth
on your own actions,
not those of your children.

William C. Martin,
*The Parent's Tao Te Ching*

--------------------------------------------------------

# 7

# REACHING AND KEEPING
# A HEALTHY WEIGHT

--------------------------------------------------------

ELEVEN-YEAR-OLD NATHANIEL ROBBINS, the protagonist in Robert Kimmel Smith's novel *Jelly Belly*, carries 109 pounds on his 4-foot-8-inch frame. "Blimpie," "Tubby," "Piggy," and "Lard-Butt" are some of the nicknames he also carries around. As the excerpt below illustrates, this boy is emotionally scarred and physically uncomfortable, not only from being fat but also from trying to lose weight:

> Right now there are probably three million kids reading this and laughing at me. I mean, you're probably saying, "Big deal—the kid misses one meal of spaghetti and a piece of blueberry pie and he runs upstairs and cries his head off." But it wasn't really that at all. I was lying across my bed, miserable and crying, because there wasn't any answer to it all. I was *always* going to be fat, I was *always* going to be on a stupid diet, and I was *always* going to be miserable. It just seemed like there was no hope. It was going to be the way it was, forever and ever. And that's why I was crying. I could take a diet for a week or a month. But the fact was that I had already been on a diet for four months and *I hadn't lost any weight.*[1]

Rather than help, Nathaniel's diets have deepened his self-loathing and hopelessness. This chapter seeks to help the countless children who identify with his misery, the overweight young people whose pain has been compounded by misguided and ineffective weight-loss advice.

Prevention may be the best course of treatment, but how do we help children who are already seriously overweight? The advice surrounding nutrition and weight loss is often contradictory and seemingly ever-changing. It tends to leave adults as confused and hopeless as the overweight children they seek to help. I'll begin by presenting the general advice I give my clients and their parents and then review other weight-management plans and programs before addressing some of the damage our dieting culture does and potential dangers associated with campaigns to reverse the obesity epidemic.

## WEIGHT MANAGEMENT AND CHILDREN

In fact and fiction, dieting to lose weight, or dreaming about the end results, is a pervasive, obsessive activity for many American children. Vanessa, age sixteen, diets and dreams, as she describes in *Fat Talk*, an ethnographic study that reports the voices of real teenage girls talking about weight, attractiveness, and dieting:

> The other day my girlfriend asked me, "Can you imagine what life would be like if we both lost fifteen pounds?" and I said, "Oh, wow! Right now, I'm a little bit chubby . . . I just know that if I lost fifteen pounds, I'd be more self-confident. I'd be able to walk past the soccer team and not feel all embarrassed. I could just walk right up to those guys and say, 'Hi, how are you doing?' I'd feel so much better about myself if I were thinner."[2]

Judi, age thirteen, a fictional character in *Fat Chance,* notes that her secret desire is "to be the thinnest girl in the entire eighth grade." Her biggest fear is "that I'll get as fat as Ms. Roth [the teacher] someday, or even fatter." Dieting is an overriding concern in her life:

> I'm going to start a new diet tomorrow. I've been on diets before, but this time I'm going to be really serious about it. You see, this is my last chance to lose weight because next year I'll be in high school, and who wants to be a fat freshman?[3]

Vanessa and Judi match the popular profile of a teenage girl growing up in the United States today. Study after study reports that dissatisfaction with weight, as well as inappropriate dieting behaviors, are pervasive, particularly among white middle-class girls. Rather than steer them toward a healthy weight, however, this preoccupation with weight loss and body image can promote extreme and detrimental behavior, fostering unhealthy eating habits and a negative self-image (discussed below). My goal is to put forth reasonable and moderate guidelines that will help steer these young people back toward healthy, balanced eating and enable them to break free from their obsession with dieting.

In whatever course I teach, talk I give, or workshop I lead, the recurrent questions about weight management programs are, what *really* works, and *how long* does it take? To both, the answer is that it depends. It depends on how we measure what works or what is effective; it depends on children's genetic background, age, and growth rate, as well as their home and social environment. There is no simple or easy answer, though many parents desperately wish there were.

I can say with more certainty what does *not* work for kids: restrictive diets. By restrictive diets, I mean eating plans that strictly curb the amount and type of food permitted. There is little, if any, evidence that they work. Most short-term weight loss cancels itself out, and restriction generally leads to nagging parents, anxious kids, and bad long-term results.

Drawing on a huge amount of research and experience in adult obesity, most experts agree that success in combating obesity depends on long-term *weight management,* not a "diet." Weight management is not just weight loss. Management also means rethinking individual behavior and choices to sustain a healthy weight with balanced eating and physical activity, day in and day out. This is much more difficult than "going on a diet" for a few weeks.

Traditionally the term *diet* referred to what we eat every day, which over time becomes an eating pattern. Using available, affordable, and acceptable foods, culture shapes our diet. In the past quarter century, however, the term took on a specific and sometimes pejorative sense of a short-term restrictive eating plan whose goal is weight loss. When most people consider obesity treatment, they mistakenly plan short-term penance, not lifelong weight management.

What follow are several questions and my answers related to dieting and weight management. These are typical of questions I field from parents, educators, and health providers as they seek to help seriously overweight youth reach and keep a healthier weight.

### Should a five-year-old overweight child be on a diet?
No, a five-year-old overweight child should eat like a five-year-old healthy-weight child, not like an eighteen-year-old basketball player.

I do not endorse weight reduction for children—except for extremely over-weight seven- to eleven-year-olds and teens with health complications—but I do support weight maintenance, which stalls excess weight gain and allows overweight children to "grow into" their weight. Children don't need diets; they need to eat for their age and be moderately active. Guidelines endorsed by the American Academy of Pediatrics say that, for overweight children ages two to seven, the goal is weight maintenance, not weight loss. If an over-weight child maintains her weight as she grows, her weight and height will come back into line.[4]

*If a nine-year-old child is so overweight that his blood pressure is high and he has sleep apnea (breathing difficulty), should he be on a diet to lose weight?*
First, the family's healthy eating and activity should stop the weight gain. Then, changes in eating and activity should aim toward a weight loss of about one pound per month.[5]

*What are the changes in eating required to stop the weight gain or to lose a pound or two a month?*
This question usually means, "I want a diet that works." I hear it from par-ents, and I hear it from lots of health professionals. "You're a dietitian; give her a diet." Again, I give my standard answer, "A seven-year-old should eat like a seven-year-old. Choose foods from all parts of the Food Guide Pyra-mid in the *amounts* recommended for her age and activity."

*That sounds too easy. Why are kids still getting fatter?*
After I find out what a child usually eats and we compare samples of the recommended amounts with his usual daily diet, I try to bring the fam-ily's idea of normal amounts in line with reality. After some probing into what and how much he ate yesterday, or any day in general, I may find that this seven-year-old overweight child has been eating like a seventeen-year old. His reported daily menu, like Dwayne's, may look something like this:

Before school: a large glass of orange juice (12 oz); Fruit Loops (¾ cup) with whole milk (1 cup); and one jelly doughnut

Snack at school (brought from home): Snapple drink (12 oz); potato chips (6 oz bag); mozzarella cheese stick

Lunch served at school: pepperoni pizza (2 slices) and whole milk (8 oz)

After-school snack: large serving of fries with three packs of ketchup; soda (12 oz)

Supper: two pieces deep-fried chicken; rice and beans (about 1 cup); three bites (1 tablespoon) carrots; two glasses of soda (20 oz)

TV time: large bowl of chocolate ice cream (1 cup)

Snack before bed: sweetened applesauce (¾ cup) and one chocolate graham cracker

Throughout the day: M&M candy (4 oz bag)

Total calories for day (approximately): 3,200

In one day Dwayne takes in foods from all parts of the Food Guide Pyramid in at least the minimum number of recommended servings (counting the fries, ketchup, and pizza tomato sauce as vegetables, the double-size orange juice and applesauce as three fruit servings). But he also takes in about 3,200 calories. The estimated daily calorie requirement is about 1,800 calories for a moderately active seven-year-old boy with a healthy weight-for-height. The range is 1,400 to 2,400 calories depending on activity and appropriate growth rate. Dwayne does not need "a diet." Dwayne needs to eat like a seven-year-old and to spend at least an hour a day in moderate to vigorous physical activity—like a seven-year-old!

Dwayne's food choices are not necessarily "bad" (though they could use improvement in the high-fat and sugar department); the main problem is they are "big." Eating the recommended number of servings in the recommended serving sizes would give Dwayne a great start for improving his daily diet and for slimming down as he grows up. Tilting his food choices toward less-calorie-packed foods would make his diet healthier and give him an excellent chance to have fewer chronic diseases as he grows up.

With a few modifications, Dwayne's daily diet can be adjusted to provide approximately 1,800 calories from foods that he finds acceptable—and that meet the guidelines for a child his age. From a nutrition education perspective, these changes appear relatively easy and painless; but Dwayne and his family may think they are very restrictive, like a "diet." The goal, then, is to include the same foods he usually eats but in smaller amounts and gradually change the type, such as moving from whole to low-fat milk, from jelly doughnuts to toast and jelly. To help him learn choices, foods are grouped as "anytime" (carrots, rice, and beans), "sometimes" (soda, ice cream) and "seldom" (fries, doughnuts, M&Ms). Dwayne and his family will decide (with guidance) how to interpret "sometimes" and "seldom." A sample day might look like this:

Before school: small glass of orange juice (8 oz); Wheaties topped with Fruit Loops or lightly sweetened Cheerios (1 oz), with 1 percent low-fat milk; toast and jelly

Snack: apple, banana, or kiwi, or 100 percent fruit juice (6 oz); water; mozzarella stick or peanut butter spread on 2 low-fat Triscuits

Lunch: vegetable (broccoli) pizza (2 slices); low-fat milk (1 cup); unsweetened applesauce (4 oz)

After-school snack: Lite canned fruit (½ cup) or 100 percent fruit juice (8 oz); chocolate graham crackers (2 squares); water

Dinner: oven-baked chicken (3 oz); rice and beans (1 cup); carrots (raw or cooked, ½ cup); green and red pepper strips; ice cream (½ cup); water

TV time (or family game): popcorn and 12 oz soda

Total calories (approximately): 1,800

### Will an overweight child like Dwayne actually eat this type of food, every day?

Yes, unless his family eats most meals from take-out restaurants or vending machines. This sample daily menu does require Dwayne's family to spend a minimal amount of time shopping for groceries and preparing meals and snacks. And with very little effort his family can adopt an eating plan similar to the one outlined above that is acceptable, affordable, and available for Dwayne. It follows nutrition guidelines that represent millions of dollars in educational development and promotional materials (the USDA Food Guide Pyramid for Young Children). But most nutrition education programs stop here. They provide the information. The best programs also tailor the information to an individual's needs and situation, and this plan does that too, for Dwayne, with modified amounts of foods he is used to and a method for choosing among the "seldom" foods that now boost his total calories into the stratosphere for a kid his age.

*What is the likelihood that Dwayne will eat according to this plan and slowly grow into his weight?*

A very small likelihood—if all we do is "give" his family the diet plan. What is required, experts claim and I agree, is learning to change behavior.[6] To support healthier food choices, Dwayne and his family need to learn skills— shopping to have snacks available rather than going to McDonald's for fries, and cooking with less grease (oven-baked chicken, homemade popcorn with minimal oil). And they need to substitute activities to replace TV time and to encourage them to apply their new skills. For Dwayne, this may involve learning to choose a goal and reward: "If I have only one 'seldom' food each day for at least five days a week, I get to go bowling with my brother" (behavioral contracting); learning to check his degree of hunger, by making a fist, imagining it as his stomach, and counting how many fingers full he feels (stimulus control); or making a chart of how many "seldom" foods he eats a day or number of times a week he turns off the TV for half an hour or more, then reviewing it with a parent (self-monitoring).

For best results, parents should work with their children to make sure the goals they choose are positive, specific, and realistic, like these:

Positive goals: "I will drink more water," not "I will drink less soda"

Specific goal actions: "I will play hopscotch and talk with Anna outside after school for about an hour, three out of five days a week," *not* "I will play more outside games"

Realistic goals: "I will eat raw carrots, which I like (I hate cooked carrots)"

*Should a child be in a weight-management treatment program even if the family is not part of it?*

The Expert Committee on Obesity Evaluation and Treatment, a group that develops guidelines for the American Academy of Pediatrics, recommends that when a family believes obesity is inevitable or resists efforts to modify activity or meals, the treatment of an overweight child should be deferred until the family is ready to change; or the family should be referred to a therapist who can address the family's readiness. "Lack of readiness will probably lead to failure, which will frustrate the family and perhaps prevent future weight-control efforts." The committee further recommends that the whole family be required to participate "in creating new family be-

**PARENTING SKILLS**

Here are wise recommendations from the Expert Committee on Obesity Evaluation and Treatment on ways parents and caretakers can support weight management, healthy eating, and physical activity. Not coincidentally, these points echo the guidelines in chapter 6.

- Use activity and time with your children—not food—as a reward for desired behavior.
- Establish times for daily family meals and snacks.
- Determine what food and when to offer it, while children decide if and how much to eat.
- Offer only healthy options: "An apple or popcorn?"
- Remove most junk-food temptations from the home, and limit less nutritious fare by buying it only in small containers. Offer ice cream, salty high-fat snacks, soda, and candy only as part of *planned* meals and snacks.
- Be a role model; improve your own eating and activity behaviors.
- Be consistent in setting limits. "Giving in" reinforces undesirable behavior.
- Find reasons to praise your children's behavior. Children are good; behaviors can be good or bad.

haviors consistent with the child's new eating and activity goals." Otherwise, regular caregivers who do not participate in these changes may undermine the treatment program.[7]

The most successful programs for kids are those that enroll both children and families.[8] In fact, one program that targeted the parents exclusively—and not the child—found that improved parenting skills brought about the child's weight loss (see the box "Parenting Skills").[9]

*Are there successful plans and programs—commercial or based in health clinics—that are safe for kids and that work over the long term?*

It is difficult to say. An untold number of obesity treatment plans for children and adults crowd the marketplace, and some are better than others (my review of a few better-known plans and worthwhile programs follows).

A specific program's effectiveness is hard to gauge. To most kids and parents, effectiveness usually means that the program enabled participants to lose weight and keep it off. To program providers, effectiveness usually means that some participants stopped gaining weight and improved one or two eating and activity behaviors. I think effectiveness should involve maintaining weight as a child grows (not weight loss) and meeting one or two realistic behavior goals each week.

### Should parents who seek to slow their overweight child's weight gain keep daily logs that detail how much the child eats and exercises?

Many weight-management programs recommend record keeping or "self-monitoring," to keep track of and then analyze the eating and exercise behavior patterns. For overweight kids, this can be a drag and a nag point for their parents. It is better to agree on a goal and reward, such as eat only one "seldom" food most days and spend time with positive activities (like Dwayne's "go bowling with my brother") rather than laborious writing. That said, record keeping relates to greater success for adults in weight management. There is no evidence for kids.

Self-monitoring involves recording what you eat; what's happening (or not happening) before and during eating; and what happens after eating. The idea is to figure out the *antecedents, behavior,* and *consequences* of your eating patterns. These are the "ABCs" of your food and eating environment. The first tells what the triggers are to what you eat ("it's there"; "Gramma insisted I eat it"). The second tells how much and what kind of food ("two slices of pizza; two 12 oz colas"). The third tells how you feel and what happens after you eat it ("I felt stuffed and mad at myself"). Learning what happens helps children handle the antecedents the next time in order to change unwanted behavior and consequences. A positive "ABC" could be "try to have watermelon in fridge," "ate a big slice," "felt full and healthy." The theory is that reinforcing this positive pattern by repeating it will lead to new, healthier behavior (it can also apply to goals for physical activity). That's the upside of self-monitoring. The downside is that such a close and continual analysis of self-behavior could lead to more obsessive and overcontrolling behavior. Parents can play to the positive parts (revelations and rewards) while discouraging the negative (fixation with every bite of food).

With those questions and my answers serving as the foundation, we can build on an understanding of weight-management strategies for children by examining in greater detail the advice from a handful of noteworthy books and programs.

When we read through the details of popular plans that offer specific nutritional and weight-loss advice, it's no wonder the public is confused about what and how much to eat. Margarine was once touted as a healthy alternative to butter, but then came the news about trans-fats. Products with fat-free labels were hailed as healthy alternatives, but then they were blamed for promoting overeating and excess sugar consumption. The public was instructed to forget about the old-fashioned "square meal" and its four basic food groups and to start eating according to the Food Guide Pyramid, but then various experts began fiddling with the pyramid—in some cases turning it upside down.

The experts continue to measure, calculate, and ceaselessly debate the recommended ratio of carbohydrates to protein to fats. They also continue to recalibrate the recommended daily amount and type of exercise needed to reap the health benefits of physical activity. Meanwhile, the public tunes out—and just gets fatter.

Sorting through this mountain of advice is not easy for parents or any consumer. An author's credentials can help. Many doctors and nutritionists have bona fide credentials, but they use them to present diets based on little or no scientific evidence and to sell products directly to their clients. Professional medical ethics require that a physician draw a distinct line between prescribing medications, supplements, and the like *and* also selling them. This principle is meant to distinguish licensed professionals from quacks who put profit ahead of the patients' well-being.

This brings us to one of the most controversial health experts, the late Dr. Robert Atkins. He was a trained and licensed cardiologist and at the same time served as executive medical director of Atkins Nutritionals, the company that sells his products. He developed a successful and lucrative weight-management practice based on the diet plan in his book, but he crossed the profession's ethical line by selling a large variety of nutritional supplements in his clinic. The Atkins plan has been dissected and debated ad nauseam, so here I add a perspective on its appropriateness for children.

### LOW CARBS OR LOW FAT?

Atkins's best-selling book, *Dr. Atkins' Diet Revolution,* was first published in 1972. Renamed *Dr. Atkins' New Diet Revolution* when reissued in 1992, it remained on the *New York Times* bestseller list a decade later. His high-fat, low-carbohydrate plan includes few starchy foods, bread, or vegetables and almost no fruit—all contrary to governmental recommendations and their source, the Food Guide Pyramid, which emphasizes several servings of whole grains and starchy foods and a minimum of five servings of fruits and vegetables daily.

In 1998 the kids' version of Atkins hit the market: *Taking the Atkins Program to the Next Generation, Feed Your Kids Well: How to Help Your Child Lose Weight and Get Healthy.*[10]

Many parents, devotees of *Dr. Atkins' Diet Revolution,* were apparently relieved to have the blessing of a famous diet doctor to restrict sugars and starchy foods in their children's diet. Several parents have told me that the whole family benefits from cutting out cookies and potato chips: "We're all on the diet and eating low-carb bars for snacks; the kids don't seem to miss fruits and vegetables." (As Atkins dieting climbed in popularity, low-carb energy bars made with nonsugar sweeteners were rushed to the market as replacements for plain energy bars to meet the "grab and go" market.) Many parents are convinced that "if Atkins is good for me, it's good for my kids."

Most health professionals raise eyebrows when kids are "doing Atkins" because those kids (and their parents) are likely to eat excessive amounts of unhealthy saturated fat while missing out on the nutrients and fiber in fruits, vegetables, and whole grains that are so essential to long-term good health. Yet a handful of pediatricians have told me, "The risk from extreme obesity in some kids far outweighs any damage from cutting carbs."

To Atkins supporters, and even to frustrated health providers who long for absolute answers from the scientific research community, one review reported in April 2003 and two studies the next month brought welcome news that the Atkins plan worked and even lowered some heart disease risk factors.[11] Dieters, all adults, on the "low-carb" diets lost more weight than comparison groups on a conventional low-fat diet.

But wait—that's not the whole story. The trouble was that neither the Atkins approach nor the low-fat diet worked very well for the dieters; their mild success was attributed to water loss in the early phase and to eating fewer calories, regardless of the type of diet. After a year, each group had gained some of the weight back, making the difference between diets insignificant. On top of that, over 40 percent of the participants dropped out during the year. In diet studies, dropouts are likely to be those who do not lose weight or cannot follow the diet plan.

My concern, from a practical standpoint, is this: even if low-carbohydrate diets were safe over the long haul (and there's no safety evidence yet), how long can a child—or an adult—go without a bun for the burger or without crust under the cheese and pepperoni pizza topping? One mother, in a reader review on Amazon.com, put it well when she expressed disappointment that Atkins for kids "is filled with lists of 'off limit' foods like fruits" and wondered what to do with the advice to feed her kids eggs every morning when her kids don't like eggs.[12]

Still, many parents are desperate to lose weight themselves and to stall weight gain in their children, so a diet for all family members is appealing because a family that gains weight together may lose or at least manage weight together. Under careful supervision by a physician and dietitian, the low-carbohydrate approach tailored to a child and family may be useful in helping severely overweight adolescent children learn to control and reduce weight. Even so, I would then argue against prohibiting nourishing foods that kids do like. Corn and watermelon (examples of carbohydrates that are limited under the Atkins plan) are among kids' favorites, both good sources of vitamins, minerals, and highly touted "phyto-nutrients." At the same time, I applaud any eating plan—including Atkins's—that reduces soda, fries, candy, and sugar-laden snacks.

A similar diet book, *Sugar Busters for Kids,* edited by Samuel S. Andrews et al., appeals to parents who themselves pursued low-carbohydrate eating with the best-selling Sugar Busters plan.[13] Proponents think the plan makes sense: prohibit the "terrible three" snacking staples of soda, french fries, and candy, and make kid-friendly recipes, ranging from whole-wheat pizza to tofu shakes. After all, the official surveys show that kids eat too much junk food. To its credit, it includes healthy carbohydrate foods—whole grains, fruits, and vegetables. But critics fault this plan of restrictive dieting for being too extreme—prohibiting favorite foods and imposing unusual and time-consuming preparations. These restrictions can lead to diet failure, and diet failure, in turn, relates to lowered self-esteem and depression. I discussed this plan and the criticism with a group of parents who were seeking ways to improve their children's diets. One parent gave the most predictable, and practical, response of all: "Never eat french fries? Never drink soda? That'll be the day! Prohibition never works with kids." I agree; moderation is the key.

At the other end of the spectrum from Atkins are low-fat plans such as that outlined by Judith Shaw in *Raising Low-Fat Kids in a High-Fat World.* Shaw's book is geared toward parents willing to put time and energy into a family shift away from the high-fat habit; she recommends having "your child as a primary focus while also considering you and your life." She provides lessons in camouflaging fat, taking the fat out, restocking your kitchen,

## KNOW YOUR FATS

To reduce the amount of fat in our diet, it's important to know that some fats are relatively "good" and others are quite "bad." All are fattening, but some types promote health while others decrease it by the way they affect the amount and type of cholesterol in blood.

All pure fats and oils are high in calories (9 per gram) compared to pure protein and carbohydrate (4 calories per gram). Fats contain about 120 calories per tablespoon and should make up 30 percent or less of daily calories.

Most foods contain mixtures of different types of fat—*monounsaturated* (mono), *polyunsaturated* (poly), and *saturated*—classified by the type that dominates the mix. (Saturated fats are usually solid at room temperature and are called "saturated" because their molecules have all the hydrogen they can hold.)

Hydrogenated oils and trans-fatty acids *(trans-fats)* are formed when unsaturated fats are *hydrogenated*—the process of adding hydrogen. Mono and poly fats can be hydrogenated until they are artificially saturated, making them solid at room temperature (food manufacturers hydrogenate oils to produce a more solid fat product and to extend the shelf life of products such as cookies and crackers; some margarines are produced this way). Trans-fats are the most threatening to health because they raise the "bad" cholesterol and triglycerides in blood and lower the "good" cholesterol.

Nutritionists recommend eating foods that contain mainly mono fats, with poly fats making up the difference, and limiting saturated and trans-fats as much as possible. Look for—and try to avoid—foods with "partially hydrogenated oil" or "hydrogenated oil" on the ingredient list.

What foods contain large amounts of these fats?

MONO FATS (CHOOSE MOST OFTEN)
Olive oil
Canola oil
Almond or hazelnut oil
Soft margarines made with the above oils
Avocados

POLY FATS (CHOOSE OFTEN)
Corn oil
Soybean oil
Sesame and walnut oil
Soft margarines made with the above oils
Salmon and other fish
Flax seed

SATURATED FATS (CHOOSE SELDOM):

Butter

Lard

Fat in beef and other meats

Palm and coconut oil

Hydrogenated oils (especially hard margarines)

TRANS-FATS (CHOOSE SELDOM):

Commercial french fries

Margarine

Vegetable shortening

Most crackers, cookies, pastries, breakfast bars

Most savory snacks and potato chips

Prepackaged desserts, puddings

No more than 10 percent of daily calories should come from saturated and trans-fats. This means children should eat about 15 grams or less of these combined fats daily; adults, 20 grams or less daily. The average American eats about 35 grams of combined saturated and trans-fats daily. Here are some examples of foods with saturated and trans-fats.

| Food | Serving size | Saturated fat | Trans-fat | Total trans- and saturated fat |
|------|-------------|---------------|-----------|-------------------------------|
| Jell-O Chocolate Pudding Snack | 1 | 1.5 g | 1.5 g | 3.5 g |
| Dunkin' Donuts glazed doughnut | 1 | 2.5 g | 4.0 g | 6.5 g |
| Nabisco Wheat Thins | 8 | 1.0 g | 2.0 g | 3.0 g |
| Big Mac with medium fries | 1 | 10.0 g | 4.0 g | 14.0 g |

and keeping (low-fat) hamburgers on the menu. Her plan resembles the Dean Ornish low-fat diet plan but with meat and chicken, tailored for families with kids. Not a diet, this is an all-out overhaul of family eating that requires command of food ingredients, food labels, and recipes as major weapons in combating the high-fat world. Health professionals generally applaud this method because it exemplifies putting knowledge into action (see the box "Know Your Fats"). Learn the tricks, hustle up the ingredients, reorganize your kitchen, and go to work! They have confidence that, in time and with effort, the family will eat the low-fat diet. Pointing to her own success, one dedicated mother who used Shaw's low-fat living suggestions to help her overweight twins claims, "These ideas work, given time, energy, skills, and an ability to handle restaurant-eating-withdrawal symptoms."[14]

Without skills, energy, and time, however, many parents find these laudable goals difficult to achieve. Selecting only one or two manageable suggestions to work on is more reasonable. Simply buying cinnamon graham crackers to stock the snack shelf instead of potato chips or replacing the soda shelf in the refrigerator with a big container of water gives copious returns for small changes in the kitchen.

## FINDING THE RIGHT BALANCE

Because of the popularity of the Atkins diet program (and its knock-offs), as well as doubts about its safety and effectiveness, pressure from the public prompted a governmental response to investigate what is really known about popular diets. The U.S. Department of Agriculture initiated a scientific review of weight-loss plans in 2000 and published the results in March 2001.[15] The study asked: is the information in these diets scientifically sound, and are popular diets effective for weight loss and/or weight maintenance? Among its other questions it touched on these diets' reported effects on the risk of heart disease or diabetes, and on levels of insulin and leptin, the long-term hormonal regulators of energy balance.

It measured the diet plans against scientific criteria from research studies and reviewed their diverse nutrient composition: Atkins's and the Carbohydrate Addict's are high fat, low carbohydrate; Weight Watchers' is a balance of carbohydrate and fat; and the Ornish diet is low fat, low animal protein, and high vegetable. After analyzing as much relevant data as could be assembled, the study concluded with a recommendation for a diet resembling Weight Watchers'—balanced carbohydrate and fat, and flexible choice from a wide variety of foods. The study's conclusion corresponds with the 2002 governmental recommendations for sources of calories: 25 to 35 percent fat, 45 to 60 percent carbohydrates, and 15 to 20 percent protein. The scientific report on weight management diet plans concluded, "A diet high in vegetables, fruits, complex carbohydrates (whole grains and legumes), and low-fat dairy is a moderate-fat, low-calorie diet that prevents weight gain, results in weight loss and weight maintenance. It is associated with fullness and satiety. It reduces risk of chronic disease. It is fast, convenient, and inexpensive. How can we convince people it works, and to try

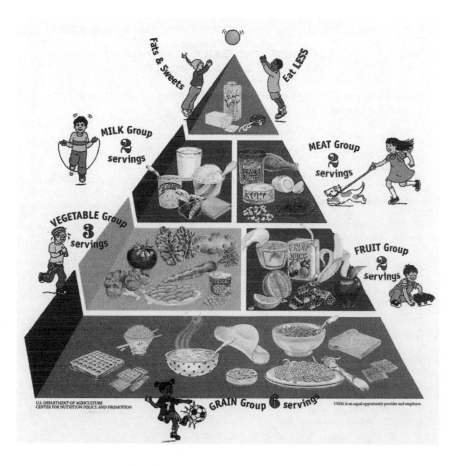

FIGURE 5. The children's Food Guide Pyramid is still the best basic guide for managing weight and promoting health. ("Food Guide Pyramid for Young Children: A Daily Guide for Two- to Six-Year-Olds," U.S. Department of Agriculture, Center for Nutrition Policy and Promotion, 1999)

it?" Making a critical point that applies to children's diets too, the report concluded: "The American public needs to be told (and believe) that diets are not followed for 8 days, 8 weeks, or 8 months, but rather form the basis of everyday food choices throughout their life."[16]

I view this report's conclusion as further proof that the USDA Food Guide Pyramid, with some fine-tuning, is still the best basic guide for managing weight and promoting health. Figure 5 presents the children's Food

## RECOMMENDED DAILY SERVINGS
## FOR CHILDREN AND ADULTS

Understanding serving sizes is essential for following the Food Guide Pyramid's recommendations. What counts as a serving?

GRAIN GROUP
*(bread, cereal, rice, and pasta—preferably whole-grain)*

1 slice of bread
about 1 cup of ready-to-eat cereal
½ cup of cooked cereal, rice, or pasta

VEGETABLE GROUP

1 cup raw leafy vegetables
½ cup other vegetables (cooked or raw)
¾ cup vegetable juice

FRUIT GROUP

1 medium apple, banana, orange, or pear
½ cup chopped, cooked, or canned fruit
¾ cup fruit juice*

DAIRY GROUP
*(milk, yogurt, and cheese—preferably fat-free or low-fat)*

1 cup milk or yogurt
1.5 oz natural cheese (such as cheddar)
2 oz processed cheese (such as American)

MEAT AND BEAN GROUP
*(meat, poultry, fish, dry beans, eggs, and nuts—preferably lean or low-fat)*

2–3 oz cooked lean meat, poultry, fish
1 cup cooked dry beans or tofu
2 soyburgers (2.5 oz each)
2 eggs
¼ cup peanut butter
⅔ cup nuts

How many servings from each food group do you need daily? It depends on your age, gender, and activity level (see opposite).

*Limit juice to one serving (4 to 6 oz) for children ages 1–6; two servings (8 to 12 oz) for children and teens ages 7–18.

| Food group | Children ages 2–3 | Children ages 4–6, women, some older adults | Older children, teen girls, active women, most men | Teen boys, active men |
|---|---|---|---|---|
| Grain | 6† | 6 | 9 | 11 |
| Vegetable | 2† | 3 | 4 | 5 |
| Fruit | 3† | 2 | 3 | 4 |
| Dairy | 2 | 2–3 | 2–3 | 2–3 |
| Meat and Bean | 2 (for a total of 5 oz) | 2 (for a total of 5 oz) | 2 (for a total of 6 oz) | 3 (for a total of 7 oz) |
| Total calories per day | 1,000–1,400 | 1,600 | 2,200 | 2,800 |

SOURCE: USDA, 1999; American Academy of Pediatrics, 2001.

†Serving size is two-thirds of regular serving.

Guide Pyramid, and the box "Recommended Daily Servings" applies alike to children and adults (it complements chapter 6's box on portions and servings). To sum up, carbohydrate-rich foods from the grain group are the diet's foundation (a minimum of six daily servings recommended). Fruits and vegetables form the pyramid's next level (three to five servings of vegetables and two to four servings of fruit); the meat group (which includes nuts and legumes) and dairy group share the third level (two to three servings each); and oils and sweets make up the pyramid's peak (with the admonishment, "use sparingly").[17]

Meanwhile, several nutritionists who are critical of the pyramid have put forth alternative versions. One proposed alternative is the Mediterranean Diet Pyramid promoted by Walter Willett at Harvard's School of Public Health, which encourages eating more whole foods and plant-based oils and less red meat and white flour. Another pyramid guide developed by the Center for Science in the Public Interest recommends eight to ten servings of fruit and vegetables—the results of extensive research by the National Institutes of Health on dietary approaches to stop hypertension.

I agree with many critics that a pyramid overhaul could first of all emphasize serving size and recommend serving sizes by age group. And it could distinguish "healthy" carbohydrates such as those found in brown rice, whole-wheat bread, beans, vegetables, and fruits from less healthy, highly refined "white carbs" such as sugar, white bread, and pastries. It could both encourage moderate use of "healthy" fats (olive, canola, walnut oil) and discourage eating processed fat, which usually contains trans-fats (margarine and hydrogenated solid fats in pastries and snack foods). Finally, it could extol the importance of daily physical activity and drinking water as the main beverage instead of drinks laden with sucrose and corn syrup. But let's not throw out the baby with the bathwater. The pyramid's foundation, structure, and basic principles remain sound.

The question that echoes in the scientific study above, "How can we convince people it works, and to try it?" addresses the desire for quick fixes among adults and children for our weight problems. When medical doctors and registered dietitians recommend a diet high in vegetables, fruits, and whole grains, with small amounts of low-fat animal products, the public questions our credentials and our advice. Why? Is it because people do not like vegetables and fruits? Is it because they have never tasted vegetables and fruits? Is it because vegetables and fruits are not available? I believe an answer lies in the strong competition from the 12,000 food products that beckon at every turn. The taste conditioning for added sugar and fat begins in childhood and gets consistent, daily taste reinforcement. Such conditioning is a very hard act to follow, no matter how strong the evidence that a balanced diet is the best bet for setting and maintaining a healthy weight. Still, I have yet to find a two-year-old seated with adults who clearly enjoy watermelon and strawberries who does not like eating them too.

What affect kids' current and future eating behavior and weight more than other factors are their parents' eating behavior and weight. Families can beat the competition from "junk foods" by exposing children to a wide variety of healthy foods and by following the pyramid's advice to eat a variety of foods in reasonable serving sizes. Healthy body weight will follow—for kids *and* adults.

### GETTING FIT WHILE HAVING FUN

Fitness books, like dieting books, crowd the marketplace and target worried parents. Motivation, fun, and long-term health are the themes. Most fitness books, like most diet books, urge parents to protect their children from diseases that befall unfit children, and then they try to show that fitness is fun and not a chore. Setting a child up for success, not failure, is the goal.

Examples in this genre include *Fit-Kids: Getting Kids Hooked on Fitness Fun!* by Mandy Laderer and *Fit Kids: The Complete Shape-Up Program from Birth through High School* by Kenneth H. Cooper et al.

I endorse these books and others that encourage fitness, even if they have a highly structured exercise program. But I am never surprised that kids do not like isolated, formal workouts that quickly become boring. What most kids want, and need, is other kids to play with. Two-year-olds learn to enjoy active play from watching older siblings or other children, and children of any age generally prefer free play and active games to structured workouts. When no active siblings are around to encourage play, then television and other passive activities quickly and easily replace movement.

My views on fitness reflect contact with boys such as Alex, an only child who was born to two very successful parents in professional careers after several failed attempts to conceive a child. By age five, Alex, so treasured by his Greek parents, spent most of his time with grown-ups, or reading or watching television on his own. He was very overweight. Because he quickly tired and had trouble running, he resisted attempts to involve him in soccer or other group activities. He disliked swimming, even with a private coach. His diet was quite healthy, but he ate large amounts and snacked frequently. His parents were anxious; they worried about his weight and, at the same time, about his getting enough food. Each would independently feed him on the side, even while trying to follow a reduced food plan. So what worked to stall his weight gain was nothing the grown-ups did, but rather the arrival of his lively cousins for an extended summer vacation. These six-year-old boy twins loved running around the yard and floating boats in a brook behind the house. They and Alex built forts and kicked balls, dug big holes and played with trucks in the dirt. Alex loved it. He was so busy that food and television lost their draw. When he started school in the fall, Alex was willing to try some of the active games and to invite a classmate to play at his house. By the next year his BMI had moved down from the "overweight" to the "at risk" category.

Like most other kids, Alex benefited from free play that meets the American Academy of Pediatrics recommendation for all children ages two to eighteen: one hour of moderate to vigorous physical activity most days. To make room in their family's life for this hour's activities, both indoors and out, parents need to limit TV and video time—regardless of any imagined (and real) time crunch—and have fun with their kids.

In some cases, a family and/or health provider may decide that a structured long-term program, involving outside intervention and support, is the best route to help an overweight child manage his or her weight. The degree to which the child's weight poses risks to psychological and physical health and the degree of support the family is able to provide may trigger the decision. What follows is a general review of a few different types of programs I recommend. (Note: I don't endorse commercial programs because comparisons of effectiveness with similar programs for kids are not available.)[18]

Committed to Kids is an integrated four-level weight management program using dietary intervention, behavior modification, and exercise. As weight management programs go, this is one of the most comprehensive, scientifically grounded, user-friendly ones available.

Targeted to a variety of age groups and families, the one-year program offers its four levels in a weekly outpatient clinical setting. A child's weight when starting the program sets the first level. "As a child loses weight, he graduates to a new level. This encourages short-term success through goal setting, feedback, and motivational techniques to improve health behaviors," states Melinda Sothern, a professor of exercise physiology and lead author of the program. The program covers all bases: medical checkups, eating plans and snack suggestions, solving problems family-style, handling emotional pitfalls, and creative ideas for physical activity. It provides workbook forms and checklists to monitor goals, activity, and food. After completing the program, children are encouraged to come to quarterly special events and evaluations free of charge and to attend classes that help prevent relapse. One report of program effectiveness cited 60 percent of participants who reduced their BMI from 32 to 28 after one year. We would only hope (dream?) to see such a program widely accessible to children and families as part of a nationwide health-care network. Sothern's Committed to Kids program is now available in book form for individuals and families as a twelve-week plan, called *Trim Kids*.[19]

Other programs develop in medical centers, with training for providers, and then are offered as commercial programs to children and families by private-practice health professionals or sold for group use in health clinics. These are packaged as program kits with a leader's manual and materials for participants. Shapedown, developed in 1979, is one such family-based program that targets children from six to eighteen years old. The program is sensitive to psychosocial issues pertinent at each stage of development.

It emphasizes improving parenting style, such as helping children find a balance between "self-nurturing and limit setting" or learning "body pride and good health" and "balanced eating and mastery living" (mastery living means achieving a balance of all the characteristics). Workbooks include case story readings, practices, food and activity records, goals, and contracts. A related book for adult weight management that expands the concepts is *The Solution: Six Winning Ways to Permanent Weight Loss* by Laurel Mellin. The Shapedown program reported its effectiveness as a significant decrease in weight and an increase in self-esteem after fifteen months.[20]

What "shaped" my opinion of Shapedown's program was a riveting session of *The Oprah Winfrey Show*, aired November 14, 2002. In it Mellin, creator of Shapedown and *The Solution*, explained her approach to Oprah and illustrated it with flashback and current film clips of children and families who had used the program—many with improved weight and lifestyles. The live interview with a mother and daughter, both overweight, was heartwrenching. First, the twelve-year-old daughter described her misery from being teased and bullied; she had no friends. Her mother then detailed her own attempts and failures to help her daughter lose weight and, in desperation, her own weight gain so her daughter would not be fat alone. Facing the family, Mellin quickly pointed out how the child had taken on the role of parent and now bullies her mother, making her miserable too. The mother and daughter were in tears, and so was I. The camera closed in on Oprah, who reminded the audience, "No child is overweight alone." In fact, that was the theme of the show—to reveal how children are enmeshed in a society that overfeeds their bodies and underserves their emotional needs.

The point is that Mellin and her Shapedown program have it right—but her solution is complicated. She suggests dealing with "emotional trash" and learning parenting skills. To become a nurturing parent takes a lot of skill, determination, patience, and support: to know where to draw the line between indulgence and limit-setting; to be accepting and constructively critical; to be balanced and not lead a chaotic lifestyle. Yes, I say, we could all benefit from learning these skills. Shapedown is a beginning, and in the hands of well-trained and sensitive health providers, it can help overweight children and families manage the social stigma of being overweight while developing eating and activity skills.[21]

The school-based Eat Well and Keep Moving is an interdisciplinary curriculum for teaching upper elementary school nutrition and physical activity. It is "a multifaceted program that encompasses all aspects of the learning environment—from classroom, the cafeteria, and the gymnasium to school hallways, the home, and even community centers," according to the handbook description by its authors, Lillian Cheung and Steven Gortmaker. Targeted at fourth- and fifth-grade children, the program includes actual classroom physical activities and health promotions through clubs and contests like "Freeze My TV," a contest that teaches kids how to log and graph TV time, come up with alternative activities, and keep a journal. Other activities focus on keeping "FitScore" and "SitScore" logs and overcoming the barriers to physical activity. This 480-page program, with illustrated activities for forty-four lessons and ready-made handouts, is clearly a valuable guide. During a large field trial in ten schools, the program's participants reduced TV time and increased fruit and vegetable consumption. The girls who participated, but not the boys, also cut their level of obesity compared with control groups. My evaluation is simple: we need look no further for sound teaching/learning materials for this important age group. Let's move on to implementing such a program in schools nationwide.[22]

There are many other programs, few with evidence of effectiveness, mainly because parents, communities, and the government do not place children's health high on the priority list for financial and public resource support—and because any attempt to compete with the excesses of the seductively sophisticated food and entertainment marketplace offerings would demand monumental energy and audacity.

In judging the various weight management methods that are on the market, we might keep in mind the following report from a leading professional guide, *Handbook of Obesity Treatment,* published in 2002. It evaluates results from seventy-eight studies on various treatment programs for children by research design, number of participants, type of diet and exercise and concludes:

Individual child and family treatments provide short-term benefits.

Very little evidence exists for long-term treatments and weight management.

The most successful programs include diet, exercise, and behavior change methods.

The most effective diet treatments cannot be identified because comparisons are lacking.

Exercise combined with diet enhances weight loss and improves maintenance.

Less structured, flexible lifestyle exercise is more effective than high-intensity.

Reducing sedentary activity, if reinforced, leads to increased moderate physical activity.[23]

Of equal note, most of the programs the *Handbook* describes required intense individual or family involvement and commitment for an extended period of time in order to be successful, even in the short term.

A lack of family support can be a major stumbling point for an otherwise well designed program. A pediatrician I know works in a clinic in a low-income urban community where 75 percent of the children are overweight or at risk of becoming overweight. He asked me to consult on a project he developed there. The program, for seven- and eight-year-olds, was held Saturday mornings and required a parent or family member to accompany the child during the sessions. The kids loved the program and clearly adored the pediatrician and other team members. But other family members were much less happy to be there, and the parents did not attend regularly. Because the multiple demands on today's families can be overwhelming—and some parents may have outside jobs on Saturday morning, while others catch up on chores, sleep, or community activities—he didn't really need an in-depth analysis to figure out why these family members were not "ready to change." I agreed with him that working one on one with kids or even with kids and family members in a weekly group program is, at best, a good start and may work for a few overweight kids. But weight management programs do not work for all families and cannot alone reverse the obesity epidemic.

Despite any advice and endorsements I made above, concerted weight management efforts—or any other campaign that targets fatness—can backfire. Negative consequences are the dieting culture's nightmare and feed its obsessions, which we consider next.

## THE DIETING CULTURE AND DYSFUNCTIONAL EATING

Obsessive dieting, like obesity, ranks as an epidemic; estimates are that at any given time as many as 60 percent of white girls are dieting. Dieting methods, parents are warned, escalate to higher levels of eating disorders such as anorexia nervosa and bulimia.

Countless magazine articles and books blame the drive for thinness on a cultural misperception that the beauty ideal of slimness delivers social status or moral superiority. They claim that this ideal drives girls to control their appetites and their body size by dieting. Some feminist writers see dieting as bondage for girls who struggle to gain their own identity but end up oppressed by an unrealistic body-size ideal. Others rage against dieting as a gimmick to sell fraudulent cures and products by first promising thinness and control and then offering other products to reward or console dieters for "being good/bad." If following our diet exactly makes us feel great—or, conversely, blowing it upsets us—then maybe we'll need to treat ourselves with new clothes/hair products from these nice folks!

The drive to diet varies by race and culture. African Americans, who suffer from higher obesity rates than whites do, are generally more tolerant of larger sizes, as evidenced by interviews conducted by anthropologists for the Teen Lifestyle Project in Tucson, Arizona. They followed white and black girls from middle school to high school and studied their perspectives of body image. Girls from the two groups summed up the differences with photos and quotes in *Newsweek:*

> [photo caption of lean white girl] "White girls think you can never be too thin. They say, 'I'm so fat. I'm so ugly.' To me, the ideal is trim and strong, athletic—but not too strong."

> [photo caption of two heavy African American girls] "Black girls think size doesn't matter—if you've got the right attitude. They say, 'It's really how you carry yourself. It's what you wear, how your hair is done and how you put it together that gets you attention.' The guys at my school don't trip on skinny."[24]

These and other studies show that black females, as well as Latinas, are less rigid in their concepts of beauty than their white counterparts; they spoke positively of "making what you've got work for you." White images of style, in contrast, encapsulate beauty ideals that can lead girls to experience dissatisfaction with their bodies and to desire weight loss as a way to be perfect and popular. One study of 4,000 fourteen- to eighteen-year-old high school girls, in equal number black and white, reported that white adolescent girls were nearly twice as likely to perceive themselves as overweight and six times more likely to engage in unhealthy weight-loss practices, such as using pills and vomiting to keep or change their weight.[25]

In recognition of the detrimental effects of dieting, guidebooks on diet and health for adults and children have changed their message over the past couple of decades. The pitch is now *diet-free* or *non-diet* healthy eating for kids and grown-ups. In the 1980s, books peddled weight-loss diets for children, but in the 1990s, the focus shifted to healthy lifestyle programs. Strict prescriptions for eating and exercise gave way to flexible alternatives to body beauty, inside and out. Losing weight to feel great became a quest of finding yourself through your talents and body movement. On closer view, the new labels feature the old tune—weight-loss and exercise suggestions are embedded within these guidelines for healthy lifestyle.

To illustrate the shift, compare the titles of two books by Frances M. Berg, a family wellness specialist and the editor of *Healthy Weight Journal.* The first, *How to Be Slimmer, Trimmer and Happier: An Action Plan for Young People with a Step-by-Step Guide to Losing Weight through Positive Living,* represents the diet book genre of the 1980s: losing weight is the path to healthy body weight and happiness. The book gave sound guidance on creating good habits—eating right, counting calories, avoiding fad diets—and a reader reported that "After ten weeks on the Action Plan, I found controlling my snacking easy, and I was able to concentrate on constructive activities instead of dreaming about a cookie."[26]

Fourteen years later Berg wrote *Afraid to Eat: Children and Teens in Weight Crisis.* Reviewers reported, "Berg serves up a feast of facts on four major problems: dysfunctional eating, eating disorders, size prejudice, and overweight." Berg condemns dieting as a major cause of the "crisis in eating and weight": "Children are possessed by fear, many children don't eat normally. They shun certain foods, they diet, and they binge. There's a new name for these eating patterns—dysfunctional eating."[27] The program Berg offers in 1997 is similar to her 1983 program; she calls for moderation in eating habits and an active lifestyle. While the pro-dieting hook in the 1980s linked dieting to happiness, the anti-dieting advice of the 1990s imparted the message that dieting leads to unhappiness and "weight crises."

One other book, written by a credentialed health professional, illustrates this shift. In *Save Your Child from the Fat Epidemic,* the registered dietitian Gayle Alleman warns: NO DIETS. "Diets in childhood may lead to disordered eating later in life." "Rather than a diet, just begin offering your child a different array of foods—ones that are low in fat, sugar, and calories."[28] One point recurs: moderation is essential.

I applaud this movement to redefine dieting as lifetime weight management and healthy living. The problem is, parents and the media continue to pass on destructive dieting messages and unrealistic body ideals to younger generations. In spite of the new emphasis on substituting lifetime weight management for dieting, one study showed that girls whose mothers diet or focus on weight control strategies at meals and in conversation were significantly more likely to have ideas about dieting than those whose mothers did not focus on dieting.[29] Clearly, a dieting culture defines this generation, passed from mothers (and fathers) to daughters—and, in some cases, to sons.

Some young people are so desperate to lose weight that they would resort to pharmaceutical and surgical procedures, even though none are approved for kids. They must get these ideas from their family and media. Consider the comments I heard from adolescent girls: "I am just going to have my fat sucked out, like my aunt did—it's called liposuction." "I'm gonna have my stomach closed up so I can't eat so much. I saw on TV that Carnie Wilson, the singer, did that and she is really pretty and skinny now." "My mom took me to this big research place where they were testing pills for kids to lose weight. I took them and this lady talked to us about eating better, but nothing worked."

I agree with those who say we should appeal to adult role models to stop complaining about their bodies or discussing their latest diet, because such comments promote unhealthy dieting and distorted body image. In no small part because of parents' attitudes, young kids link success and self-esteem to body image. Comments they overhear—"I'm so fat" or "So-and-so has really put on weight"—condition them to worry about their weight and make fun of others who are heavy. Children need role models who affirm their self-worth in other ways. We should focus on making balanced, moderate eating a way of life, not a diet, and make physical activity fun and desirable for children, not competitive.

A nationwide campaign to reduce obesity and to heighten awareness of obesity's risks might inadvertently trigger young children's lifelong obsession with body weight, be they fat or thin, and promote fat discrimination. Berg and others have brought important attention to this concern, and they argue that society's view of body size is what needs to change:

> Our culture's obsession with a beauty narrowly defined and the destruction left in its wake are evidenced in stories, journals, and books of girls and young women. Women and girls of all sizes, bone thin to full fleshed, tell stories of shame and abuse, struggles and sorrow, hollow victories and full-bodied failures. They speak of bingeing and purging, weight gain and weight loss, dieting and stomach pain; of feeling cold, sick, and

exhausted; of flinging themselves on the bed sobbing. They lament the wasted years and the talent and energy spent on obsessing over weight and appearance.[30]

Those in the fat acceptance movement would argue that the answer is to embrace *all* body types and therefore accept obesity. Given the health risks and discomfort associated with being seriously overweight, however, I do not believe this is a viable option. The risks of obesity outweigh the risks of fighting it; therefore, we must proceed with efforts to reverse the fatness epidemic. The very real challenge is to ring the alarm bell on obesity's risks and to campaign against fatness in a way that does not worsen disturbed body image, perpetual dieting, eating disorders, and fat discrimination.

### EATING DISORDER AWARENESS

Obesity's link to eating disorders is complex and controversial. My view on this matter has been influenced by the work of Mimi Nichter, an anthropology researcher and author of *Fat Talk: What Girls and Their Parents Say about Dieting*. She claims the media have led people to believe that eating disorders are far more common than they actually are: Though "1–3 percent of girls do suffer from eating disorders; the other 97 percent demonstrate a wide range of attitudes and behaviors toward their bodies."[31] Because most statistics about teenage girls and their eating habits come from surveys that report a general concern about body size, we tend to assume that dieting is prevalent too.

Nichter's in-depth studies question the assumption that there is an epidemic of dieting among teenage girls. She asks, "Do girls actually lose weight from their diets? Given the cultural imperative to be thin, are girls *over-reporting* their dieting on surveys because they feel they should be dieting? If *everyone* is dieting, why do studies continually report that American youth are becoming increasingly overweight?"[32] She found that for many teenage girls, activities that focus on health—including the "work" of eating—were closely aligned with beauty work. Dieting seldom meant restrictive eating; it was, rather, part of body-talk language. "I'm so fat" is a way of communicating feelings, about themselves and their bodies. Boys, too, worry about their bodies, especially size. Size, according to another writer, "is a kind of involuntary self-definition. Short kids were called Mouse, String Bean, Little J., Leprechaun, Shortie, Half Pint, Spaghetti."[33]

Evidence from other surveys does indicate widespread dieting among girls but does not directly connect dieting and eating disorders. For example, a 1996 National Institutes of Health study of nine- and ten-year-old girls reported that 40 percent were trying to lose weight.[34] A 1997 Commonwealth Fund survey of the health of adolescent girls reported 58 percent of high school girls had dieted, one in four regularly counts calories, and nearly one in five said she had binged and purged.[35] A statewide study of high school students in South Carolina reported that 13 percent of white and 9 percent of black girls said they dieted to lose weight, and 2 to 3 percent in each group reported vomiting to lose weight.[36] Yet no study reported any cases of eating disorders, as diagnosed by meeting the full criteria. In all three studies, the researchers urged health professionals to capitalize on the concern of those who reported dieting or vomiting and to provide "proper weight control information."

That advice is good. Because the rate of obesity is higher by several magnitudes than diagnosed eating disorders, the important lesson from Nichter's work and the survey reports is that dieting, personally defined by individual girls, is part of our culture and is likely to continue to be a kind of lifestyle code for worrying about body size. Rather than fight it, we can join it and steer the interest and concern toward healthy eating.

I furthermore agree with health professionals and educators who say we must loosen our rigid standards of beauty and help our children accept the diversity of human appearance. And yet school-based programs to spread eating disorder awareness and promote body-size diversity may make bad matters worse. Programs to affirm acceptance of diverse body size and thus prevent disordered eating studies report little progress.[37] A Stanford University study of third- through sixth-graders who participated in a program to accept a diversity of body sizes found that 42 percent of girls and 35 percent of boys still wanted to look thinner; 6 percent of girls and 20 percent of boys wanted to look heavier.[38] Older girls with body-size concerns may have reduced risk of eating disorders such as bulimia.[39] Eating disorder prevention programs have no place in elementary schools because young girls understand very little about dieting.

These results may seem contrary to my call for increasing awareness of the health risks of obesity along with awareness of the health risks of dieting. But we do not have good methods for dealing with these contradictory societal messages: "have a perfect body" versus "eat, eat, eat." As parents and health providers, we must know the health risks associated with these contradictory messages. Pursuit of a perfect body leads to disordered eating; eating too much leads to obesity. But we should not *over*emphasize these risks to our children, because such awareness campaigns can heighten rather than lessen their preoccupation with their body image.

The debate about dieting as a danger to children's well-being is likely to continue between the non-diet advocates of body-size acceptance who claim dieting leads to reduced self-esteem, or worse, eating disorders, and the traditional medical view that dieting to reduce excess weight is important to improve health. Rather than push on with that debate, all of us—parents and health-care workers alike—need to support healthy living by our own moderation in eating, moderation in sedentary recreation, and moderation in high-pressure time commitments. And above all, by moderation—and one day, perhaps, elimination—of discrimination against fat children.

The following chapter takes a closer look at ways to combat fat discrimination and to encourage more flexible concepts of beauty—such as those voiced by the African American teenagers above—while simultaneously encouraging overweight youth to achieve a healthier size.

## SUMMARY

This chapter aimed to show why restrictive diets generally do more harm than good for overweight children. Overweight kids do not need to "go on a diet"; they need to eat for their age and be moderately active in order to grow into their weight and develop positive eating habits and active lifestyles.

Sifting through the spectrum of weight-loss and nutritional advice available to children and adults, I endorsed a diet high in vegetables, fruits, whole grains, and other complex carbohydrates, with moderate amounts of fat and protein. The government's Food Guide Pyramid is a valuable model of balanced eating for life, which can help everyone rein in the over-inflated serving sizes that have become so common in homes and restaurants. We examined some of the professional programs available to families of overweight children, as well as obesity's link to eating disorders, both of which highlighted the family's critical role in any child's success—or failure—at reaching and keeping a healthy weight. Too often parents, along with the media, pass on and reinforce unhealthy concepts of dieting and unrealistic notions of the beauty ideal. Fighting the fatness epidemic should be a matter of health and wellness, *not* personal appearance.

So far we have learned a great deal about one-on-one treatment, but the explosion of overweight kids calls for group intervention programs and populationwide prevention programs. Support and assistance at home and school are essential. Even so, constant messages from the media and the marketplace *to eat* and *to remain seated* (at the TV, at the computer, or in the car) are so strong that the most effective childhood obesity program would also update those messages.

In a perfect world, a utopia of universally healthy children, we know what we could do without: destructive media messages; thousands of readily available fast-food products; sugar-laden soda always within arm's reach; the need for two or three cars in every family. In that world of Absolute Knowledge and Perfect Practice, an ideal weight management program for parents and children would exist—free of cost and with one simple rule for prevention, one rule for treatment, one rule for maintenance. We are very far indeed from this, and perhaps the only truth we can know absolutely is that putting theory into practice inevitably has costs. Once again, our search for ideal weight management calls for a spirit of moderation to balance our expectations and our limitations.

The following example of an ideal program is absurdly simple in theory and amazingly difficult in practice.

Premise: equal energy *in* (as food and drink) and *out* (as physical activity) results in a healthy weight.

Prevention: to beat a fifty-calorie energy imbalance, eat fifty calories less *or* move fifty calories more—every day, for life; OR to beat a one hundred–calorie energy imbalance, eat fifty calories less *and* move fifty calories more—every day, for life.

Treatment: (slow) eat one hundred calories less *and* move one hundred calories more—every day, to a healthy weight; OR (fast) eat two hundred calories less *and* move two hundred calories more—every day, to a healthy weight.

Maintenance: after passing treatment, go back to prevention.

Program strength: lifelong healthy weight.

Program weakness: time, effort, and commitment—every day, for life.

# 8

---

# SLOWING THE VICIOUS CYCLE
# OF FAT DISCRIMINATION

---

ON THE WAY HOME from a family reunion in an isolated town in the western Rockies, I thought about a cousin's granddaughter—a bright, pudgy ten-year-old who preferred to talk with adults rather than play with other kids. Her parents were planning home schooling because she was unhappy among peers. She told me about a classmate who was fat and teased for hiding candy in his desk; it was clear that she related closely to him. Her reading interests were broad and already at a very advanced level, so I decided to shop for a book she might appreciate.

Back in New York City, I walked into the Bank Street Bookstore and asked for a novel or two about children who are teased because of their size. What an eye opener! Two staff members said in unison, "Get *Blubber*." And they were able to tell me details about each book on an extensive list of books about fat children, by age group, which seemed to suggest that they field many requests for these stories. Heart wrenching, comical, and always inspiring, the novels give voice and feeling to kids who bear fat discrimination and bullying in different ways.

Much of this chapter deals with fatness and fat discrimination as portrayed in children's literature. Fat discrimination is an often-overlooked dimension of the obesity epidemic. A deeply rooted cultural stereotyping about fatness fuels much of the unhealthy food behavior examined throughout this book, the consequence being a deadly alliance that attacks the most innocent among us, our children, to degrees previously unimagined.[1]

A 2003 study found a high level of implicit anti-fat bias among health professionals who treat obesity but associated obese people with "bad" and thin people with "good" and expressed strong stereotypes that fat people are lazy, stupid, and worthless. The authors concluded, "Even professionals whose careers emphasize research or the clinical management of obesity show very strong weight bias, indicating pervasive and powerful stigma."[2] Weight bias can prevent early detection of disease. There is no mistake about how deeply discrimination against fat adults—and children—afflicts our society when it pervades even those who are trained as experts in dealing with obesity.

Turning around fat discrimination is an important part of helping overweight children achieve and maintain a healthy weight, because society's intolerance of fat bodies makes overweight or "at risk for overweight" children even fatter. An immoderate, intolerant, zealous "food police" attitude makes its victims miserable as it feeds a vicious cycle. It encourages their peer tormentors and discourages their own best efforts by presenting them with impossible expectations. Children's fiction bears witness to the teasing and bullying that reinforce the cycle of overeating, reduced physical activity, and lower self-esteem. The question for parents, educators, and health providers is, how do we fight fat discrimination and break down unrealistic and rigid concepts of beauty yet also heighten awareness of obesity's risks and help our overweight children achieve a healthier size? Parents struggle with two contradictory messages to impart: "Size doesn't matter" and "Size matters." To help them navigate the highly sensitive topic of weight and body image with their children, this chapter reinforces our main theme of moderation as an approach to the problem. Moderation means sensitive understanding, a spirit of caring that prompts an informed approach to a serious issue. Here and elsewhere, as our society confronts its varied afflictions from overconsumption, the task in working with kids is to help them make reasonable and balanced choices. Their need for help from adults rings out clearly from the children's novels examined here.

## SOCIAL STIGMA AND WEIGHT GAIN

Linda is the main character in Judy Blume's popular novel *Blubber* (1974), written for sixth-grade readers. She has a weight problem. The girls in school know Linda is on a diet; they overheard the school nurse tell Linda she should lose some weight because "you are ninety one pounds . . . that's too much for your height." Wendy, a classmate, hands out copies of a How to Have Fun With Blubber list. "School isn't as boring as it used to be. . . . We made Linda say, 'I am Blubber, the smelly whale of class 206.' We made her say it before she could use the toilet in the Girls' Room, before she could get a drink at the fountain, before she ate her lunch and before she got on the bus to go home. There are some people who just make you want to see how far you can go."[3]

Humiliations like those Linda endures have real-life parallels from long before 1974. Classic 1960 studies illustrate the social stigma of obesity. In a seminal article published in 1961, children and adults were asked to select the child they would find easiest to like from six drawings of children with physical difficulties, such as having one hand or being in a wheelchair or obese. Regardless of the age, sex, social, economic, or racial background of those asked, everyone liked the obese child least.[4] These preference tests applied even when children who were themselves overweight ranked their peers. When this study was dramatized in a 1995 television documentary called *Fat,* one reviewer noted, "Five-year-olds still prefer to lose an arm than be fat."[5]

Over four decades later, reports of negative attitudes toward obese children and reduced self-esteem among them suggest that the force of discrimination is even stronger today. In ever larger numbers, children now associate obesity with a variety of negative characteristics, such as laziness and sloppiness. Several studies report that school-age children rate fat figures as possessing numerous negative traits: poor health, friendlessness, ugliness, meanness, laziness, argumentativeness, dirtiness, stupidity, and sadness. Preschool children also demonstrate prejudicial attitudes and behavior toward obesity; they ascribe more negative characteristics than positive ones to fat rather than to normal figures, and more to fat female than to fat male figures.[6]

The most notable evidence among these studies has come from the prominent obesity researchers Janet Latner and Albert Stunkard. They decided to replicate the classic 1961 study and see if the discriminatory situation had changed. Their title states the conclusion: "Getting Worse: The Stigmatization of Obese Children." They carefully show through analysis of responses, from students who included 458 fifth- and sixth-grade boys and girls attending upper-middle- and lower-middle-income U.S. public schools, how stigmatization has increased in the last forty years. Noting the "steep rise in prevalence and severity of childhood obesity," they conclude—

regardless of students' gender or socioeconomic status—"The most important finding of this study was that children were most strongly biased against the obese child and that this bias was even stronger in 2001 than it had been in 1961." As they note, "Anti-fat attitudes may begin in children as young as 3 years old," increasing steadily with age. The authors do not trace the cause of this attitude, only saying that it is overall an unsurprising result because it agrees with other evidence of strong bias. They call for "education, prevention, and intervention" to attack the discrimination.[7]

Analysis of why individuals, especially white American women, value thinness girds and motivates a large literature. One researcher noted, "Slenderness represents restraint, moderation, and self-control—the virtues of our Puritan heritage. White culture considers obesity bad and ugly. Fat represents moral failure, the inability to delay gratification, poor impulse control, greed, and self-indulgence."[8] Slenderness may indeed relate to social status. The duchess of Windsor and Gloria Vanderbilt—both of them rich and thin—supposedly remarked (or one did), "You can never be too rich or too thin."

The blatant discrimination obese adults face in our society has been well documented. Susan Bordo, for example, observes that "People avoid sitting next to obese people (even when the space they take up is not intrusive); comics feel no need to restrain their cruelty; socially, they are considered unacceptable at public functions." She interprets this overt hostility against obese people as caused by a social perception of "their defiant rebellion against normalization."[9]

If we take this discrimination against *difference* into the future, increasing knowledge about genetics raises questions and ethical dilemmas about dealing with undesirable characteristics. In *Born That Way: Genes, Behavior, Personality,* William Wright describes a frightening case of fat discrimination: "A group of young couples were asked if, knowing that their fetus has a fifty-fifty chance of becoming an obese adult, they would abort. Over three-quarters said they would. If such thinking is typical, Kate Smith, Gertrude Stein, or Luciano Pavarotti's chances for survival would have been, well, slim."[10] Surely, society would suffer the loss of great talent if a fat-fearing society decided to use genetic information to select them out.

History teaches us that when we meet a new health crisis, scapegoating is self-destructive. The initial American response to the AIDS epidemic is only one illustration of this response. Irrational condemnations of those afflicted distract a society from the challenge of attaining its containment or cure. In the instance of our childhood obesity epidemic, social discrimination is markedly counterproductive. Yet this is precisely the attitude that our public accepts or encourages.

## THE VICIOUS CYCLE

Discrimination against overweight children by other children and adults often pushes them to eat more and exercise less. And numerous studies document how fat kids, victims of discrimination and bullying, often respond by withdrawing from peers or by becoming bullies themselves. Bullying is a topic of research with applications far beyond overweight children and adults. Two excellent books by William S. Pollack, *Real Boys* and *Real Boys' Voices*, analyze bullying as part of a "vicious cycle" that "begins and ends" with what Pollack describes as the "Boy Code, the strict rules of masculinity that punish boys who seem feminine, weak, or gay to their peers."[11]

A large governmental study of child development reported that about one-quarter of all middle-school children were either perpetrators or victims (or, in some cases, both) of serious and chronic bullying. Bullying behavior included threats, ridicule, name calling, punching, slapping, jeering, and sneering.[12] Is this aggressive behavior just part of growing up, an experience that toughens a child? Or is it a serious manifestation of violence and disrespect that should be stamped out entirely? These questions are under study, especially after recent episodes of school violence that involved bullying, some for being "fat or pudgy."[13]

Getting teased about being overweight often occurs during times when children are engaging in physical activity, such as during physical education class or recess. Kids who can't run fast or whose heavy thighs are on display draw attention. One of my graduate nutrition students in 2001, now a healthy weight, wrote this after a class discussion on the stigma of being overweight:

> It came to the point where I was somewhat of an athlete—a racer. Yet I had no sprinter's body, no warm-up suit. The one thing I had was the fear of embarrassment, of someone seeing my nude fat body as I suited up for gym class. I raced to the gym to get changed before anyone else. . . . Coaches couldn't believe how quickly I got on the playing field. They thought I just loved the sport. My motivation was to beat the competi-

tion in getting suited up before everyone else. I did increase my talent, but they were already the victors on the field.

Overweight children who are less able to cope with teasing spend less time and energy in physical activity and enjoy it less than children with better coping skills. This was the conclusion of a study that measured the minutes spent by obese and non-obese children in mild to strenuous leisure time physical activity as well as their degree of sports enjoyment, then related their activity levels to scores on a scale that measured "coping skills for teasing."[14]

These study results are no surprise to anyone who has observed overweight children in a playground for several minutes. Though many heavy kids get labeled "lazy," it is their size that actually limits their active capabilities. The extra weight results in reduced endurance and leg pain from stressed joints. Physical activity is taxing. Less ability to move, combined with reduced skill and confidence, results in continued weight gain. A diagram of this vicious cycle (Figure 6) comes from a weight management program reviewed in the previous chapter, Committed to Kids.

Anyone working with overweight children could fill in the vicious cycle with more details of ways a child is caught at each turn of the wheel. For instance, bullying in the lunchroom leads to poor eating patterns and unhealthy food behaviors—hidden food, emotional eating, binge eating.

How can parents help break the cycle? Perhaps we can foster ways other than eating—such as talking, writing in a journal, or doing artwork—to cope with emotional wounds inflicted through teasing. It is also crucial to make sure that overweight kids feel encouraged, not embarrassed, in physical activity. We readily shower praise on the kids in our neighborhoods and schools who excel at sports, yet those on the sidelines are often the ones who most need our attention and support.

I recall watching a jump rope contest involving mostly African American kids from Harlem. These kids were big, but very active. The parents were cheering the contestants: "Way to go, big girl! Go, girl!" The winner of the final Double Dutch round—a heavy girl who looked to be age fifteen—would not likely be chosen for the cheerleading squad in an upscale suburban high school just a few miles away, but here she was definitely the star of the day. These kids were supported by community activities and by affirmation for their participation, regardless of body size. This kind of parental and community support for active play will help them grow into their large size and help counter the forces making them fat. Now splice in

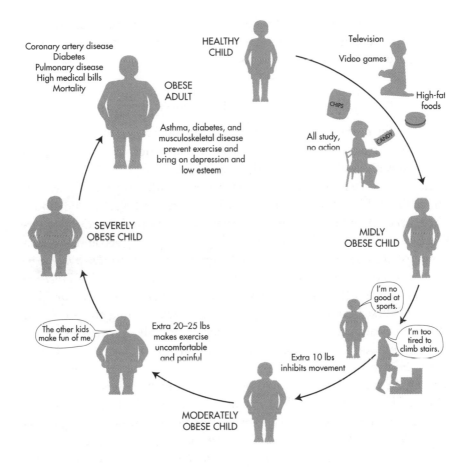

FIGURE 6. Fat discrimination feeds the cycle of overeating, reduced physical activity, and lower self-esteem. (Adapted from "The Vicious Cycle of Childhood Obesity," Committed to Kids, www.committed-to-kids.com, 2002)

a sound track with voices heckling them because their fat jiggles when they jump rope. No need to guess what happens next: they retreat indoors, take comfort in snacking in front of the TV set, and conclude that jumping rope is only for skinny kids.

We do see some signs that obsession with skinniness is weakening and the attraction of fitness is growing as some women are more accepting of their bodies and taking better care of them through exercise and balanced eating.[15] Yet deeply ingrained body dissatisfaction goes on from one generation to the next. Yes, some parents are learning to break the vicious cycle for themselves and their children, yet body dissatisfaction continues to be a huge problem that fuels the extremes of restrictive dieting and poor eating and physical activity patterns.

## DOCUMENTING DISCRIMINATION

As the twin problems of childhood obesity and fat discrimination have grown in America, neither has received much attention in the most extensive and well-known commentaries on children. Robert Coles, the much acclaimed professor of child psychiatry at Harvard, has probably written more about children since the 1960s than any other scholar, but not about these issues of child obesity and its related forms of discrimination.[16] During the 1990s Jonathan Kozol wrote a series of compelling accounts of crises among children in the United States: *Savage Inequalities: Children in America's Schools* (1991); *Amazing Grace: The Lives of Children and the Conscience of a Nation* (1995); *Ordinary Resurrections: Children in the Years of Hope* (2000). These books dramatically document the appalling afflictions and discriminations suffered by our children, especially in areas of urban poverty, yet nowhere is obesity or fat discrimination an issue, even though they affect more youth than the scourges of asthma or AIDS, especially among the inner-city black and Hispanic children he observes.

Other books on the health problems of American youth focus on eating disorders such as bulimia and anorexia; examples are the best-selling books by Mary Pipher, *Reviving Ophelia: Saving the Selves of Adolescent Girls* (1994), and Sara Shandler, *Ophelia Speaks: Adolescent Girls Write About Their Search for Self* (1999). Though "food addiction" and eating behaviors come in for analysis, obesity and fat discrimination again go unmentioned.

Finally, Myriam Miedzian, in *Boys Will Be Boys* (1991), and William Pollack, in *Real Boys' Voices* (2000), have listened to the voices of American boys on the issues of drugs, violence, and bullying, and, in Miedzian's terms, "breaking the link between masculinity and violence."[17] Once more, they largely overlooked obesity and the violent bullying of fat children. But fat kids are the most frequent targets. One sixteen-year-old male, reflecting on the ceaseless, blatant bullying that tormented him as a child in school, recalled in a *New York Times Magazine* article, "When I was fat, people must have gone home and thought of nothing else except coming in with new material the next day. They must have had *study groups* just to make fun of people who were overweight."[18]

Even specialists in the field of childhood obesity overlooked the subject of fat discrimination as late as the 1990s. A conference on the prevention and treatment of childhood obesity occurred in Bethesda, Maryland, in March 1993, and a collection of its papers under the conference title duly appeared.[19] Its forty-three scholarly papers represent over one hundred specialists in this area and offer a wealth of data on topics ranging from the epidemiology of childhood obesity in the United States to influences on children's eating behavior and the fear of obesity in childhood (earlier chapters draw on some of this valuable material). Yet notably, among these numerous studies there is no mention of fat discrimination. By 2001, however, the situation at a childhood obesity conference in San Diego, California, had changed, with the subject of fat discrimination prominently represented by a distinguished contingent of scholars and activists. This development provided one indication that academic analysis of fat discrimination has begun to catch up with its longstanding expression in children's fiction.

My point about the experts' books mentioned above is that if they related fat discrimination to the problems they address, they could further resolution of them all. Each author discusses problems of American youth. Yet to omit any mention of being overweight and its discrimination at this time, in this society, leaves a significant gap in our understanding of a problem that deserves careful attention from writers who focus on children.

Given the paucity of academic material about discrimination against fat children, those few scholars who have taken up this particular cause deserve attention. Among the recent articles and books on fat discrimination, Sondra Solovay's *Tipping the Scales of Justice* is uniquely distinguished for its thorough analysis of how this form of prejudice attacks obese children in our society. She expresses well the challenge before us:

> Fat kids will suffer objectifying and stigmatizing events because of their weight. The discrimination is entirely predictable and the resulting devastation is foreseeable as well. These experiences result in lower self-esteem, alienation, and denial of the benefits of activity while unnecessarily curtailing the kids' future opportunities. Protecting every fat child from all harassment is impossible, but some basic improvements need to be made. Specifically, parents and the public need to be educated and to educate themselves about fat prejudice in order to alleviate some of the intense cultural pressure put on children to lose weight no matter what the cost. It is unfair that children be treated differently by their families, peers, caregivers, and teachers just because they come in "a larger package." Improving the quality of life for fat children must become a priority for all people interested in a just society."[20]

Fighting fat discrimination may improve the quality of life for fat children by improving their psychological well-being, but would their risk of physical disease owing to being overweight remain high? The answer is that improvement of one leads to improvement of the other. Children who feel comfortable and act constructively with others, whether in the classroom or on the playground, and who participate freely in extracurricular activities or other opportunities for achievement, usually find a balance in eating and sedentary activity.

This healthy balance is the goal expressed consistently in the children's literature discussed below. Yet the power of these books stems from much more; it comes primarily from a common cry against the injustice of social discrimination. To combat intolerance here, as we have with issues of race and gender, should be our main aim, because discriminating against fat children will make the problem of being overweight worse. The very existence of this genre of fiction derives directly from the growth of unchecked discrimination. It is an index of prejudice in America.

## INSIGHTS FROM CHILDREN'S FICTION

The [fifth-grade] classroom door opened and a woman and a fat blond girl walked in. Sharon sits behind me and I heard her say, "Ugh." Diane sits beside me and she whispered, "I hope that she isn't going to be in this room . . ." Elsie was gross. Her eyes were squished above cheek bubbles of fat. Her chins rippled down her neck. She really didn't have a waist except where her stomach bulged out below her chest. Her legs looked like two bed pillows with the ends stuffed in shoes. I knew everyone hated having Elsie in our room.

*Jenny describing Elsie (both age 10),*
*in* Nothing's Fair in Fifth Grade *by Barthe DeClements*

An indispensable source that documents the crisis of obesity and fat discrimination, and the relation between the two—a source unmentioned in academic or scientific writings on fatness and discrimination—is children's fiction. Often literature manages to express social attitudes more exactly and more eloquently than personal interviews can, and to a remarkable degree scholarly research now reinforces its themes of fat discrimination during the last half century.

Children's fiction has the distinct advantage that, unlike scholarly writings, it is readily and compellingly accessible to those suffering from fat prejudice as well as to those of any age who may wittingly or unwittingly perpetuate the stigmatization of fat children. For these reasons, knowledge and use of children's literature can help parents and educators illuminate and undo the emotional pain caused by anti-fat attitudes.

Children's literature today routinely reinforces or reflects the social stigma attached to fat kids. This negative representation of the overweight body began to appear with frequency in children's fiction during the middle to late twentieth century; before that, an overweight body was not viewed as a problem at all. As noted in part 1 of this book, childhood obesity too rose to its present worldwide scale during the last half-century.

In nineteenth-century fiction and earlier, children were regarded as unhealthy, pathetic, or even humiliated for being too thin, as, for example, in Charles Dickens's *Oliver Twist* (1838) and Charlotte Brontë's *Jane Eyre* (1847). In the relatively few cases when overweight children are mentioned, they are usually privileged. An exception is a minor character in Dickens's *Pickwick Papers,* a young servant who is designated throughout only as "the fat boy" and is spoofed for his insatiable appetites and sloth.

In twentieth-century England, fat discrimination in children's literature becomes noteworthy in the writings of Frank Richards (the pen name of Charles Hamilton, 1875–1961), who created the character of Billy Bunter. Richards wrote thirty popular books about this character in the first half of the century. But Billy Bunter, a greedy little fat fool, is not a powerfully drawn stereotype. He only dimly signals the fat discrimination that will burst forth later in William Golding's character Piggy in *Lord of the Flies* (discussed below). There is an evident difference between Richards's spoof and the brutal humiliation directed at obese children depicted in fiction more recently.

Fast-forward to J. K. Rowling's immensely popular Harry Potter stories, which typify the disrespect fat kids get. Harry's heroic qualities shame those of his cousin, Dudley Dursley, a stupid, cowardly bully, endlessly pampered by his parents and constantly tormenting Harry. But Dudley's worst attribute, which follows him from early childhood to adolescence, is his fatness. In several episodes that obviously target the humor induced by such stereotypes but ignore the hurt they may inflict on fat children as readers, Dudley's obese eating behavior attracts ridicule and punishment. This characterization of a fat child never wavers. None of the extensive commentary on the Harry Potter volumes, though sometimes critical of their religious implications, mentions the author's portrayal of Dudley and the blatant discrimination it represents. Presumably such discrimination is deemed amusing or unremarkable in the way that anti-Semitism or racism was in the United States a century ago.

In the first book of the series, we meet Dudley's family. He is born to a father who is a "big beefy man with hardly any neck"; Dudley is a child with "a large pink face, not much neck, small watery blue eyes and thick, fat head . . . Harry often said that Dudley looked like a pig in a wig." Rowling carries the pig simile to a magical conclusion by having a wizard give Dudley a pig's tail. It seems a just punishment for the sin of gluttony.[21]

The fourth book in the Harry Potter series, *Goblet of Fire*, also dwells on Dudley's fatness. The boys are now in early adolescence and, Harry relates, "Dudley's diet isn't going too well" because he is constantly "smuggling doughnuts into his room." His parents try vainly to replace "Dudley's favorite things—fizzy drinks and cakes, chocolate bars and burgers"— with fruits and vegetables. But in the end "Dudley had reached roughly the size and weight of a young killer whale." A few pages later Harry comments that Dudley "had finally achieved what he's been threatening to do since the age of three, and become wider than he is tall." Rowling is clearly determined to mine the joke of Dudley's body size for all it's worth—as she continues to do in the fifth volume. But her humor is not funny: no child makes such a determination. In reality, the culprits are not children of any size or persuasion, but rather ignorance and insensitivity from an uncaring and uninformed society.

As in the first volume, Dudley's humiliation comes swiftly, again the consequence of his gluttony. This time, Harry's young wizard friends trick Dudley into consuming a toffee that contains an "engorgement charm." Suddenly Harry sees Dudley "kneeling beside the coffee table, gagging and sputtering on a foot-long, purple slimy thing that was protruding from his mouth," which turns out to be his tongue. In the midst of the merriment that follows, a sympathetic wizard saves Dudley, but Harry regrets that he has to leave early because he "didn't want to miss the fun."[22] Fun, indeed, to watch a fat kid get his just desserts.

Enough time passed between Rowling's fourth and fifth volumes for my granddaughter, Mia, to have her first big birthday party just after the publication of *Harry Potter: The Order of the Phoenix*. Our family had waited in a long line at the Bank Street Bookstore for an early copy so we would be ready to discuss it at the party. As Mia greeted Joe, a smart eight-year-old, he naturally had a copy of the book, just in case the party lagged and he could cram in another chapter. I seized the opportunity for another interview.

"What page are you on, Joe?"

"410."

"What do you think of Dudley in this one?"

"The same. He's 'demented,' like the first chapter says."

"Okay, but why don't you like him?"

"He's fat and ugly."

"Would he be as ugly if he weren't fat?"

Joe was unaware of being interviewed but not of standing next to a boy who was decidedly overweight.

"Well, like, ya know, all that blubber isn't very cool, is it?"

"But he tried, he went on a diet."

"His parents forced him."

"And then he became his school's heavyweight boxing champion."

"Junior heavyweight, just so he could bully Harry more."

"How about that time he almost got killed fighting with Harry?"

"So what? I wish he were dead, tortured first, then starved to death."

By this point the games had started and there was no way Joe could ever see the likes of Dudley as a player. The interview ended as it had begun, on a note of fat intolerance, as common to kids as birthday cake.

I confess that after the party I wondered, as I often do when talking with kids about fat discrimination, had I in some way put words in Joe's mouth? So I returned to the novel's depiction of Dudley, to check if it fit the characterization of the detested fat child that had leaped at me from its pages. The facts are just as Joe recalled: the first chapter's title is "Dudley Demented." As in the earlier books, the opening pages describe Harry as "skinny" and then quickly reinforce the old stereotype of Dudley, still Harry's juvenile tormenter, as a relentless fat bully. A change is that while "Dudley was as vast as ever," the "hard dieting" imposed by his fat father and his mother had turned him into his school's junior heavyweight boxing champion, and so better able to beat up on Harry (just as Joe said). Harry, who has turned surprisingly mean in his adolescence, teases Dudley by calling him "a pig that's been taught to walk on his hind legs" and provokes a fight between them. Also as in previous episodes, magical forces of one kind or another bring Dudley down. Harry's allies include Mrs. Figg, who "shrieked at Dudley, still on his back in the alley. 'Get your fat bottom off the ground, quick! . . . Get up, you useless lump, get up.'" Dudley is defeated, humiliated, but Harry and Mrs. Figg take pity on him. Despite his "massive arms," and "sagging slightly under his weight," they manage to lug him home.[23]

How may millions of young readers respond to this characterization of Dudley's agony? Presumably as Joe does, with a mix of disgust, laughter, and ridicule. But in a culture suffering from a plague of obesity joined with a fierce fat phobia, how many readers will look in the mirror and see an image of Dudley? The Harry Potter books are just one current example from those that routinely associate fatness with rude, offensive behavior by ugly brats who are justly punished precisely because of their food habits. The clear message is that fat kids must finish last. Insidiously, social discrimination appears as humor but carries a lethal message: making fun of fat kids—and in extreme cases, physically bullying and hurting them—is acceptable and safe because they deserve it. This portrayal only worsens the problem of childhood obesity by creating stereotypes and undermining the self-esteem of those very kids who most need constructive attention and assistance as they modify eating and physical activity behavior.

## THE PIGGY PARADIGM

The fundamental change of attitude about fat children from the nineteenth century to the twentieth stands out vividly in two renowned novels written exclusively with kids as the main characters, R. M. Ballantyne's *The Coral Island* (1857) and William Golding's *Lord of the Flies* (1954). Both became instant classics, regarded as the best of the many books each author wrote, and have remained in print since their initial publication. A fascinating aspect about comparing these two novels is that Golding deliberately constructs his story as an explicit response to Ballantyne's book because it records basic changes of attitude toward human nature and society.

Both novels have the same physical setting, a South Pacific island, where a group of English boys has been stranded. While Ballantyne's group quickly and confidently emerges as a band of young British Victorian heroes who triumph gloriously over every adversity or enemy, Golding turns his kids into lethal little killers as they inexorably descend into an awful savagery that climaxes with the murders of two of their own. The main point for our purpose is the way Golding portrays the one fat child in his group. Whereas Ballantyne nowhere even implies fatness among his stalwart youth, Golding wastes no time in making the contrast between Ralph, the "fair boy," and his antithesis, nicknamed "Piggy"—"shorter than the fair boy and very fat." Golding does not ridicule Piggy; he lets the other boys perform that cruelty, thus making him the only pathetic and bullied character, deliberately murdered after unbearable humiliation. It is striking how Golding will not let the reader forget Piggy's fatness: the nickname seems insufficient because in the first four pages alone, Golding refers to Piggy as "the fat boy" a dozen times. He then highlights this presence throughout the book as the boys gang up against him, screaming as Piggy tries desperately to save himself, "You shut up, you fat slug."[24]

Golding deserves recognition for introducing a genre of children's "fat fiction" because a flood of novels following *Lord of the Flies* featured overweight kids as pitiful as Piggy. The character traits are unmistakable regardless of the plot: the fat child, male or female, is victimized, persecuted, or irremediably misunderstood, usually by peers and parents alike. Obese girls like Linda in Judy Blume's *Blubber* (1974), Lara and Molly in Cherie Bennett's *Life in the Fat Lane* (1998), Emma in Louise Fitzhugh's *Nobody's Family Is Going to Change* (1974), Judi in Leslea Newman's *Fat Chance* (1994), Marcy in Paula Danziger's *The Cat Ate My Gymsuit* (1974), or Elsie in Barthe DeClements's *Nothing's Fair in Fifth Grade* (1981) relate the same sort of self-hatred, peer ridicule, and parental alienation as obese boys like Bobby in Robert Lipsyte's *One Fat Summer* (1977), Simon in Chris Crutcher's *Whale Talk* (2001), Bertie in Toby Forward's *Pie Magic* (1995), Eric in Chris Crutcher's *Staying Fat for Sarah Byrnes* (1993), and Stanley in Louis Sachar's *Holes* (1998). Mercifully, none of these obese children meets the terrible fate of Piggy. Yet horrendous discrimination and heart-wrenching confessions of self-recrimination scream from these pages, all directly related to childhood obesity.

Much of this genre deals with bullying. Bobby, age fourteen, in Lipsyte's *One Fat Summer* is tormented by schoolmates, by his father, even by five-year-olds who call him "fatso." But his worst experience comes with bullying by Willie, a local teen at the beach who taunts Bobby, drums up accusations, and physically beats him up. In a horrifying scene Willie and his cohorts, boys and girls, inflict the punishment Bobby fears most: "I felt a hand on my belt buckle. 'NO.' I turned and tried to run. Someone tripped me, and they were suddenly all on top of me, laughing, pulling at my clothes. All I could think of was that they would see me naked, without any clothes, stark naked." Left alone in his humiliation, Bobby contemplates death, thinking to himself: "Poor fat Bobby Marks. . . . Slob. Better off dead."[25]

The worst effect of bullying on fat kids is self-denigration. This particular form of cruelty is often identified with boys, but these novels demonstrate vividly that girls are equally adept at peer torture. As noted above, Blume's *Blubber* skillfully relates the process that turns Linda, overweight and insecure, into the victim of her fifth-grade class led by the bully, Wendy, who forces Linda to say with tears in her eyes, "My name will always be Blubber."

In the end, Bobby does emerge as a hero—a character development foreshadowed in Golding's treatment of Piggy. Though brutalized, Piggy appeals to common sense and tries to reason with the mob even as it attacks him. At the book's conclusion Ralph, the fair boy, weeps for his "true, wise friend called Piggy." The little fat kid who begins as an object of ridicule ends as a heroic figure, vindicated as the wisest of all.

Golding thereby provides a paradigm of fat heroism for subsequent children's literature about overweight kids. *Nobody's Family Is Going to Change* by Fitzhugh typifies the compelling theme of an obese adolescent's self-transformation from victim to hero. This novel features Emma, age eleven, whose father and brother call her "Piggy" (a common name for these kids, found in several of the other novels, with no implied reference to *Lord of the Flies*). As the story begins, she stares with "hatred at her own reflection in the mirror." "'Monster,' she whispered to herself.' Disgusting. You are truly and completely disgusting'," this "fat brown girl with funny hair." Yet, surprisingly, she has the "audacity to smile" because "You're smart. You're smarter than all of them. . . . You'll show them all." The glory of the story is that Emma does indeed show them through her irrepressible will and intelligence. She turns her father's cruel ridicule of her obesity and her classmates' discrimination completely around through acts of determined self-transformation. Rather than label herself a "fat black girl who hates the world," "some big fat loser," she finally comes to understand that her weight problem "is your problem, not mine." She reasons to herself, "What's wrong is trying to change them. They are not going to change. But I can change. I can change myself."[26] Seeing self-worth in something other than size, Emma's example surely influences those around her, as she leads a dynamic group of classmates who name themselves the "Changelings." The heroism of Emma, as well as Bobby's in *One Fat Summer* and Brian's in Ian Bone's *Fat Boy Saves the World,* calls on values of courage and empathy any heroic character types in America should possess. We need to reexamine carefully and critically the traits we admire in children. By reading this children's literature together, as a family exercise, we may define together what we value in one another.

Reading aloud together about fat kids makes sense for several reasons. First, the children's fiction with overweight characters is easily accessible and inexpensive, well written, and replete with controversial issues that often relate to the whole family. Second, many of the novels address family dynamics. A family-style reading would at least give parents a chance to learn how parents are portrayed critically and to talk about it.

Fathers generally come off worse in these stories, especially when confronting their daughters. In *Nobody's Family Is Going to Change,* for example, Emma's father is brutal throughout the book, telling his eleven-year-old girl: "'You're so fat and spoiled you wouldn't know what life is about if it came up and hit you in the face!' The word *fat* went through Emma like an ice pick . . . Emma couldn't believe the hatred she saw in his eyes." Mothers, meanwhile, are usually submissive to their spouses. They are gentler to their overweight children but almost always unhelpful, as in the instance when Emma's mother begs her, "And, honey, you *must* diet. You don't want to grow up to be a big fat woman, do you?"[27]

Parents never emerge as heroes in these novels of children who struggle with self-esteem in the face of fat discrimination. They are not up to the task of positively reinforcing their children, much less giving freely the unconditional love that psychologists such as Robert Brooks urge. Must we interpret this children's literature as ammunition for kids in what Sylvia Hewlett and Cornel West call "the war against parents"?[28] I prefer to view the stories as both a useful critique and creative compendium of "do's and don'ts" for all of us who try to end discrimination against overweight children. Talking about children's fiction that confronts fatness can air tensions and resolve conflicts. No family should miss this opportunity for learning.

Unlike restrictive dieting for children—which does not establish healthy lifelong patterns—reading and talking about body size and feelings toward others who tease or bully help children deal with their own unique body size and shape. From another perspective, equally apparent in this literature, parents should convey contemporary knowledge and concern about bulimia and anorexia. The age-old practice of reading children's literature to kids may easily include a parent's counsel.

The dynamic of family reading means urging your kids to read to themselves, to their siblings, and to you as parents, and then talking with teachers about expanding class sessions that require each student to read aloud.

Of course, some families or classrooms may already practice this dynamic, but we may be sure that a powerful appetite for it does exist among children. Regardless of J. K. Rowling's fat discrimination, she exposed an immense thirst for children's literature. America, like Britain, is wild about Harry, as kids charge into their local bookstores so that they can spend long hours reading thousands of pages, in preference to sitting before the tube. The fact that publishers and parents alike find this amazing is one measure of our underestimation of the intense pleasure that comes from reading children's literature.

As parents of two enthusiastic readers, and now grandparents of another three, my husband and I speak with the experience of over four decades of reading children's literature to our kids. We have found in reading aloud classics from nursery rhymes and Dr. Doolittle to Dickens and *Lord of the Flies* that endless treasures abound in them for family entertainment and discussion that we usually fail to find in television. Even after thirty-five years, we have vivid collective family memories of choking up in the midst of reading *Lord of the Flies,* and then asking ourselves, as Piggy dies, why are we all crying? Or at the book's end, how can Ralph conclude that Piggy, a little fat object of group ridicule at the beginning of the book, was really the wisest of his friends? How many times I had to pry my son away from Tolkien's *Lord of the Rings* to eat dinner, and how often we imagine our granddaughters will soon come under that same magic spell. As we see now from Harry Potter, this spell holds an even larger and more enthusiastic audience. As with every age or era, there are different opportunities always for different kinds of questions, such as, why should we laugh at Dudley Dursley? Do you or would you like to have friends like him? Such discussions need not take the form of preaching but rather sharing sentiments and ideas. Experience with my cousin's granddaughter, the chubby preteen I wanted to find books for—or with some of my own students—shows the difficulty of talking to teenage girls about weight.[29]

Reading may pave the way to discuss this touchy topic. It can give a family an opportunity to read and talk in a way that television seldom allows. Eliminating TV from a child's routine is an impractical measure, but an even distribution of time in a family schedule that includes daily tasks, homework, and reading aloud or alone together is a measured, practical recommendation that can maximize quality time of parents with children. My appeal is for moderation and balance. (The box "Insights from Children's Fiction" includes all the titles mentioned here.)

My emphasis on reading to kids is meant to suggest a range of activity

## INSIGHTS FROM CHILDREN'S FICTION

The genre of fat fiction offers important insights into childhood obesity and its relationship to fat discrimination. The following excerpt gives voice to the experience of discrimination.

> I hate my father. I hate school. I hate being fat. . . . All my life I've thought that I looked like a baby blimp with wire-frame glasses and mousy brown hair. Everyone always said that I'd grow out of it, but I was convinced that I'd become an adolescent blimp with wire-frame glasses, mousy brown hair, and acne. . . . What does a blimp know about communication? How could she know what it feels like to be so fat and ugly that you're ashamed to get into a gymsuit or talk to skinny people? Who wants to say, "This is my friend, the Blimp"?
>
> Marcy, age 13, in *The Cat Ate My Gymsuit*

The following books may give older children, teens, and their parents an introduction to the subject of childhood obesity.

Cherie Bennett, *Life in the Fat Lane*

Judy Blume, *Blubber*

Ian Bone, *Fat Boy Saves the World*

Chris Crutcher, *Staying Fat for Sarah Byrnes* and *Whale Talk*

Paula Danziger, *The Cat Ate My Gymsuit*

Barthe DeClements, *Nothing's Fair in Fifth Grade*

Louise Fitzhugh, *Nobody's Family Is Going to Change*

Toby Forward, *Pie Magic*

William Golding, *Lord of the Flies*

Benjamin Hoff, *The Tao of Pooh*

Robert Lipsyte, *One Fat Summer*

Leslea Newman, *Fat Chance*

J. K. Rowling, the Harry Potter series

Louis Sachar, *Holes*

Sapphire, *Push*

Robert K. Smith, *Jelly Belly*

that may enhance family communication. The appeal of reading lies, of course, in our wish to become enchanted or enthralled through storytelling. The act of reading a book, in the hands of a gifted storyteller, need not be restricted to the text itself. It can be embellished in many ways, and grandparents may excel in such excursions, by recollecting how the child's father or mother behaved in a particular situation. T. Berry Brazelton endorses the unique role given to grandparents as a source of keeping family values alive through inventive storytelling.[30] There is an ideal place where the oral tradition complements the written, especially for young children thirsty for knowledge of their own parents' upbringing. A reading session, therefore, could involve a multi-generational family reciting and performing a scene from Shakespeare, or it might make an old nursery rhyme come alive for a four-year-old by personalizing it with a favorite family anecdote about how Mommy acted when she was little. The main point is that in this creative, intimate, imaginary land of storytelling lies vast potential for sentiments to be shared, values conveyed, and prejudices aired or even dissolved. It is a place and a path to forge trust and make connections, the key prerequisites to overcoming discrimination where it most often begins, in the family.

## TEACHING TOLERANCE

As we move from the family setting to schools, teachers and parents alike will be familiar with the Winnie the Pooh series by A. A. Milne, complemented by Isabel Gaines's *Winnie the Pooh First Readers.* In adolescence and adulthood there is Benjamin Hoff's wise interpretation, *The Tao of Pooh,* which explains with incomparable clarity the philosophy behind the series.[31] These books teach tolerance, understanding, and compassion to a range of ages through their compelling diversity of lovable characters. It is significant that the hero is an overweight, adorable, irresistible bear.

Educators know they can learn from and use novels like *Winnie the Pooh,* but they may be less acquainted with children's fiction that specifically deals with fat discrimination. These frequently portray school teachers in ways that underline the crucial roles played by these figures in our children's lives, for good and ill. For example, Ms. Finney, Marcy's ninth-grade English teacher in *The Cat Ate My Gymsuit,* is uniquely understanding and appreciative of Marcy's intelligence—a model teacher who seems instinctively nondiscriminatory, outwardly indifferent to Marcy's large size. Her approach fosters body-size satisfaction in a way that leads to healthier youth. Similarly, Mrs. Hanson, in *Nothing's Fair in Fifth Grade,* is a model of fairness. When all of Elsie's classmates attack her mercilessly, Mrs. Hanson sets an example that eventually moves one of the others, Jenifer, to extend a hand of friendship. Urged by her teacher toward insight, Jenifer finds Elsie in tears, "sad and hopeless and alone." "I had never thought of Elsie as a human being," she confesses. "Just a fat girl."[32]

In my own classroom experience of teaching college students, no single novel dealing with the issue of discrimination matches the emotional power of *Push* by Sapphire.[33] This is the account an obese African American teenager called Claireece Precious Jones retells: the agonized adolescence of a sixteen-year-old growing up in Harlem and raped repeatedly by her own father. As the novel opens, Precious records her humiliation when a Harlem hospital nurse found she was pregnant at age twelve and weighed over 200 pounds.

The abuse Precious gets from her parents, peers, and society at large seems as endless as it is outrageous. When she discovers she has contracted AIDS, her situation appears irredeemable. But her high school teacher, Miss Rain, has the insight to perceive her "island of competence," a gift for creative writing. As this capacity begins to flower, Precious learns to appreciate Alice Walker and Audre Lorde, to recognize in them companions for life who will not hold her hostage to color or obesity. *Push* is a rare novel that manages to convey at once the terrible depths of discrimination and the seeds of a solution. It captures fiction's profound and eloquent relevance to reform of social attitudes about obesity in America.

The novelist Susan Richards Shreve, in an essay in the *New York Times,* writes of how reading stories inspired her as a young girl and concludes now, as a professional writer, "Fiction is a glimpse at our common humanity, a reminder of it, a generous engagement between the reader and the imagined world of a book."[34] The value of many of these novels is to inspire an empathic awareness like Jenifer's in *Nothing's Fair in Fifth Grade.* The link so many of them make to a teacher's achievement as catalyst also reaffirms the value of education and collaboration by children's novelists and schoolteachers to promote "a glimpse at our common humanity."

The novels discussed above represent only a small fragment of their genre. All published since 1954, they reveal the virulence of this epidemic and its corresponding discriminatory abuse. Teachers and parents can use these books to promote empathy with the problems overweight children and teenagers face so that young people as well as adults are motivated to make discrimination based on being overweight unacceptable.

## SUMMARY

This chapter showed how the social stigma of obesity worsens the vicious cycle of poor eating and lessened physical activity that first led to obesity. Turning around fat discrimination is an important part of helping overweight children achieve and maintain a healthy weight, because society's intolerance toward fat bodies can make fat children even fatter.

Fighting fat discrimination is tricky because in helping children form values, parents struggle with contradictory social messages about beauty versus social tolerance: "Size matters" and "Size doesn't matter." One way toward a solution is to read books for young adults from the fat fiction genre and discuss with children, fat and thin, their feelings toward characters who absorb and inflict the hurt of being fat—for instance, asking how they feel about this one or that, whether they know similar kids, and who would be a friend and why or why not. Asking and discussing how these stories touch children is a powerful solvent of discrimination. Another approach is to support good teachers and school texts that help kids discover and develop values of tolerance for diversity. Encouraging children of all sizes toward emotional health and a sense of self-worth smooths and speeds their path to physical health.

We have seen how the Harry Potter novels—appealing to both children and adults—and other fictional accounts depict discrimination against fat children. They highlight the swift rise of childhood obesity and its consequences within our society. As evidence, consider the testimony of Lara, the "two hundred pound–plus teenage blimp" of Cherie Bennett's novel, *Life in the Fat Lane,* who says in despair to a fat friend: "If you ask a thin girl with no talent or brains if she'd rather be her or you, she'll pick her. Skinny girls who chain-smoke four packs of cigarettes a day would rather get lung cancer than get fat. Being fat is the worst thing in the world. Everyone knows it. So no matter what you say, the world wins. And we lose."[35] Lara's sentiments, and their context of intense self-hatred because of her obesity, had no place in either fact or fiction before the last half-century. Young girls and boys among us with feelings like Lara's therefore face a new era of problems.

Nothing short of a nationwide campaign that reaches the highest level of government and the smallest family member is likely to slow the vicious cycle related to obesity. Chapter 9 picks up the idea of a campaign to create a community based on tolerance. Rabbi Joseph Telushkin captured its spirit when he proposed a "Speak No Evil Day" as an act of Congress. It envisions "a day when a fat adolescent will not have to fear a biting comment about his weight from parents or peers."[36]

# 9

## MOBILIZING TO HELP OUR OVERWEIGHT CHILDREN

SOME MIGHT ARGUE that the solution to the childhood obesity epidemic is not rocket science. It boils down to commonsense rules: "Go out and play." "Eat your vegetables." "Come home for dinner."

Yes, we should follow that old-fashioned advice, but the rise in overweight and obesity and the epidemic's related costs impel us to do much more. Children and their families cannot alone combat the forces that propel the growing rate of childhood obesity; the problem—and the remedies—reach far beyond the home.

That point was made abundantly clear at the national nutrition summit held in May 2000.[1] "Communities can help when it comes to health promotion and disease prevention," Surgeon General David Satcher said in a statement when the summit ended:

> When there are no safe places for children to play, or for adults to walk, jog, or ride a bike, that's a community responsibility. When school lunchrooms or workplace cafeterias don't offer healthy and appealing food choices, that is a community responsibility. When new or expectant parents are not educated about the benefits of breast-feeding, that's a community responsibility. And when we don't require daily physical education in our schools, that is also a community responsibility.[2]

The summit put the obesity epidemic high up on the national agenda and marked a turning point in efforts to improve the nation's eating and activity. Organized by the U.S. Department of Health and Human Services and the Department of Agriculture, it was the first government-sponsored summit on food, nutrition, and health since the landmark 1969 White House conference. By late 2001 a report titled *The Surgeon General's Call to Action to Prevent and Decrease Overweight and Obesity* was available.[3] Noting that the total direct and indirect costs attributed to overweight and obesity amounted to $117 billion in the year 2000, the "call to action" listed dozens of worthwhile strategies and steps that schools, communities, private industry, and government should take to help overweight Americans reach and maintain a healthier weight.

A sister summit took place in April 2000, one month before the national nutrition summit, and held equally vital research information and creative approaches to an "epidemic of poor lifestyle."[4] The meeting featured experts from academia, government, industry, advocacy groups, and health professions; its funding came mainly from food corporations. One of its working groups studied a question I probe in this book: "What environmental and societal factors affect food choice and physical activity?" The group—using research information from health care, anthropology, community planning, economics, and public policy—examined large-scale social change in several countries, including the United States. In the use of tobacco, recycling, seat belts, infant car seats, and breast-feeding, it confirmed, people's patterns of behavior are very sensitive to the physical environment (public space) and the marketplace environments (advertising, availability). The group correctly concluded that preventing obesity will require many stakeholders to cooperate in changing social behavior and industry practices that influence individual behavior. Bottom line: individuals cannot be expected to carry the entire burden of behavior change; institutions and industry have big roles to play as well.

The leaders of both summits wisely urged everyone to move beyond assigning blame for the obesity epidemic. "If we knew whom to blame, we would identify a villain, which would help us focus a social campaign," wrote James O. Hill and others. "We would have a target for fixing the problem, and of course we would know where to send the bill. There is no clear single villain; everyone owns a piece of the responsibility. Therein lies the challenge."[5]

Raising awareness is a first step. Awareness through education can motivate and lead to action. Yet we need to face the fact that the public keeps getting fatter in spite of the abundance of information publicized year after year that poor nutrition, overeating, and inactivity lead to obesity. The time is overdue to change the environment—the schools, neighborhoods, marketplaces, and workplaces—in ways that will amend children's (and adults') eating and activity.

## WHAT SCHOOLS CAN DO

Our overweight children's improved health is still far from the top of the long wish list of most schools. As we observed in chapter 5, the availability and promotion of junk food on campus, the unpopularity of government-regulated school lunches, and the steady reduction of physical activity in the academic schedule give schools a part in the epidemic. Academic standards, safety concerns, and budget shortfalls push students' health lower on schools' lists of priorities. "If Johnny can't read by first grade, parents are going to be up in arms," says Connie Holt, a dietitian. "But if he gains five pounds in first grade and doesn't eat well, nobody's going to say anything."[6]

Even if schools want to become part of the solution and make obesity prevention a high priority, they face significant hurdles. Surveyed and asked to name the barriers to changes on campus that would help prevent and treat obesity, school administrators had answers: 49 percent named lack of trained personnel; 43 percent, lack of materials; 40 percent, lack of classroom time; 40 percent, lack of funds; and 34 percent, lack of staff time, especially in less affluent school districts.[7]

A chief cause of the problem is money, mainly lack of money to support kids' needs for healthy food and physical activity and at the same time meet parents' and teachers' expectations for academic achievement (that now requires kids to sit still with books and computers). California provides a telling example of just how dependent schools are on junk-food revenue. Initial legislation there to ban the sale and serving of junk food on campus was "opposed not only by the soft drink and food industries but by the California Teachers Association, which feared the loss in educational funding."[8] It's time to ask ourselves if student achievement must come at the expense of their health.

Here are actions schools can take—with the support of parents, the community, and state and local funding:

**1** *Phase out junk food on campus and offer healthier alternatives.*
Two dozen states introduced legislation in 2002–03 to regulate school vending machines or set new nutrition standards such as bans on candy and soda,

according to the national conference of state legislatures. California school boards did not renew lunch contracts with Pizza Hut and found healthful juice and water alternatives for school vending machines. In fall 2003 New York City enforced regulations that ban the sale of soda, chewing gum, and hard candies in schools by using a central contract in purchasing vending machines.[9] School districts nationwide might well emulate their acts.

There is considerable opposition to outright bans on selling these food items from those who believe children should learn (and have the right) to choose healthy food and drink and those who believe the source of revenue is crucial to education. Besides, they say, kids will just buy these foods elsewhere. Not surprisingly, the National Soft Drink Association says obesity is "about the couch and not the can."[10] And I say school classrooms are the one place kids can read, think, and learn without nonstop eating—a place to uncouple other activities from food. Nourishing snacks should be available at reasonable, scheduled intervals throughout long, and often erratic, schooldays. Vending machines stocked with healthy alternatives to candy and soda, and available at planned snack breaks, could provide a learning laboratory for healthy eating and—if controlled by school officials— reasonable school revenue. A ban on vending machines or a switch to healthier fare in them cannot reverse the obesity epidemic. But it is a good way to find out if modifying accessible snacks decreases kids' calorie consumption and obesity.

School stores that sell foods of "minimal nutritional value" also came up for review in some school districts. The snack bar at Aptos Middle School in San Francisco used to sell items such as extralarge cheeseburgers, Slim Jims, and Hostess cupcakes. "I'd see kids coming in with $2 and buying a 20-oz caffeinated soda and a giant bag of chips every day," the principal told the *San Francisco Chronicle*. "I almost felt like a criminal selling this stuff to them." But then the snack bar revolutionized its food offerings after the school district passed a resolution calling on schools to phase out unhealthy foods. Now the snack bar menu carries items such as chicken vegetable soup, pasta, and sushi, while the vending machines dispense bottled water. Pizza is sold by the slice rather than whole. "We have not seen kids bringing in their own junk food or quarts of soda. It has worked really well," one parent reported.[11] As with most changes, a positive response to banning junk food in vending machines and school stores requires attractive replacements. It is clear that changing the food culture at school is challenging, but given the eating environment outside the school gate and in many homes, it is the one place to "learn [healthy eating] by doing."

**2** *Overhaul the school lunch program to make it more appetizing, nutritional, and popular.*

What a concept—ask the students! Over 135,000 high school students around the country participated in student-led dialogues in nearly 250 high schools early in 2003 to identify their top ten concerns about schools, communities and the world in which they live. Most concerns were with school; school lunch policies were number one, ahead of poor-quality teachers and lack of clean and accessible bathrooms. Students everywhere were concerned with the cost and quality of lunch and advocated longer lunches and improved nutritional value. As one student in Philadelphia put it, "They've been serving the same food in my high school since my mother was a student there, and it was bad back then."[12]

Even if vending machines are banned from schools, some appetites for fast food are so strong that, according to Nancy Rice, nutrition services director in Griffin, Georgia, "Some kids won't eat at all until after school, saving their money for McDonald's." Even so, her school tried some of the students' recommendations from a survey by the National Foodservice Management Institute and did raise lunch participation. These recommendations include sandwiches and a fresh fruit bowl served every day and express carts that help speed up the serving lines with only one choice per line. Ready-to-go salads packed in "see-thru" containers have been a sold-out success in many schools.[13] And a scheduled lunch of at least twenty minutes from "sit down" time improves the lunch experience.

An inspiring model is Opelika, Alabama, where parents and school officials in this rural community decided that nutritious school lunches were nonnegotiable and increased financing to buy fresh fruits and vegetables from local farms, and to prepare them in the school kitchens. Kids there eat and like fresh sweet potatoes, butter cream peas, and black-eyed peas.[14]

Just as inspiring is the 54,000-student, urban school food revolution example in Oakland, California, which after nearly two years of planning and nudging began to serve nutritious lunches. Overcoming resistance from school officials, in 2002 the Oakland Unified School District banned soda and "junk food" snacks and formed a nutrition task force that negotiated improvements, including buying from local merchants nutritious prepared food that kids like and can buy from easy-access carts. Here were their goals:

> Identify foods that are nutritious and popular with students, such as vegetable wraps, tasty grilled chicken, soy burgers, salads, and fruit juice.

Serve enjoyable and culturally familiar foods; expose students to new foods, such as "yam sticks."

Improve the quality of food service workers by working with their unions in training them and developing career ladders.

Work proactively with parents and the school board to fund the purchase and preparation of fresh foods *and* to drop any ideas that the school food program should not only pay for itself but make money for other activities (in Oakland and many other districts this goal would be the most difficult to implement).

Seek cooperation from teachers and school officials to buy into the idea that learning about food and health is important curriculum content.[15]

Putting these goals into practice required widespread grassroots organizing and work that touched on the budget, the classroom course work, and the expectations of what the product of an education should be.

Still, innovations may not please every palate; many Oakland students go to the local Burger King for fries and to the corner store for soda and chips. The point is, schools must provide attractive alternatives to these foods. If they don't, and parents can't, who will? School is the place to learn about and practice what we all know: nutritious food is the foundation for healthy living—and learning. With half a chance, nutritious food at school will go a long way toward slowing down the runaway obesity epidemic.

All of these ideas turn what some view as negative regulation into positive action. The *Surgeon General's Call to Action* urges schools to enforce existing USDA regulations against serving foods of minimal nutritional value during mealtimes in school food service areas (or from vending machines). In other words, close the student stores and put vending machines off-limits during the lunch hour so students eat the nutritionally superior cafeteria food. It's high time to make the cafeteria an attractive "dining destination" for all students.

In spring 2003 the SchoolFood Plus coalition, a group formed to improve the New York City school nutrition programs, reported that the major players were in line to turn school lunchrooms into attractive places with tasty and nourishing food—and hence into popular dining destinations for students. This goal is now within reach, freshly fueled by a reorganized New York City Department of Education, by the grassroots advocacy of the

Community Food Resource Center, a direct service organization, and by impressive groundwork already laid by some individuals and groups—to set up pilot Cookshop programs that include classrooms with community gardens, demonstration "schools that cook," and a "vegetable of the month" program in every school.

One challenge requires attention in order to ensure that all children regardless of economic level have access to nutritious, tasty food: to erase the stigma attached to subsidized lunches available based on economic need. Prepayment, with the same coupons for all students, is one potential remedy. Getting rid of separate lines for free or reduced-price lunches and a la carte items will let all students order from the same menu as equals. This is a crucial issue if the overall goal is (and it should be!) that "no child goes hungry."

Doubtless parents and others concerned with children will be instrumental in changing the image of the sixty-year-old nationwide school lunch program. A dizzying array of resources is available to help the effort. To get started, go to the resource group initiated by the surgeon general (www.ActionForHealthyKids.org). Its virtual folder on "health-promoting foods in our schools" has fact sheets, data, research reports, tools, and programs that work. There is even a slide presentation for "making the case" to school officials. When a PTA wants to do something about overweight kids, I say, "Start with lunch!"

### 3 Reinstate daily recess and physical education, and promote physical activity throughout the day.

Junk food is only one of the two culprits in the rise of overweight among children. Instead of only taking away, let's bring back recess in elementary and middle schools and add a variety of attractive physical activities for children in physical education classes, grades K–12. We need to restore the opportunity for PE before children have lost the ability to move at all.

Over the last half century school districts across the country have been quietly eliminating recess, or "unstructured play," from their elementary schools. Some schools don't even have playgrounds. The reasons range from safety concerns to an obsession with raising standardized test scores. Recess used to be an opportunity for kids to run, play, and socialize. Many experts fear that cutting recess time is another step toward an increasingly lonely and sedentary—and overweight—childhood. "Daily school recess is essential; it's founded on problem solving," argues Rhonda Clements, an education professor at Long Island's Hofstra University. Studies show that children who have midday recess are less sluggish, perform better in class, and are more attentive.[16]

Some schools argue that physical education (itself an endangered species) can fill the recess void. Both PE and recess are essential but different. Recess is unstructured time and provides for creative play, social learning, and blowing off steam. The New PE described in chapter 5 applies to individual kids and aims at fitness for life. The Web site www.PE4Life.org offers ideas on how to make PE for Life work for schools. Adopting this new approach to physical education and reclaiming recess are vital to a child's development and major tools for preventing obesity.

Even non-PE teachers can do their part to promote physical activity within the school throughout the day. For example, Take 10! is a classroom program that includes physical movement in short spurts to increase study efficiency. Teachers or students choose a Take 10! lesson card that includes a physical activity, a cool down, a few questions from the "OrganWise Guys" (geared to reinforce a topic in language arts, math, or science), and stickers to record completion of the session on a tracking chart (see www.ilsi.org/activities for additional details).[17]

The National Association for Sport and Physical Education offers these guidelines:

Elementary school–age children should accumulate at least thirty to sixty minutes of age-appropriate and developmentally appropriate physical activity from a variety of activities on all, or most, days of the week.

They should try to accumulate more than sixty minutes, and up to several hours per day, of activity.

Some daily activity should last ten to fifteen minutes or more and include moderate to vigorous activity.

Children should not have extended periods of inactivity.[18]


To meet the requirement of a minimum of thirty minutes daily, a variety of activities at school could be provided for all children regardless of their varying abilities, sizes, and shapes. This may help keep them from falling asleep in the classroom or quell the urge to reach for a caffeinated soft drink.

Guidelines for adolescents call for physical activity daily as part of play, games, sports, work, transportation, recreation, physical education, or planned exercise, in the context of family, school, or community activities. Adolescents should engage in three or more sessions per week of at least twenty minutes of moderate to vigorous activities.[19] And let's not forget that the USDA's Dietary Guidelines for Americans, which form the basis of all federal nutrition education and health promotion activities, tell everyone—children, teens, and adults—to aim for sixty minutes of moderate physical activity most days of the week, preferably daily.

**4** *Encourage walking to school.*
Of trips to and from school that are one mile or less, children make only 31 percent by walking; children within two miles of school make just 2 percent of school trips by bicycling. Parents and schools should support the nationwide Kidswalk-to-School initiative, a coalition of several governmental agencies and volunteer organizations spearheaded by the CDC.[20]

Kidswalk-to-School is a program to promote safe routes for walking to school. One aspect involves organizing "walking trains" with volunteer leaders to ensure safe passage by foot. Another aims to consolidate bus stop pickups by having children walk in groups accompanied by adults to one central bus stop in a neighborhood. The program offers a step-by-step plan to involve kids, parents, school officials, police officers, and community members in organizing events to make walking not only "cool" but also enjoyable. It gives everyone a greater chance to experience the neighborhood as pedestrians. This program has reduced car trips and increased daily physical activity among children—and adults—in several communities nationwide. Parents concerned about safety have found many ways to ensure safe routes to school (www.saferoutestoschools.org). A "walkability checklist" is helpful in getting a program started (www.walkinginfo.org).

Ensuring safe public spaces for "walking trains" as transport to school requires supervision. Parents can volunteer, or traffic can be rerouted. I believe the best method to reduce "gratuitous" car use for kids who live less than one mile from school is to mount a grassroots type of movement to encourage more general communitywide walking and biking, with kickoff events, pedometer giveaways, and prizes for accumulated miles. The 10,000 Steps a Day program, initiated in Colorado, is promoted nationwide to get everyone moving by tracking steps with pedometers that motivate more daily walking—for an accumulation of at least 10,000 steps throughout each day (www.pbs.org/americaswalking).

One way to change the status quo and encourage walking to school is through regulation, such as the use of license plates or stickers on vehicles for alternate-day use only. In Mexico City heavy fines are levied on car owners whose plate does not indicate legal use that day. In the spirit of moderation, I say that a version of car-use regulation within a mile of schools is reasonable to thwart the rise in childhood obesity by boosting the use of the "walking train" or "big sister and brother" programs for walking to school. A positive side effect would be cleaner air for children in the school playground. A parent group in Denver mounted an appeal to drivers waiting in vehicles for children after school to turn off their motors at the school gate. Better yet, it added, park the car several blocks away from the gate and meet children on foot.

At the end of the day, if anyone still needs to be convinced of the value that walking programs have for school kids, ask the teachers. Some report that children who walk to school are more alert and better behaved than those who ride the bus or arrive by car. It makes sense that kids who get some physical activity and fresh air between lying in bed and sitting at a desk are likely to have better appetites for both breakfast and learning.

**5** *Improve teacher training and use interdisciplinary intervention to reduce youth obesity.*

Parents and school boards must identify nutrition and health as priorities and, in turn, support teacher training to put healthy food and fitness behaviors into the daily curriculum. A schedule could feature classroom discussions about varying body size, as suggested in chapter 8, and sensitive methods of encouraging physical activity.

One useful way to engage the attention of parents, school officials, and teachers is to measure each child's fitness level, rather than weight and BMI, as the indicator of health. This refocuses support on *all* children—fat and thin—in schoolwide initiatives to improve health (and fight obesity).

In 2001 the Department of Education in California measured children using a "Fitnessgram" that reported aerobic capacity and body composition. The results—25 percent of California kids were unfit; up to 54 percent in some districts—were then analyzed according to state assembly districts to provide policymakers and school officials with a clear picture of childhood fitness in their districts and communities. As a wake-up call and motivator, reporting fitness levels of kids spotlights the need for supporting schools as a place to counter obesity and promote health without singling out fat kids. Parents and school officials readily connect fitness to health and overall school performance.[21]

Schools ready to take action and looking for a complete program do not need to reinvent the wheel. If the value of and need for improved food and physical activity are recognized as a priority, several programs are available for adapted use in the curriculum and in after-school programs. A program tested for two years in public schools in four ethnically diverse Massachusetts communities, Eat Well and Keep Moving, has been used for four years in fourteen city schools in Baltimore and in other schools across the country. Its development and evaluation were supported with grants from the National Institutes of Child Health and Human Development, the Centers for Disease Control, the Harvard School of Public Health, and sister institutions. Unlike traditional health curricula, Eat Well and Keep Moving is a multifaceted program that encompasses all aspects of the learning environment—classroom, cafeteria, gymnasium, school hallways, community centers, and home. Using sophisticated learning and behavior choice theories, interdisciplinary approaches, and market research, the program fits into an existing school curricula in four major subjects and physical education classes. The sessions focus on decreases in screen time and high-calorie foods with increases in fruit and vegetable intake as well as moderate and vigorous physical activity. They use activities such as "Freeze My TV," which tracks hours of screen time and generates alternative and related activities of graphing, making charts, and writing in journals. A parallel activity charts a "FitScore" and a "SitScore," while "Get 3-at-school and 5-a-day" has a kit with cards about fruits and vegetables in a classroom game that takes kids from one "produce" box to another for several minutes of physical activity. Though the program's goal is to improve food and physical activity choices, it worked in the two-year study phase to lower the rate of obesity, especially for girls in the program. Both girls and boys reduced television hours and increased fruit and vegetable consumption as compared to the children in schools that did not have the program.[22] This program is a model for schools nationwide to adopt. It succeeds in training teachers to apply personal fitness and healthy eating goals. Healthy, motivated teachers are good role models.

We all must support teaching with higher pay and more respect and encourage our young children to value teaching as an indispensable profession. Teachers, from kindergarten to university, have many opportunities to urge responsible social choices, including choices that affect our health, in accord with what educator Carol Gilligan aptly conceptualizes as the "ethic of care." From the perspective of a parent and grandparent, Gilligan's ethic rings even truer to me today than when I first read it two decades ago, because of the emphasis she places on the responsibility each of us has for all of our children—and, by extension, for our many overweight children. What more responsible role may a person assume in direct interaction with a child?

**6** *Keep schools open longer on a daily and annual basis for after-school activity.*

Every forum on improving children's health that I have ever attended always ends with the same recommendation for action: provide improved, energetic, and attractive after-school and summer programs for children. Though these programs are optional, they are essential for parents whose work hours collide with the gap between school and "after-work" for their children. Quality supervised after-school physical activities in school facilities for all children who need them require as many, though different, resources as the regular school program.

The budget, the personnel, and the supervision all require commitment from school boards, parents, and taxpayers. And when those are all in line, the real challenge is to devise energetic and attractive activities for kids. One resource is to encourage and train older peers who are enthusiastic and like leading their younger peers. There is plenty of evidence that peer and older youth leaders themselves benefit from "walking the talk" when working with others. Training children to be leaders of after-school activities is a valuable resource that rewards the participants, the leaders, and the resource budget. Less supervision is required while the quality and energy of the activities goes up. One possibility is to develop "service learning" as part of the regular curriculum and include training volunteer leaders for after-school programs as an attractive component.[23]

A tested and ready-to-go active recreation program is SPARK—Sports, Play, and Active Recreation for Kids ages five to fourteen. Developed and tested at San Diego State University, this program includes training for youth leaders, teachers, after-school staff, and parents in strategies that motivate participants. (See the box "How Parents Can Help Schools Counter Obesity among Students.") The program focus is on relaxed, inclusive activities: cooperative and aerobic games, multicultural dances for all ages, modified sports to incorporate all skill levels and both sexes, challenging competitions without elimination, and nutrition awareness (www.foundation .sdsu.edu/projects/spark).

## HOW PARENTS CAN HELP SCHOOLS
## COUNTER OBESITY AMONG STUDENTS

- Actively participate on school food committees to advocate nutritious, accessible offerings, upgraded food service worker status, and a positive eating environment for meals and snacks at school.

- Organize "walking trains" for students to walk to and from school in groups, and/or organize an alternative drop-off/pickup point farther away from campus for drivers so their children can walk part of the way.

- Demand inclusive physical education that is rewarding for children of all sizes, shapes, and abilities.

- Organize parent groups to lobby school officials to remove fast food and soda companies' products and logos from campus and promote healthy alternatives.

- Participate in and encourage citizen participation in movements to allocate budget resources that support active, attractive after-school programs.

- Encourage school sports teams and other school clubs to sell nonedible items—such as school supplies or T-shirts and water bottles with the school logo—rather than candy for fundraisers. Or, better yet, sell students' talents and skills; for example, to lead active games at birthday parties for younger children or (with sponsors) to provide musical or drama entertainment to groups of seniors in retirement communities or nursing facilities.

- Advocate the removal of Channel One from classrooms, since it encourages passive, sedentary learning through television watching and beams in commercials for junk food. Alternatively, initiate classroom projects to use it for developing critical analysis of commercials and "TV turn off" activities.

- Lobby administrators to fix broken water fountains and install additional ones as alternatives to soft drinks.

- Support curriculum content revisions and teacher training to incorporate learning activities in the academic program that empower students to choose and enjoy healthy food and physical activity.

- Encourage classroom reading and discussion of books that portray overweight youth in ways that teach tolerance and empathy.

Somewhere along the line, when a child is clearly struggling with obesity and his or her family is unable or unwilling to help, community members—neighbors, health professionals, civic and religious leaders—must step forward and provide support. Community facilities and institutions—such as recreational centers and city hall, with its power to allocate resources and design public places—must also do their part to help create an environment that promotes health and not obesity.

The highly publicized case of Anamarie Martinez-Regino, the extremely overweight toddler who was taken away from her parents' custody in 2000 by New Mexico state authorities because the family couldn't control her weight, provides a stark lesson in how a community can first fail to help an obese child and her parents and then intervene in an insensitive and inappropriate manner. Anamarie weighed 6 pounds at birth but zoomed to 110 pounds at three years old and 4 feet 6 inches tall. At 130 pounds, she was hospitalized and put on a liquid diet for weight loss; at 123 pounds, she was released to her family and a supervised day-care program. When she was found to be out of compliance with her strict diet, she was taken away from her family on the basis of child abuse.[24] There is no question that her weight threatened her health but the family, very concerned and eager to help, needed sensitive guidance and supervision, not charges of child abuse.

Parents of obese children generally sort into three groups. The first includes families who identify incorrect feeding and physical activity patterns and then show a high degree of self-efficacy and cooperation as a family to improve these behaviors. They seek out opportunities for their children to eat in a healthier manner and to be more physically active. Parents in the second type suffer from overwhelming stress, perhaps from time and work pressures or from addictive behaviors including eating disorders and alcoholism. Or they may be overprotective and feel guilty and helpless about their kids' weight. Those in the third explain their children's overweight as a biological predisposition and feel little responsibility for the problem or the remedy. Families in the second and third groups are likely, though this is not always true, to have difficulties related to poverty, single parenthood, or psychological problems. The first group is often fairly successful at encouraging healthier behaviors, while the second and third groups need outside help.[25]

Here are actions that people and institutions in communities should take to help our overweight children:

**1** *Encourage the flexible use of public facilities for high-quality youth programs, and support these programs through community volunteers and public funds.*

Opening up community centers, churches, and school gyms for positive, supervised activities after school and on weekends counterbalances watching television at home. School and community programs that offer alternatives to sedentary activities and unhealthy eating help children in obesity-prone living conditions get out of the cycle of overweight and inactivity. Parents do not always have the time, know-how, or resources to support activities that would combat the excess sedentary activity, overeating, and "emotional eating" that lead to excess weight gain.

We all have a stake in financing and training those who work with children to provide high-quality supervision that starts in day care, intensifies in schools, and continues after school and year-round in our communities. For citizens who want to make a difference in the child obesity epidemic, volunteering or recruiting volunteers beyond home and school to take part with children in "any activity but TV and binge eating" is a positive step.

Acting on the premise that reducing nationwide obesity starts in neighborhoods, the National Heart, Lung, and Blood Institute and the National Recreation and Park Association developed Hearts N' Parks. It organizes regular activities to improve lifestyle choices through park and recreation departments and other community-based agencies. And it gives community organizations a chance to gain public recognition for encouraging healthy behaviors as well as developing partnerships to further enrich children's activities. The program offered "FunFit" events in many cities during summer 2003 featuring field games, swimming, and prizes in a healthy lunch contest. More than fifty Hearts N' Parks sites called "magnet centers" were active in eleven states in 2003. A performance report from thirty-six sites in 2002 shows that children learned or would "like to play again" an average of five activities and "got better at" seven activities (www.nrpa.org and http://emall.nhlbihin.net).

Programs shown to promote healthy weight have already been developed for targeted groups of children. One example is Go Girls! This African American community program for preteen and teen girls emphasizes physical movement, such as dancing or group walks, for girls of all sizes and shapes.[26] Another example is Just for Kids, a ten-session program for children ages five to ten. Kids meet as a club once a week after school to work with a health professional, teacher, or trained volunteer. Besides physical activity and food experiences, each session includes a group discussion on feelings about body size, eating, friends, and teasing. The program helps develop limit setting and self-nurturing skills through role playing, problem solving, and expressing feelings, which in turn help the children learn how to modify eating and physical activity behaviors.[27] Programs like these can take place in community facilities, if community members are willing to bring children in and get activities going.

An inspiring model for ways that local people can share their talents and skills with children who, in turn, will inspire other children is captured in a public broadcasting documentary, *Who's Dancin' Now?* This award-winning film is about children in the New Mexico public school system who were introduced to a one-year dance program by New York City Ballet principal dancer Jacques d'Amboise using school facilities and volunteers. It shows children without rhythm or confidence in their appearance learning movement skills and then, at the culminating performance for parents and the public, enjoying their own remarkable achievement. As they find commitment, discipline, and resilience through dance, these American Indian kids also learn hope. D'Amboise's work with children in this minority group—whose rates of obesity are the highest in the country—does not take direct aim at the obesity epidemic but certainly represents an inspired way to help thwart it.[28]

**2** *Reclaim the streets for play and community activities.*
A big leap beyond "traffic calming" with old-fashioned speed bumps is what David Engwicht, an international leader and innovative thinker in the fields of transportation, urban design, and community development, describes as street reclaiming. Among the dozens of ideas he provides for psychological and physical street reclaiming in *Street Reclaiming: Creating Livable Streets and Vibrant Communities* are roping off street sections on scheduled days or placing "islands of furniture and play equipment" in selected street areas for sitting and playing. The intent behind his ideas is to widen recreation areas and narrow streets, to slow car traffic and signal the importance of street use for recreation as well as transportation.[29] Through street reclaiming, a street might become a premier playground for children, with supervision a community responsibility. And we might also reduce traffic volume, pollution, and the sale of drugs.

Moreover, Engwicht argues against the notion that children need private backyards, organized sports, and family rooms in the house, because these lead to an impoverished environment where kids lose the spontaneity of exchanges among other kids. Along with increasing physical activity, spontaneous play is essential training for citizenship and social skills.

Street reclaiming for jump rope, hopscotch, freeze tag, bike and scooter riding, and roller-skating is a first step in efforts to raise healthier kids. Street life and attractive public spaces offer stimulation and opportunity for safe physical activity when the stresses within the home build to explosive levels—places for children to be with others, rather than withdraw into a world where comfort comes only from screen images and where food is the only friend.

**3** *Encourage "smart" growth that decreases urban sprawl and dependence on cars.*

Urban sprawl is a major culprit in the obesity epidemic. Expansive suburbs with no walking destinations such as stores, restaurants, and movies require more and more car travel, less walking and biking. Street cul-de-sacs with no way out but onto major highways prohibit children from playing with friends across the highway or in the next cul-de-sac. And research indicates a link between communities' layout and their inhabitants' body weight. People who live in counties and cities with walkable neighborhoods walk more and weigh less than their car-dependent counterparts.

Walking and biking paths are prescribed by urban planners to counter the car culture in existing suburbs. Changing zoning laws is essential to allow apartments and commercial activities near single-family homes in new urban housing developments. Dan Burden, director of the advocacy group Walkable Communities Inc., says, "The ideal community for walking is the place that is compact. It's got great public space and allows a lot of people to know a lot of people. The key is mixed use."[30] Yet, even in Southern Village, a "New Urbanist" community in Chapel Hill, NC, built with extra streets, trees, sidewalks, alleyways, front porches, corner stores, and parks, people are just beginning to get around their new neighborhood on foot rather than hopping in the car for every little trip.

We know the difficulty of changing behavior from studies of stairway use in existing buildings; to encourage people to climb stairs, building designers and property owners made stairwells more accessible, safe, and attractive but still had to campaign for a switch from elevator to stair use. And we need parallel major campaigns to speed the progress away from our car culture.

**4** *Promote and support nongovernmental organizations that provide healthy alternatives for youth.*

In the summer of 2001 President George W. Bush visited a YMCA camp and mentioned an informal movement he is fostering to encourage Americans to do more on their own to take care of their neighbors and neighborhoods. Referring to America as "a country that values family and friendship, a place where people learn values and character," he described the youth camp as a "community of character," a place that encourages parents and children to spend more time together.[31] And of course, we already do support community programs and camps like those sponsored by the YMCA. But I challenge President Bush to buttress his appeal to us all with the necessary financial support for basic facilities, training of qualified leaders, and assistance for those who cannot afford to take the first step toward participation.

Other programs for those who cannot spend time together as families deserve our support. One example is the Fresh Air Fund in New York City, which provides inner-city children summer camp experiences and a chance to spend time with suburban and rural families. When my family lived in the suburbs of New Jersey, we had a rewarding experience for many summers and some additional holidays with two brothers from Bedford-Stuyvesant in Brooklyn, New York. From the time Jeff and Greg were eight and nine, the same ages as our sons, they enjoyed our backyard and camped, swung on ropes and space trolleys, gathered around bonfires, and played with our pets. The whole neighborhood looked forward to their month-long visit every summer, and especially to the dancing in our living room when all the kids were preteens. Jeff and Greg had the naturally big appetites of growing boys and were always on the move. One summer the program leader asked us to invite Joey, a very pudgy, sedentary nine-year-old redhead. Constant access to our neighborhood outdoor activities and healthy meals left little time for snacking and TV. Joey learned to swim and ride a bike.

In 2002 more than 6,000 children took part in the Friendly Town program, sponsored by New York City's Fresh Air Fund, with visits to volunteer families lasting from one week to a full summer in suburban and rural areas in thirteen eastern states and Canada.[32] Here is just one example of a nongovernmental organization with a long track record of solid accomplishment. It and programs like it give us reasons for optimism in our efforts to improve all of our children's quality of life.

**5** *Improve the availability and affordability of nutritious food offerings in low-income neighborhoods.*

Improved access to "green markets"—farmers' markets and other outlets with abundant varieties of fruits and vegetables—is a priority recommendation in the surgeon general's call to action against obesity. Evidence from large governmental studies confirms that increased fruit consumption results in lower body weight.[33] The fact is that such foodstuff, much of it organic, attractively and conveniently displayed in salad bars and to-go containers, is a hallmark of affluent suburbs, trendy villages, and cosmopolitan college towns. In contrast, in impoverished neighborhoods, grocery stores typically offer produce of lower quality and less variety, tucked away in a produce section and overshadowed by the markets' attention-grabbing displays of highly processed, high-calorie foods from major manufacturers. How can communities help make fresh, affordable produce and better-quality, minimally processed food more available—and popular—in the neighborhoods that need it most? All customers, including those paying with food stamps, are in the same boat.

One worthwhile program enables participants in the Women, Infants and Children program to use a "slide card" to purchase farmers' market produce and facilitates payment to farmers from a governmental fund. This is a great program for making produce accessible to women and children and, at the same time, supporting farmers who raise fruits and vegetables for local markets. Expanding such a program to others, using available stores, would be an excellent way to supply subsidized fruits and vegetables to a large number of people.

Another fast-growing movement is home delivery of organic produce, becoming available in more and more neighborhoods. (An Internet search for "organic produce home delivery" yields many resources for this service nationwide.) This delivery service is a welcome addition to neighborhoods because it provides what is seasonally fresh; the box of produce is relatively affordable and usually comes with suggested recipes. Neighbors can order this service collectively, splitting the cost and sharing the produce so none of it goes to waste.

**6** *Health providers: intervene when children are at risk of becoming overweight, and offer sensitive, ongoing support.*

In 2000 Dr. Ronald Sokol, a well respected British pediatric obesity expert, pinpointed the need for health professionals, especially pediatricians, to be more proactive and sensitive in working with families whose children are overweight: "It is now time for a 'call to arms' to bring together pediatric health-care providers in mounting an all-out battle against childhood obesity and to begin to approach it as the most common chronic illness in childhood. It is no longer acceptable to refer a family with an obese child (the adult family members are also frequently overweight) to a nutritionist and abdicate the responsibility for dealing effectively with this chronic, frustrating disease."[34]

In August 2003 the American Academy of Pediatrics developed its first-ever policy statement on the specific problem of childhood obesity. Though most pediatricians already track children's height and weight, the new policy urges them to look for unusually rapid growth, a signal of increased risk of obesity. The new policy also encourages pediatricians to do the following:

Identify and track patients at increased risk because of family history, ethnic, or cultural factors

Routinely encourage physical activity and promote the academy's existing recommended limit of no more than two hours of television or video viewing daily

Encourage parents or caregivers to promote healthy eating

Encourage breast-feeding because studies have shown it may reduce children's risk of becoming overweight or obese

Actively promote anti-obesity programs in their communities, for example by discouraging the sale of sugary sodas at schools and encouraging physical education programs that focus on person fitness, not just team sports[35]

According to Dr. Marc Jacobson, a pediatrician at New York City's Schneider's Children's Hospital and coauthor of the new policy, the aim is to avoid stigmatizing youngsters who already are overweight and to focus less on labeling them than on advocating healthful activities for all kids. "It's not just pediatricians who can solve this, it's going to be the whole society."[36]

One positive action comes from the College of Family Physicians of Canada. Doctors across Canada write physical activity prescriptions for their patients as a more effective way of tackling obesity through active counseling, especially for children and young people. They use simple evaluations to assess fitness capacity to support these prescriptions, including a Step Test Exercise Prescription.[37]

To learn healthy eating behavior, parents and caregivers need skillful, sensitive guidance, lots of practice, and praise to build confidence. Children need precisely the same things. Here is where intervention on the part of health educators and health providers is critical. Families can use skills, not just advice.

Health educators generally teach a new skill or behavior by first motivating their students: they extol its reward (feeling healthy and confident) or threaten dire consequences (being unhealthy; having an unhealthy child). Then they teach how to do it. The problem is that this sequence can seem backwards to the learner. Hearing advice to prevent obesity is no guarantee that parents will follow it; they need to learn *how* to do it, not just why. They need guidance, practice, and praise to make it work.

A case in point involves a young couple I worked with who learned the hard way that a positive, authoritative feeding relationship with their child is easier to establish in theory than in practice. They took a parenting class while expecting their first child and were frustrated that the class focused mainly on why to breast-feed, rather than on how to do it. They wanted to nurse their new baby because they already believed breast-feeding would help prevent obesity and give their child the best nutritional start in life, but they became overwhelmed by the "hard sell" approach of the class; they worried that if they failed, their child would not get off to a healthy start. They tried to breast-feed their new baby, Jennifer, but after a week they gave up because the baby was screaming with apparent hunger, they feared dehydration, and the mother's breasts were painful from attempts to get the baby to "latch on." They had only a brief session with a lactation consultant in the hospital, and to visit one after leaving cost way more than their insurance covered. They were motivated, but they lacked the skill and support they needed.

The couple's challenges mounted during the first eight weeks when little Jennifer became colicky. Her sleep-deprived, exhausted parents ordered in high-fat, high-calorie, low-vegetable meals and fell into a pattern of eating haphazardly rather than coming together as a family at mealtimes. Jennifer settled down but only with lots of bottles—milk and high-sugar juice, and an extended period of foods only from jars.

Two years later the family was still at a loss about how to manage food choice and mealtimes. Their attention was focused on how to manage Jennifer's "terrible twos"—her food and eating tantrums, demands for soda instead of milk, refusal of all vegetables, screams for attention in restaurants. At age three she started day care, and though her parents were admittedly relieved to get a break, they worried that juice was given instead of water and that Jennifer did not like the snacks and meals.

## HOW OUR COMMUNITIES CAN FIGHT OBESITY

- Organize and promote a variety of physical activities in neighborhoods, such as scavenger hunts, kite flying, tag, Frisbee tossing, hopscotch, jump rope, badminton, ice skating, Rollerblading, and dancing.

- Lead, join, or support the grassroots movement America on the Move to make small changes in physical activity for everyone—walking 2,000 extra steps each day (AmericaontheMove.org).

- Work to increase the availability of school facilities and public spaces and safe streets after school and on weekends for spontaneous play and worthwhile programs. Volunteer to supervise these activities; work with law enforcement and neighborhood patrols to help keep streets and parks safe.

- Support farmers' markets in lower-income neighborhoods. Pressure major supermarket chains not to "abandon" lower-income neighborhoods and to offer produce and other healthy foods there in greater variety and quality.

- Invite health professionals to serve on advisory boards of service organizations to plan and implement ways to support health promotion events and activities.

This case illustrates what may happen if children's most valuable "teachable moments"—their infancy—slip away unused by parents. Prenatal care and "anticipatory guidance" for parents is essential, but continued coaching and support are just as vital during their children's early years and at each challenging milestone of physical and psychological development to adulthood. The point is that parents may accept the wisdom of standard nutrition and health guidelines, but they are likely to deviate from that sound advice in spite of their good intentions. Health professionals can help. As with Anamarie, the extremely overweight child removed from her parents' care, health professionals need to mine all available resources from social services, health agencies, and public programs to put parents in touch with support networks. They may shift some of their intensive prenatal health care and parental support, within health coverage reimbursement guidelines, to more postnatal services. Ideally, as citizens we all need to rethink our health-care priorities and put our money on prevention (see the box "How Our Communities Can Fight Obesity").

The marketplace, worksites, and media all loom as large factors in what and how much food children consume, as well as in shaping their ideals of body size and activity. In the wake of the McDonald's lawsuit, which highlighted the complicit role of the food industry in the obesity epidemic, corporate leaders, their workers, and their customers are concerned with the role of private industry in the obesity epidemic.

Major food companies are on the defensive. The Grocery Manufacturers of America, the powerful food-trade group whose members sell close to $500 billion of food products a year, urged a congressional panel not to blame individual foods as the cause of America's weight gain. Soft drink industry representatives have said they were "shocked to see their product singled out and demonized as the main culprit behind the obesity problem."[38] But some companies are shifting to the offense. "PepsiCo—whose biggest product is fat-laden Fritos—went out and hired Kenneth Cooper, father of aerobics, to help it promote 'nutrition, fitness, and wellness.'" And "Kraft Foods . . . rejected a television ad for Double Stuf Oreo cookies because it portrayed teens as too sedentary."[39] These last two are positive actions. Stay tuned for the results.

Voluntary change by big players in the food industry could head off further cases such as the McDonald's lawsuit. But lawsuits are necessary, some people argue, to get the public's attention about the role of fast food in childhood obesity. Lawyers apparently have their sights on "big food" and hope to do to Mega Gulps what they did to Joe Camel. Once again, I plead a case for moderation. I believe most people do not make a conscious choice to become obese or make their children obese. Improved marketing concepts can benefit everyone by enhancing, rather than undermining, their ability to choose food wisely. Lawsuits are extreme remedies we should reserve for a last resort. Let's pressure the food industry in other ways—by voting our preference with our spending dollars; by supporting reasonable governmental regulation; by making our voices heard—and compel the industry to become a partner rather than an adversary in fighting obesity.

There is one other heavyweight factor on the horizon: Wall Street analysts say the big food companies are facing serious financial risks because of soaring obesity rates. One report ranks large companies by their percentage of unhealthy, "less good food" products and suggests that "Wall Street is at least handicapping the effect that the public health debate could have on the corporate bottom line."[40]

Here are actions corporate America could take to demonstrate its concern about our overweight children and willingness to do something about it:

**1** *Take leadership in promoting "reality-size" food servings and healthy alternatives to high-calorie meals, drinks, and snacks.*
To start, how should fast-food companies target America's growing "waist-land"? The major immediate action is this: use a big chunk of their advertising millions to offer and promote smaller "reality-size" servings rather than "super-size value" meals. They can rightly claim they are doing so in the spirit of saving America's health. People who eat three super-size meals a week can potentially add sixteen pounds of extra body weight a year. (Many claim they share the big, economic value-size servings, and I say that's great. But far too many kids don't share. And suppose companies advertised the idea of sharing meals. If too many people did so, wouldn't companies have to come up with an "extra bag" charge to make a profit?)

Another action, to modify ingredients and menu items, is already in place at some restaurant chains. The use of healthier fats and other ingredients (such as all white meat for chicken nuggets) or healthier menu items (veggie burgers, salads, chicken BLT sandwiches, vegetable/whole-grain soups, and fresh fruit) are examples. But remember the McLean burger? To make sure lack of popularity doesn't get these new healthier items thrown off the menu too, companies have to spend big money on advertising them, especially to kids, as hip and cool.

Following the "McFrankenstein" episode (as the judge in the McDonald's lawsuit labeled Chicken McNuggets), there is great pressure on companies to make information on ingredients, nutritional content, and calorie value of products more clear to consumers through labeling and brochures that "do not require a magnifying glass to read." Many companies will do this.

My other personal and professional recommendation comes from accompanying many children to fast-food restaurants: promote free ice water (at no charge for the cup) without grumpy looks from employees. With my rule of "one soft drink per child, seconds are water," holding the line on obesity-promoting sugary drinks would be much easier with water at hand.

In an ideal world, these changes by fast-food companies would help parents and kids pick foods to make a dent in the obesity epidemic. Fast-food restaurants could provide a learning laboratory with healthy choices as well as clear and accessible information about the food products; parents in turn could encourage the choice within limits and themselves demonstrate the behavior they want their children to learn.

The reality is that lots of kids eat fast food without supervision and guidance. Many of us don't think about eating healthy foods when "eating out." And even at home, take-out fast foods are common. Otherwise upscale healthy restaurants copy them on kids' menus. (Is there a kids' menu nowadays *without* chicken nuggets, fries, or a hot dog?)

One promising development is that many fast-food chains are already moving into the slightly more upscale family restaurant business, where it is possible to choose a variety of healthier foods and eat more slowly. Remember, eating slowly is one weapon against obesity.

**2** *Set standards on what and how products are marketed to children; modify media ads and product tie-ins to promote healthy food choices and reality-size high-calorie foods and drinks.*

Big food makers find every imaginable way to put their brand names in front of children. For example, McDonald's golden arches uniform is on Barbie dolls; Barbie earns her spending money working there. I would like to see a Barbie who eats fruits and vegetables. The promotional message? "Barbie stays fit by eating Barbie-size meals with plenty of fruits and vegetables." (Perhaps one day Mattel will offer a "reality-size" Barbie too.)

Because of a backlash to advertising and promotion, some marketing and product tie-ins are changing. The British Broadcasting Corporation no longer allows the use of its Teletubbies children's television characters in fast-food sponsorships. But there is a very long way to go. Burger King has a "Big Kids Club" aimed at kids ages four to twelve. The club's Web site uses the slogan, "Start livin' large at Burger King." It's time to stop glorifying overeating—especially for children.

Self-regulation is only a start. Professor Walter Willett at the Harvard School of Public Health notes, "We don't sell children guns, alcohol or drugs, but we do allow them to be exploited by food companies."[41] Setting standards on marketing to children is essential. (See point 3 under the "What Government Can Do" section below for information and ideas on regulating the media.)

**3** *Provide corporate support to employees through "reality-based" work-life schedules and benefits.*

From on-site gyms to healthy food in their cafeterias, some companies have taken great strides toward providing worksite wellness and weight management programs and opportunities for physical activity and healthy snacks during the workday. This is a start, especially for parents to be fit role models for their children. Even so, what parents really need is more flexible, balanced work-life schedules so they have more time to be involved in their kids' lives, be physically active with their kids, and prepare healthy meals at home.

In fact, a National Bureau of Economic Research analysis of the economics of obesity concluded in 2002 that the growth of fast food accounted for 68 percent of the rise in American obesity (no news there) *and* tied the rise to women's putting in more time at paid work and less at cooking.[42] Fast-food restaurants rushed in to fill the vacuum—offering cheap, convenient meals dense with fat and calories. Given this added burden to carry—blame for the rise in obesity—what are women to do? Particularly low-income, single head-of-household, twelve-hour-a-day working mothers?

Employers who provide strong benefits and flexible working schedules are taking a big step toward improving our children's health. Of course, droves of soccer moms also make fast-food stops as they dash around town in cars on tightly programmed schedules with no time to cook. We all need balance rather than blame in finding solutions for the rising rate of obesity (see the box "Strategies to Effect Change in Private Industry").

As a direct result of rising medical concerns about the nutritional health and increasing obesity of American youth, several states have tried assertive legislation to eliminate or regulate unhealthy food consumption in schools. The attempt represents a big step toward safeguarding the future health of our children. But government at all levels needs to do more—through public education, incentives, regulation, and taxation—to fight obesity.

While the number of overweight children has more than doubled in the past thirty years, estimates on state and federal governmental spending per child per year to counter the rise are minuscule: for preventive measures, $1.21; for disease treatment, $1,390.00.[43] The Improved Nutrition and Physical Activity Act, a U.S. Senate bill that aims particularly at reducing obesity among children and adolescents, was introduced in June 2003. It calls for funding of $60 million in 2004 to set up a demonstration program in community organizations to conduct activities that have shown some benefit for curbing obesity.[44] If it passes, it will not necessarily level the playing field when $60 million must compete with McDonald's (or many other companies') billion-dollar food-promotion budgets.

Meanwhile, in addition to the funds we spend on medical treatment for obesity-related chronic diseases, millions of dollars go into commercial diet products to treat obesity among children and adults—some are costly, some are dangerous, and most are unsuccessful. Isn't it time to pay for the proverbial "ounce of prevention," instead of the "pound of cure"? Here are actions that should be a priority of local, state, and federal government:

**1** *Legislate and support—through incentives such as tax breaks or subsidies—the actions in schools, communities, and the private sector advocated above.*
Many may resist a "nanny" government taking action on this front. Champions of free choice, who oppose legislation and regulation affecting food choice, claim that soft drinks and fries are not dangerous: "It's not the food, it's the lifestyle that is to blame."[45] My answer to them is "yes, but." We are dealing with children's health here, and children are innocent. They don't have a "choice"; their parents and their environment dictate what they eat and whether they live active or sedentary lives. Just as government legislates and regulates to protect kids from secondhand smoke and to prevent them from using tobacco or drinking alcohol as a minor, so too it should

take action to protect children from the health consequences of becoming seriously overweight.

A powerful scholarly critique of the food industry and the case for regulation is Marion Nestle's *Food Politics*. Nestle's study bristles with insights that bear directly or indirectly on prospects for the kind of legislation I urge here. In her conclusion, she writes about the need to begin action for the sake of children:

> If the roots of obesity are in childhood, then marketing of foods to children deserves substantial public opposition. Banning commercials for foods of minimal nutritional value from children's television programs and from schools, and preventing such foods from replacing more nutritious foods in school lunches, are actions ripe for advocacy—school by school, district by district, state by state.[46]

To improve food choices, she advocates manipulating prices to influence buying decisions by subsidizing the cost of fruits and vegetables. Price supports would compensate in part for the low economic added value (profit margin) of these foods—and parallel those in place for dairy foods and sugar.

Nestle's proposals are not unrealistic or nebulous. She is aware that various interested agencies will vigorously oppose them (and, yes, some proposals have drawn criticism). But price supports for fresh fruits and vegetables to increase healthy food availability as alternatives to high-fat, high-calorie foods will encourage improved meal and snack choices. Price supports to promote fruits and vegetables as attractive, "cool," and tasty foods will help them compete with fast-food offerings—especially in low-income neighborhoods. Governmental subsidy support that pays local farmers to grow fruits and vegetables will bring the consumers' price down. These are good and viable methods to reduce the rise of obesity among kids.

### 2 *Levy a tax on food products of minimal nutritious value, and use the revenue to fund healthy weight initiatives.*

Where will the money come from for healthy weight initiatives? One answer is a tax on junk food. Suggestions for a "Twinkie tax" have been argued since 1994, when Kelly Brownell, a psychology professor and obesity researcher at Yale University, introduced the proposal to tax unhealthy junk foods that contribute to obesity as one of "16 Smart Ideas to Fix the

World."[47] It is undeniably controversial, as evidenced by Supreme Court Justice Clarence Thomas's statement that taxing junk food denies freedom of choice. Others worry that taxing high-fat foods disproportionately affects poor people without necessarily changing their eating habits. Okay, a tax on junk food is a regressive tax, but it's a price worth paying if it steers consumers toward healthier choices.

The idea is not as radical as it sounds. Eighteen states already have a tax on high-calorie, low-nutrient food (soda, gum, and snack foods), and it raises nearly $1 billion annually—imagine what a boon it would be to health promotion campaigns!—an amount close to what McDonald's alone spends on marketing.[48] Unfortunately, the states neither earmark the tax revenue for public health messages and education about food and physical activity nor use it in campaigns to reduce the rate of obesity among children. And it has not apparently reduced consumption of the taxed foods. Funding is necessary, but not alone sufficient, to thwart the rise in obesity. Creative initiatives with cooperation from all stakeholders in children's health are also necessary.

Robert Frank, a professor of economics, ethics, and public policy at Cornell University and the author of *Luxury Fever*, argues persuasively for a tax on luxury items that would generate revenue for investment in public services and reduce wasteful consumption. Objecting to such a tax because it deprives people of the right to decide how best to spend their money makes no more sense, he argues, than objecting that a tax on pollution deprives polluters of the right to decide for themselves how much toxic waste to dump into the environment. "The same logic that leads us to instruct our elected representatives to alter incentives regarding pollution also provides a reason to instruct them to alter our incentives regarding consumption spending."[49] For our purposes here, the same logic applies to controlling obesity. A "health tax" on "luxury foods" such as high-fat snacks and sugary drinks consumed especially by kids would help finance programs and educational campaigns for better nutrition.

A June 2003 survey sponsored by the Harvard Forums on Health revealed the good news that Americans are willing to fight obesity in children by paying higher taxes, supporting more physical education, and limiting the products school vending machines can offer. Four of ten Americans polled said they would be willing to pay up to $100 a year in additional taxes if funds were used to curb obesity rates in children. "People recognize that children need help to make the right choices," said David

Blumenthal, a professor of medicine and health policy at Harvard Medical School.[50]

**3** *Require the media to create and present public health messages equal in air time to food promotion ads.*

Imagine if Channel One television, brought right into most U.S. classrooms courtesy of corporations with products—mainly food—to peddle, were required to match every food ad with a motivational healthy food or physical activity ad. In the United States, where overeating is a big part of the rising rate of obesity, food is the most heavily advertised commodity. The food industry spends about $33 billion a year encouraging people, mainly children, to buy their products; the National Cancer Institute spends less than $100,000 promoting fruit and vegetable consumption.[51] It's time to correct this imbalance.

The length, timing, and placement of high-fat, low-nutrient food advertisements that sell food mainly as entertainment, emotional comfort, and rewards should be matched by public service ads for healthy alternatives. For example, ads that promote the benefits of drinking water, accompanied by efforts to make clean, cold drinking water more widely available in public buildings, could help curb the public's seemingly insatiable thirst for soda. Promotions to encourage breast-feeding and campaigns for "reality-size" food servings are clearly good projects. A far-reaching public education campaign to combat the childhood obesity epidemic is urgently needed, and the media must do their part to get the word out.

One advertising campaign worthy of greater and continued support is VERB: It's What You Do. Initiated by the CDC to combat childhood obesity, VERB encourages children ages nine to thirteen to choose a verb—such as "run," "bike," or "dance"—that they can use as a starting point to become more physically active. The commercials, developed by a top advertising firm, feature computer-generated girl and boy figures whose bodies are formed of action verbs such as "pass" and "slide." In one spot, a girl jumps off the diving board and swims through water filled with words such as "twist," "run," and "jump." A voice-over says: "Everywhere you go, everywhere you look, there are verbs out there just waiting for you to get into" (www.verbnow.com).

Criticized for not addressing the "fast-food crisis," the CDC apparently steered clear of fast-food content because kids would not respond to a negative message, according to a CDC spokesman. "A campaign about 'don't do this' and 'don't do that' just sounds too much like lecturing."[52] Yet perhaps top advertising creators will come up with a positive message about "reality" serving sizes of favorite foods. I am sure they could.

**4** *Allocate funds for training health professionals in methods to prevent and treat childhood obesity and for reimbursing these services in health-care coverage.*

Health management organizations and insurance companies are asking who will, and who should, pay for needed obesity-related services from coalitions of medical, nutrition, behavioral health, physical therapy, and exercise physiology professionals. Because obesity itself has not been traditionally recognized as a disease by medical and insurance organizations, reimbursement for treatment is generally out of pocket for the patient. (An IRS ruling in March 2002 recognized obesity as a disease and allowed deductions for selected weight-loss methods—with documentation from a doctor and only if medical expenses exceeded 7.5 percent of annual gross income—but not for preventive services. It did not say whether a person who loses weight and drops below the obese category can continue to deduct the cost of maintaining the weight loss.)[53]

Many people who stress individual or family responsibility believe bills for treatment should go directly to families of obese children. They believe the family is the source of the problem and should pay for the results of apparent gluttony and sloth. Other people believe the manufacturers and sellers of excessive food and drink support the gluttony and sloth and thus should pay. I argue against blame and for a solution: widespread public and corporate expenditures (and expertise) to stall and, in time, reverse the childhood obesity epidemic and its complications.

The time has come for the government and grassroots groups in partnership to consider—and realize—the potential of a national campaign to prevent obesity.

## A NATIONAL CAMPAIGN TO PROMOTE HEALTHY BODY WEIGHT

Altering the environment to encourage behaviors that prevent obesity may seem to be an insurmountable challenge. Yet we faced an equal challenge in the 1960s to reduce cigarette smoking. We succeeded by changing the environment. Smoking is no longer an attractive and seductive behavior for the majority of Americans. Partnerships among educators, government, and industry have led to substantial reductions in the number of people who use tobacco. A similar strategy to decrease the prevalence of obesity—especially in children—is required. Both efforts involve available healthy alternatives and social support from family, friends, the media, and the marketplace. Both require governmental action. At stake are children's lives and untold billions of dollars in managing obesity-related illness.

Here in outline is a nationwide campaign to help children achieve and maintain a healthy body weight.

1. The surgeon general publishes definitive evidence that obesity is unhealthy, especially in children, because it is closely associated with diabetes, hypertension, and cancer.

2. Parents become concerned and—responding to widely publicized guidelines—reduce purchases of large-size, high-fat, high-calorie food, while the public and private sector make healthier snack foods available and extol the benefits of plenty of fruits, vegetables, and water.

3. Companies curb their media advertising of soda and fast food as more public health spots air on healthy eating and physical activity.

4. Schools ban sales of soft drinks and fast food and serve healthy and attractive school meals featuring fruits and vegetables every day.

5. School districts mandate physical activity and include it in daily school schedules, along with adequate resources for schools to offer low-key, noncompetitive recreational activities—like creative cultural dance, swimming, and imaginative games—for kids of all sizes and shapes.

6. Local building codes require sidewalk networks and bike paths in all new residential areas and close alternate streets or selected street locations to vehicle traffic during peak play hours.

7. Farmers' markets and other healthy, low-calorie food suppliers receive subsidies, and restaurant chains serving these foods receive tax breaks when they develop their business in low-income areas.

8. The government levies a tax on foods with no or few nutrients per calorie, such as soda, fries, potato chips, and similar packaged snacks, thereby discouraging consumption of junk food and helping fund healthy weight programs.

9. "All-you-can-eat" restaurants and "food court" dining in crowded environments lose their appeal as the public taste favors attractive eating environments, extended dining periods, and leisurely conversation.

10. Fast food gives way to slow food and sedentary living yields to active living. Obesity rates among children (and adults) decline significantly.

Is this campaign feasible? Any analogy is necessarily imprecise, but there are valid points of comparison between anti-smoking campaigns and the campaign to reduce obesity. America has perhaps the largest core of health-conscious people in the world. Even more than heavily addicted smokers want to quit, obese people themselves usually desire a healthy weight. In fact, their desire is often so strong that studies show they would trade almost anything for a normal weight—a date with someone they admire, a promotion, or even a pension. Many obese people, children and adults, have tried to lose weight, and some have succeeded, but all face the ongoing stimulus to overeat and pressure to sit behind desks or computers. From childhood on they have to endure the rampant fat discrimination we observed in the previous chapter.

Just as smokers labeled the anti-smoking campaign "anti-smokers' rights" and themselves victims of it, so too may some fat people see this proposed campaign as "anti-fat people" and themselves as victims, not beneficiaries. Hence we should direct the campaign for children's future well-being toward healthy bodies and minds—free of stigma over their varying body sizes.

Setting boundaries generally helps children carry out their goals. Thus the majority in our democratic society agrees that no one can light up in a nonsmoking section of a restaurant or public building. In this vein, the goal for modifying eating behavior will be to reach a majority agreement that some places (such as school classrooms, gyms, playing fields, public transportation) are off-limits for eating. Appropriate places for eating will then become more inviting and attractive, encouraging children (and adults) to slow down and enjoy food.

Public action against smoking has reduced its prevalence and related health costs; public action to reduce the rising number of our overweight children is no less important. Will the model work for childhood obesity? Yes, if we launch a comprehensive campaign to stress the positive, immediate, and lifelong benefits of a healthy weight, together with available healthy foods, attractive opportunities for physical activities, and reasonable regulation, it may first stall, then reverse the dramatic increase in childhood obesity. Starting now is critical, or we may lose any chance to ward off this enormous threat to the future health of our citizens.

## WORKING FOR A BRIGHTER FUTURE: A CARING ABOUT CHILDREN CORPS

To run this campaign for healthy body weight among our children we need an energetic and enthusiastic force, a cadre that supports all our children as they grow up and manage their lives.

Over and again we learn firsthand the very hard job of meeting a parent's multiple demands. Parenting is a tall order. And support for high-quality parenting is scarce, though our society expects parents to know how to raise healthy kids—and then blames them when the product does not meet standard specifications.

Imagine there were young adults trained and available to help parents raise healthier kids and carry out the national campaign outlined above— young adults trained to lead after-school activities, promote street games, model team leadership, and "be there" when parents cannot. Imagine we could train eighteen- or nineteen-year-olds in the basics of helping healthy children grow through a program like the Peace Corps in structure and support, like Teach for America in ongoing supervision, and like both in inspiration. This is my proposal: supported with public and private funds, to show these young people who are just becoming adults themselves how to help younger children become more physically fit and more confident of their skills at healthy eating and activities. The process is bound to help the trainees themselves learn and improve these skills too. I call these trainees the Caring About Children Corps, or CACC.

Teach for America is a model that benefits both the young volunteer teachers and the children they teach. Through private funding from corporations and foundations, this program trains enthusiastic college graduates to teach in mainly urban schools, instructing and inspiring children across America. These recent college graduates are drawn to public service, some because they want to address the societal injustice of educational inequality, others because they hope to bolster their résumé and application to medical or law school.

The CACC could be open to all high school graduates and college students as a "gap year," or—as in the Teach for America program—after graduation with recruitment, training, and stipends similar to the Peace Corps'. The trainees would be young people who are likely to become parents, and it would develop their potential to relate to younger children as they give guidance after school to kids who would otherwise be home alone or in unsupervised places.

Trainees might be young people who now go to military service because they are looking for direction and training. Compared to the national military goal of *protection through preparedness (to fight),* the proposed goal of the Caring About Children Corps would be *health through training (to live).* The outcome would be healthy young adults trained in skills that many parents do not have today: to guide young children through the challenges of growing up, giving the children and themselves a shot at healthy living and a healthy body weight.

One year's CACC training could start with several weeks of learning the basics of healthy behaviors and self-management, then on to apprenticeships in child care, education, and health promotion. Apprenticeship, guidance, and leadership would be available from qualified trainers already at work as teachers, day-care providers, camp supervisors, or community health youth officers (whose jobs, of course, would be supported, respected, and well paid). Trainees would develop problem-solving skills useful in parenting or at least an understanding of the importance of helping kids grow and become resilient. The potential settings for training in the CACC are endless; after-school activity programs for every age group are crying out for young, energetic leaders and workers. Public and private day-care programs, including Head Start, are burgeoning with opportunities to learn how children grow and to observe the guidance and management they need. Day camps on weekends and school vacations would benefit from a whole cadre of energetic young leaders, themselves learning as they teach.

The emphasis would be on developing skills and "islands of competence" among the trainees *and* the children they teach. Activities could range from physical movement of all kinds; music and dance; games both creative and traditional; cookshops to learn how to grow, cook, and eat healthy foods; and group "homework" projects at school centers. School teachers and recreation program supervisors, serving as trainers, would benefit from a boost in pay from CACC funding, ongoing training, and respect; the trainees would gain in self-development, career planning, and, of course, résumé building. Most of all, the investment in future parents and their children would provide immeasurable rewards for themselves and society. Preventing a further rise in childhood obesity would be a major result, but the benefits would reach beyond weight management and physical fitness. The trainees and the children they work with—who are the employees and employers of tomorrow—would learn much about raising children, the needs of parents, and how to meet those needs. The CACC could be the small beacon leading to a brighter future for our overweight children.

Responding to the astonishingly rapid increase of overweight in British children, a letter from a doctor in Glasgow lamented, "childhood lies dying."[54] Are our children losing their childhood? In a sense, yes. Consider this: when parents say to children, "Sit still. Be quiet," what they have in mind is appropriate, moderate behavior—to sit quietly during a car trip or at a restaurant, not to sit for long hours in front of television or with video or computer games. But many of today's children sit quietly for much too long—isolated at home with their games and comfort foods.

Is this the childhood we want for the next generation? I see a brighter, healthier, more active future. I see children who are jumping and laughing in our streets, eating in moderation, and leading rewarding lives. This future calls for actions we can start today.

## CONCLUSION

This final chapter on how society can help our overweight children—at school, in communities, in the marketplace, and through governmental action—holds a road map for a national campaign, rather like the anti-smoking movement, and a proposal for an energetic and enthusiastic force to fuel the campaign. To reverse the epidemic, we urgently require action from the public and private sectors. However, we must be clear about this: any remedy begins with widespread recognition of the problem, awareness of its dimensions, and, above all, assumption of personal and social responsibility. Only then may we effectively take up the task this book advocates: to make healthier lifestyle choices for our lives and our future, as individuals and as social beings.

Many hope that research and experimentation in science and medicine will lead us out of this epidemic. Until that time comes, though, denial is dangerous to our children's health, and assumption of responsibility is imperative. The plea here is for moderation, but of a kind that demands a major realignment of attitudes in our country about food and physical activity, to safeguard our children's present and future welfare.

The values of love and tolerance remain alive today in child rearing and social responsibility. These values make the diagnosis and remedy clear: we do not need either another medical miracle or a cultural revolution to learn how to care for our children. We need rather to think sensibly and act decisively, at several levels, from the family to the highest reaches of government, to correct our everyday lifestyle problems that promote obesity.

Change can start with small actions in our families, schools, and local governments. Demanding "reality-size" restaurant food servings may stir a movement toward smaller "value" meals. Requesting water in restaurants and requiring water fountains in public spaces could foment a healthy hydration revolution and cut down on liquid calories for thirsty kids. No "food police" are needed for these corrections. But just as we legislated and regulated to reduce nicotine use, especially among our children, so too can we reduce unhealthy food consumption.

The challenge is bigger than any one of us. Yes, families are at the forefront of this campaign for children's well-being. But if they are ill-prepared to raise healthy children and if the fattening environment outside their front doors remains the same, they are fighting an uphill battle. A brochure from Weight Watchers, "Getting Kids to Eat Well and Be Active," reminded me of this point. It offers "essential talking and listening skills parents need." The brochure's litany of advice to parents—be a role model, create a supportive home environment, boost the child's self-esteem, pursue healthy eating habits and active lifestyles, present the child with healthy alternatives, help the child to get in touch with his or her feelings, discuss strategies for including favorite foods in the child's diet, avoid being a food cop, make physical activities enjoyable, and go see a doctor—is all valuable and commendable, if overwhelming.[55] Yet if brochures like this imply that parents in general can succeed on their own in "getting kids to eat well and be active," they are misleading. Getting *all* kids to maintain a healthier weight through nutritious eating and physical activity requires a groundswell of effort, attention, and concern comparable to the public health campaigns aimed at large-scale crises such as AIDS/HIV, teen pregnancy, and smoking. Advice costs much less than real assistance.

The plight of our overweight children appears everywhere today in the media and in scholarly journals. Testimony from many of those reports and studies appears in these pages and helps explain the epidemic's scale and severity. Yet in the end, I hear the voices of those who prompted me to begin this project. They include the pediatrician who told me, "It's so frustrating for everyone when a child doesn't lose weight," and the mother who mentioned to me, quietly, "We talk—a friend and I: her daughter is heavy like my Sally—we talk about their weight to each other, but to no one else."

I hope this book gives heart to those people and all who share their concerns. It registers and responds to your voices of frustration and desperation. Help is on the way.

# BODY–MASS INDEX BY HEIGHT AND WEIGHT

| | BMI | | | | | | | | | | | | | | | | | | | |
|---|---|---|---|---|---|---|---|---|---|---|---|---|---|---|---|---|---|---|---|---|
| | 13 | 14 | 15 | 16 | 17 | 18 | 19 | 20 | 21 | 22 | 23 | 24 | 25 | 26 | 27 | 28 | 29 | 30 | 31 | 32 |
| HEIGHT (INCHES) | | | | | | | WEIGHT (POUNDS) | | | | | | | | | | | | | |
| 20 | 7 | 8 | 9 | 9 | 10 | 10 | 11 | 11 | 12 | 12 | 13 | 14 | 14 | 15 | 15 | 16 | 16 | 17 | 18 | 18 |
| 21 | 8 | 9 | 9 | 10 | 11 | 11 | 12 | 13 | 13 | 14 | 14 | 15 | 16 | 16 | 17 | 18 | 18 | 19 | 19 | 20 |
| 22 | 9 | 10 | 10 | 11 | 12 | 12 | 13 | 14 | 14 | 15 | 16 | 16 | 17 | 18 | 19 | 19 | 20 | 21 | 21 | 22 |
| 23 | 10 | 11 | 11 | 12 | 13 | 14 | 14 | 15 | 16 | 17 | 17 | 18 | 19 | 20 | 20 | 21 | 22 | 23 | 23 | 24 |
| 24 | 11 | 11 | 12 | 13 | 14 | 15 | 16 | 16 | 17 | 18 | 19 | 20 | 20 | 21 | 22 | 23 | 24 | 25 | 25 | 26 |
| 25 | 12 | 12 | 13 | 14 | 15 | 16 | 17 | 18 | 19 | 20 | 20 | 21 | 22 | 23 | 24 | 25 | 26 | 27 | 27 | 28 |
| 26 | 12 | 13 | 14 | 15 | 16 | 17 | 18 | 19 | 20 | 21 | 22 | 23 | 24 | 25 | 26 | 27 | 28 | 29 | 30 | 31 |
| 27 | 13 | 14 | 16 | 17 | 18 | 19 | 20 | 21 | 22 | 23 | 24 | 25 | 26 | 27 | 28 | 29 | 30 | 31 | 32 | 33 |
| 28 | 14 | 16 | 17 | 18 | 19 | 20 | 21 | 22 | 23 | 24 | 26 | 27 | 28 | 29 | 30 | 31 | 32 | 33 | 34 | 36 |
| 29 | 16 | 17 | 18 | 19 | 20 | 21 | 23 | 24 | 25 | 26 | 27 | 29 | 30 | 31 | 32 | 33 | 35 | 36 | 37 | 38 |
| 30 | 17 | 18 | 19 | 20 | 22 | 23 | 24 | 26 | 27 | 28 | 29 | 31 | 32 | 33 | 34 | 36 | 37 | 38 | 40 | 41 |
| 31 | 18 | 19 | 20 | 22 | 23 | 25 | 26 | 27 | 29 | 30 | 31 | 33 | 34 | 35 | 37 | 38 | 40 | 41 | 42 | 44 |
| 32 | 19 | 20 | 22 | 23 | 25 | 26 | 28 | 29 | 31 | 32 | 33 | 35 | 36 | 38 | 39 | 41 | 42 | 44 | 45 | 47 |
| 33 | 20 | 22 | 23 | 25 | 26 | 28 | 29 | 31 | 32 | 34 | 36 | 37 | 39 | 40 | 42 | 43 | 45 | 46 | 48 | 49 |
| 34 | 21 | 23 | 25 | 26 | 28 | 30 | 31 | 33 | 34 | 36 | 38 | 39 | 41 | 43 | 44 | 46 | 48 | 49 | 51 | 53 |
| 35 | 23 | 24 | 26 | 28 | 30 | 31 | 33 | 35 | 37 | 38 | 40 | 42 | 43 | 45 | 47 | 49 | 50 | 52 | 54 | 56 |
| 36 | 24 | 26 | 28 | 29 | 31 | 33 | 35 | 37 | 39 | 40 | 42 | 44 | 46 | 48 | 50 | 52 | 53 | 55 | 57 | 59 |
| 37 | 25 | 27 | 29 | 31 | 33 | 35 | 37 | 39 | 41 | 43 | 45 | 47 | 49 | 51 | 52 | 54 | 56 | 58 | 60 | 62 |
| 38 | 27 | 29 | 31 | 33 | 35 | 37 | 39 | 41 | 43 | 45 | 47 | 49 | 51 | 53 | 55 | 57 | 59 | 61 | 64 | 66 |
| 39 | 28 | 30 | 32 | 35 | 37 | 39 | 41 | 43 | 45 | 47 | 50 | 52 | 54 | 56 | 58 | 60 | 63 | 65 | 67 | 69 |
| 40 | 30 | 32 | 34 | 36 | 39 | 41 | 43 | 45 | 48 | 50 | 52 | 55 | 57 | 59 | 61 | 64 | 66 | 68 | 70 | 73 |
| 41 | 31 | 33 | 36 | 38 | 41 | 43 | 45 | 48 | 50 | 52 | 55 | 57 | 60 | 62 | 64 | 67 | 69 | 72 | 74 | 76 |
| 42 | 33 | 35 | 38 | 40 | 43 | 45 | 48 | 50 | 53 | 55 | 58 | 60 | 63 | 65 | 68 | 70 | 73 | 75 | 78 | 80 |
| 43 | 34 | 37 | 39 | 42 | 45 | 47 | 50 | 52 | 55 | 58 | 60 | 63 | 66 | 68 | 71 | 73 | 76 | 79 | 81 | 84 |
| 44 | 36 | 38 | 41 | 44 | 47 | 49 | 52 | 55 | 58 | 60 | 63 | 66 | 69 | 71 | 74 | 77 | 80 | 82 | 85 | 88 |
| 45 | 37 | 40 | 43 | 46 | 49 | 52 | 55 | 57 | 60 | 63 | 66 | 69 | 72 | 75 | 78 | 80 | 83 | 86 | 89 | 92 |
| 46 | 39 | 42 | 45 | 48 | 51 | 54 | 57 | 60 | 63 | 66 | 69 | 72 | 75 | 78 | 81 | 84 | 87 | 90 | 93 | 96 |

# BMI

| HEIGHT (INCHES) | 13 | 14 | 15 | 16 | 17 | 18 | 19 | 20 | 21 | 22 | 23 | 24 | 25 | 26 | 27 | 28 | 29 | 30 | 31 | 32 |
|---|---|---|---|---|---|---|---|---|---|---|---|---|---|---|---|---|---|---|---|---|
| | | | | | | | WEIGHT (POUNDS) | | | | | | | | | | | | | |
| 47 | 41 | 44 | 47 | 50 | 53 | 56 | 60 | 63 | 66 | 69 | 72 | 75 | 78 | 82 | 85 | 88 | 91 | 94 | 97 | 100 |
| 48 | 43 | 46 | 49 | 52 | 56 | 59 | 62 | 65 | 69 | 72 | 75 | 78 | 82 | 85 | 88 | 92 | 95 | 98 | 101 | 105 |
| 49 | 44 | 48 | 51 | 55 | 58 | 61 | 65 | 68 | 72 | 75 | 78 | 82 | 85 | 89 | 92 | 95 | 99 | 102 | 106 | 109 |
| 50 | 46 | 50 | 53 | 57 | 60 | 64 | 67 | 71 | 75 | 78 | 82 | 85 | 89 | 92 | 96 | 99 | 103 | 106 | 110 | 114 |
| 51 | 48 | 52 | 55 | 59 | 63 | 66 | 70 | 74 | 78 | 81 | 85 | 89 | 92 | 96 | 100 | 103 | 107 | 111 | 114 | 118 |
| 52 | 50 | 54 | 58 | 61 | 65 | 69 | 73 | 77 | 81 | 84 | 88 | 92 | 96 | 100 | 104 | 107 | 111 | 115 | 119 | 123 |
| 53 | 52 | 56 | 60 | 64 | 68 | 72 | 76 | 80 | 84 | 88 | 92 | 96 | 100 | 104 | 108 | 112 | 116 | 120 | 124 | 128 |
| 54 | 54 | 58 | 62 | 66 | 70 | 74 | 79 | 83 | 87 | 91 | 95 | 99 | 103 | 108 | 112 | 116 | 120 | 124 | 128 | 132 |
| 55 | 56 | 60 | 64 | 69 | 73 | 77 | 82 | 86 | 90 | 94 | 99 | 103 | 107 | 112 | 116 | 120 | 125 | 129 | 133 | 137 |
| 56 | 58 | 62 | 67 | 71 | 76 | 80 | 85 | 89 | 93 | 98 | 102 | 107 | 111 | 116 | 120 | 125 | 129 | 134 | 138 | 142 |
| 57 | 60 | 65 | 69 | 74 | 78 | 83 | 88 | 92 | 97 | 101 | 106 | 111 | 115 | 120 | 125 | 129 | 134 | 138 | 143 | 148 |
| 58 | 62 | 67 | 72 | 76 | 81 | 86 | 91 | 95 | 100 | 105 | 110 | 115 | 119 | 124 | 129 | 134 | 138 | 143 | 148 | 153 |
| 59 | 64 | 69 | 74 | 79 | 84 | 89 | 94 | 99 | 104 | 109 | 114 | 119 | 124 | 128 | 133 | 138 | 143 | 148 | 153 | 158 |
| 60 | 66 | 72 | 77 | 82 | 87 | 92 | 97 | 102 | 107 | 112 | 118 | 123 | 128 | 133 | 138 | 143 | 148 | 153 | 158 | 164 |
| 61 | 69 | 74 | 79 | 85 | 90 | 95 | 100 | 106 | 111 | 116 | 121 | 127 | 132 | 137 | 143 | 148 | 153 | 158 | 164 | 169 |
| 62 | 71 | 76 | 82 | 87 | 93 | 98 | 104 | 109 | 115 | 120 | 125 | 131 | 136 | 142 | 147 | 153 | 158 | 164 | 169 | 175 |
| 63 | 73 | 79 | 85 | 90 | 96 | 101 | 107 | 113 | 118 | 124 | 130 | 135 | 141 | 146 | 152 | 158 | 163 | 169 | 175 | 180 |
| 64 | 76 | 81 | 87 | 93 | 99 | 105 | 110 | 116 | 122 | 128 | 134 | 140 | 145 | 151 | 157 | 163 | 169 | 174 | 180 | 186 |
| 65 | 78 | 84 | 90 | 96 | 102 | 108 | 114 | 120 | 126 | 132 | 138 | 144 | 150 | 156 | 162 | 168 | 174 | 180 | 186 | 192 |
| 66 | 80 | 87 | 93 | 99 | 105 | 111 | 117 | 124 | 130 | 136 | 142 | 148 | 155 | 161 | 167 | 173 | 179 | 185 | 192 | 198 |
| 67 | 83 | 89 | 96 | 102 | 108 | 115 | 121 | 127 | 134 | 140 | 147 | 153 | 159 | 166 | 172 | 178 | 185 | 191 | 198 | 204 |
| 68 | 85 | 92 | 98 | 105 | 112 | 118 | 125 | 131 | 138 | 144 | 151 | 158 | 164 | 171 | 177 | 184 | 190 | 197 | 203 | 210 |
| 69 | 88 | 95 | 101 | 108 | 115 | 122 | 128 | 135 | 142 | 149 | 155 | 162 | 169 | 176 | 182 | 189 | 196 | 203 | 209 | 216 |
| 70 | 90 | 97 | 104 | 111 | 118 | 125 | 132 | 139 | 146 | 153 | 160 | 167 | 174 | 181 | 188 | 195 | 202 | 209 | 216 | 223 |
| 71 | 93 | 100 | 107 | 114 | 122 | 129 | 136 | 143 | 150 | 157 | 165 | 172 | 179 | 186 | 193 | 200 | 207 | 215 | 222 | 229 |
| 72 | 96 | 103 | 110 | 118 | 125 | 132 | 140 | 147 | 155 | 162 | 169 | 177 | 184 | 191 | 199 | 206 | 213 | 221 | 228 | 235 |
| 73 | 98 | 106 | 113 | 121 | 129 | 136 | 144 | 151 | 159 | 166 | 174 | 182 | 189 | 197 | 204 | 212 | 219 | 227 | 234 | 242 |
| 74 | 101 | 109 | 117 | 124 | 132 | 140 | 148 | 155 | 163 | 171 | 179 | 187 | 194 | 202 | 210 | 218 | 225 | 233 | 241 | 249 |
| 75 | 104 | 112 | 120 | 128 | 136 | 144 | 152 | 160 | 168 | 176 | 184 | 192 | 200 | 208 | 216 | 224 | 232 | 240 | 247 | 255 |
| 76 | 107 | 115 | 123 | 131 | 139 | 148 | 156 | 164 | 172 | 180 | 189 | 197 | 205 | 213 | 221 | 230 | 238 | 246 | 254 | 262 |

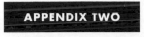

# BODY–MASS INDEX BY AGE

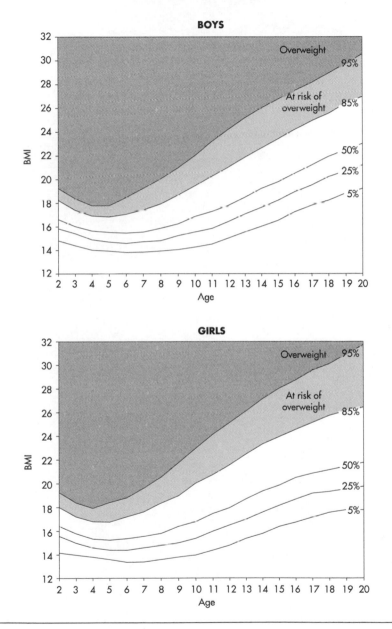

**BOYS**

**GIRLS**

Source: Adapted from Dalton 2002.

# NOTES

## INTRODUCTION

1. C. I. Ogden, K. M. Flegal, M. D. Carroll, and C. L. Johnson, "Prevalence and Trends in Overweight among US Children and Adolescents, 1999–2000," *Journal of the American Medical Association* [hereafter, *JAMA*] 288 (2002): 1728–32.

2. In order of their occurrence in this paragraph's text, I refer readers to R. P. Troiano, K. M. Flegal, and R. J. Kuczmarski, "Overweight Prevalence and Trends for Children and Adolescents: NHANES Surveys, 1963 to 1991," *Archives of Pediatrics and Adolescent Medicine* 149 (1995): 1085–91; R. P. Troiano and K. M. Flegal, "Overweight Children and Adolescents: Description, Epidemiology, and Demographics," supplement, *Pediatrics* 101, no. 3 (1998): 497–504; C. L. Ogden, R. P. Troiano, R. R. Breifel, R. J. Kuczmarski, K. M. Flegal, and C. L. Johnson, "Prevalence of Overweight among Preschool Children in the United States, 1971 through 1994," *Pediatrics* 99 (1997): e1–e4; S. S. Guo, W. C. Chumlea, A. F. Roche, et al., "The Predictive Value of Childhood Body Mass Index Values for Overweight at Age 35 Years," *American Journal of Clinical Nutrition* 59 (1994): 810–19; R. C. Whitaker, J. A. Wright, M. S. Pepe, et al., "Predicting Obesity in Young Adulthood from Childhood and Parental Obesity," *New England Journal of Medicine* 377 (1997): 869–73; and J. Foreyt and K. Goodrick, "The Ultimate Triumph of Obesity," *Lancet* 346 (1995): 134–35.

3. M. E. Eisenberg, "Adolescents Teased about Their Weight May Be More Likely to Report Suicidal Thoughts and Suicide Attempts," *Archives of Pediatrics and Adolescent Medicine* 157 (2003): 733–38.

4. W. H. Dietz, "Health Consequences of Obesity in Youth: Childhood Predictors of Adult Disease," *Pediatrics* 101 (1998): 518–25.

5. Dietz, quoted in G. Critser, "Let Them Eat Fat," *Harper's,* March 2000, 42.

6. R. Carmona, "Federal Perspectives on Child Obesity" (presentation at childhood obesity conference, "Making an Impact Now: Environmental, Family and Clinical Approaches," 6–8 Jan 2003, San Diego, CA).

7. California Center for Public Health Advocacy, "An Epidemic: Overweight and Unfit Children in California Assembly Districts," Legislative District policy brief no. 1, 2002, Davis, CA, www.publichealthadvocacy.org.

8. D. Barboza, "Rampant Obesity, a Debilitating Reality for the Urban Poor," *New York Times,* 26 Dec 2000, F5.

9. Federal Trade Commission, Bureau of Consumer Protection, www.consumer.gov/weightloss (accessed 10 Nov 2002). This Web site offers a checklist for judging commercial weight-loss programs by evidence of effectiveness and safety.

10. J. Elliot, "Children's Diets Worsen since WWII," *Guardian,* 15 Jun 2000, 12.

11. R. J. Sokol, "The Chronic Disease of Childhood Obesity: The Sleeping Giant Has Awakened," *Journal of Pediatrics* 136 (2000): 713.

12. Remarks from David Satcher, MD, PhD, assistant secretary for health and surgeon general, at summit "Promoting Healthy Eating and Active Living: Developing a Framework for Progress," *Nutrition Reviews* 59, no. 3 (2001): S7.


1. COMING TO TERMS

Notes to chapter 1 box, "Sensitivity Matters," p. 18.

*"I took offense":* B. R. Morris, "Letters on Students' Weight Ruffle Parents," *New York Times,* 26 Mar 2002, F7.

*"If we have information":* J. Loviglio, "Schools Encourage Parents of Obese Children to Instill Healthy Habits," AP online, 22 Mar 2003.

*One study showed:* V. R. Chomitz, J. Collins, J. Kim, E. Kramer, and R. McGowan, "Promoting Healthy Weight among Elementary School Children via a Health Report Card Approach," *Archives of Pediatrics and Adolescent Medicine* 157 (2003): 765–72.

Notes to chapter 1.

1. S. E. Barlow and W. H. Dietz, "Obesity Evaluation and Treatment: Expert Committee Recommendations," *Pediatrics* 102 (1998): e29–e40; also S. Parker, M. Nichter, and M. Nichter, "Body Image and Weight Concerns among African American and White Adolescent Females: Differences That Make a Difference," *Human Organization* 54 (1995): 103–11.

2. Barlow and Dietz, "Obesity Evaluation and Treatment," e30.

3. J. D. Turnbull, S. Heaslip, and H. A. McLeod, "Pre-school Children's At-

titudes to Fat and Normal Male and Female Stimulus Figures," *International Journal of Obesity and Related Metabolic Disorders* 24 (2000): 1705–6.

4. For the British sources, see J. J. Reilly and A. R. Dorosty, "Epidemic of Obesity in UK Children," *Lancet* 354 (1999): 1874–75; for the American, see W. H. Dietz and S. L. Gortmaker, "Do We Fatten Our Children at the Television Set? Obesity and Television Viewing in Children and Adolescents," *Pediatrics* 75 (1985): 807–12.

5. Barlow and Dietz, "Obesity Evaluation and Treatment," e20.

6. Centers for Disease Control and Prevention [hereafter, CDC] press release, 2 Jun 2000, www.cdc.gov (accessed 21 Sep 2000).

7. Overweight children and adolescents: recommendations to screen, assess, and manage, www.cdc.gov.growthcharts. Because infants' and toddlers' weight and length should progress at the same rate, measuring their BMI may not be useful. Traditionally, the concern for children under two was for adequate growth, not overweight.

8. N. Stettler, B. S. Zemel, S. Kumanyika, et al., "Infant Weight Gain and Childhood Overweight Status in a Multicenter, Cohort Study," *Pediatrics* 109 (2002): 94–99.

9. CDC press release, 2 Jun 2000.

10. L. H. Eck and R. C. Klesges, "Children at Familial Risk for Obesity: An Examination of Dietary Intake, Physical Activity and Weight Status," *International Journal of Obesity and Related Metabolic Disorders* 16 (1992): 71–78.

11. J. Jackson, C. C. Strauss, A. A. Lee, and K. Hunter, "Parents' Accuracy in Estimating Child Weight Status," *Addictive Behaviors* 15 (1990): 65–68; and A. E. Baughcum, L. A. Chamberlin, C. M. Deeks, et al., "Maternal Perceptions of Overweight Preschool Children," *Pediatrics* 106 (2000): 1380–86.

12. D. Young-Hyman, L. J. Herman, D. L. Scott, et al., "Caregiver Perception of Children's Obesity-related Health Risk," *Obesity Research* 8 (2000): 231–38.

13. Baughcum, Chamberlin, Deeks, et al., "Maternal Perceptions."

14. A. Jain, S. N. Sherman, D. L. Chamberlin, et al., "Why Don't Low-Income Mothers Worry about Their Preschoolers Being Overweight?" *Pediatrics* 107 (2001): 1138–46.

15. G. B. Schreiber, M. Robins, R. Streigel-Moore, E. Obarzanek, J. A. Morrison, and D. J. Wright, "Weight Modification Efforts Reported by Black and White Preadolescent Girls: National Heart, Lung, and Blood Institute Growth and Health Study," *Pediatrics* 98 (1996): 63–71.

16. J. S. Stern, "Parents' Perception of Child Weight Issues" (presentation at American Obesity Association conference, 15 Sep 2000, Washington, DC).

17. Ibid.

18. E. Goodman, B. R. Hinden, and S. Khandelwal, "Accuracy of Teen and Parental Reports of Obesity and Body Mass Index," *Pediatrics* 106 (2000): 52–58.

19. J. Dausch, "Determining When Obesity Is a Disease," *Journal of the American Dietetic Association* 101, no. 3 (2001): 293.

20. IRS policy information, www.obesity.org/subs/tax/taxguide.shtml.

21. S. Solovay, *Tipping the Scales of Justice: Fighting Weight-based Discrimination* (Amherst, NY: Prometheus Books, 2000), 130.

22. L. H. Newburgh and M. W. Johnston, "Endogenous Obesity—A Misconception," *JAMA* 3 (1930): 815–25. The findings from their classic studies of energy balance hold true today: obesity results not from "gland dysfunction" or other "endogenous" problems but rather from "various human weaknesses such as over-indulgence and ignorance" and "lessened activity." Their advice, to change established food habits, echoes in today's governmental dietary guidelines: "Balance the food you eat with physical activity—maintain or improve your weight."


## 2. GAUGING OBESITY'S TOLL

Notes to chapter 2 box, "Childhood Obesity around the World," p. 32.

*An estimated 28 percent:* United Nations Development Program, *Human Development Report 2002* (New York: Oxford University Press, 2002), 165, 173, 177.

*the World Health Organization:* E. R. Shell, "New World Syndrome," *Atlantic Monthly,* June 2001, 50–53. Obesity and undernutrition often coexist; for example, 60 percent of households in Kyrgystan (formerly in Russia) have an underweight family member and an overweight one. To explain the difference, researchers speculate about variation among family members and effects of the 1990s political and economic upheavals. The thrifty gene theory suggests that a short-term "famine" may trigger a conservation of energy (fat) in children who are genetically susceptible to weight gain. Then when food is more abundant they become fat.

*Parts of Europe, Asia and South America:* M. De Onis and M. Blossner, "Prevalence and Trends of Overweight among Preschool Children in Developing Countries," *American Journal of Clinical Nutrition* 72 (2000): 1032–39. J. J. Reilly, A. R. Dorosty, and P. M. Emmett, "Prevalence of Overweight and Obesity in British Children: Cohort Study," *British Medical Journal* 319 (1999): 1039–43.

*rising obesity rates among urban Asian children:* S. Mydans, "Clustering in Cities, Asians Are Becoming Obese," *New York Times,* 13 Mar 2003, A3.

*Among preschool children:* De Onis and Blossner, "Prevalence and Trends"; C. A. Marteiro, M. H. d'Avenico, W. L. Conde, et al., "Shifting Obesity Trends in Brazil," *European Journal of Clinical Nutrition* 54 (2000): 342–46.

*A large study in Thailand:* N. Sakamoto, S. Wansorn, K. Tontisirin, and E. Marui, "A Social Epidemiologic Study of Obesity among Preschool Children in Thailand," *International Journal of Obesity and Related Metabolic Disorders* 25 (2001): 389–94.

*Among elementary school children in . . . Montreal:* J. O'Loughlin, G. Paradis, G. Meshefedjian, et al., "A Five-year Trend of Increasing Obesity among Elementary Schoolchildren in Multiethnic, Low-income, Inner-city Neighborhoods in Montreal, Canada," *International Journal of Obesity and Related Metabolic Disorders* 24 (2000): 1176–82.

*A large study of schoolchildren in Belgium:* M. De Spiegelaere, M. Dramaix, and P. Hennart, "Influence of Socioeconomic Status on the Incidence and Evolution of Obesity during Early Adolescence," *International Journal of Obesity and Related Metabolic Disorders* 22 (1998): 268–74. Europeans refer to children above the 85th percentile as obese and severely obese; Reilly, Dorosty, and Emmett, "Prevalence of Overweight."

Notes to chapter 2

1. R. H. Epstein, "As Diabetes Strikes Younger, Children Get Lessons in Defense," *New York Times,* 20 Feb 2001, F7.

2. National Center for Health Statistics, "Prevalence of Overweight among Children and Adolescents: United States, 1999–2000," www.cdc.gov/nchs/hestats.

3. C. L. Ogden, K. M. Flegal, M. D. Carroll, and C. L. Johnson, "Prevalence and Trends in Overweight among US Children and Adolescents, 1999–2000," *JAMA* 288 (2002): 1728–32. In earlier surveys of preschool children, girls had been consistently more overweight than boys; by 2000, preschool Mexican American boys were more overweight than girls. Data from low-income families show parallel increases in prevalence of overweight for boys and girls (Z. Mei, K. S. Scanlon, L. M. Grummer-Strawn, et al., "Increasing Prevalence of Overweight among US Low-Income Preschool Children: Centers for Disease Control and Prevention Pediatric Nutrition Surveillance, 1983–1995," *Pediatrics* 101 [1998]: e1–e12).

4. K. M. Flegal, M. D. Carroll, C. L. Ogden, and C. L. Johnson, "Prevalence and Trends in Obesity among US Adults, 1999–2000," *JAMA* 288 (2002): 1723–27; also A. H. Mokdad, E. S. Ford, B. A. Bowman, et al., "Prevalence of Obesity, Diabetes, and Obesity-related Health Risk Factors, 2001," *JAMA* 289 (2003): 76–79.

5. K. M. Flegal, M. D. Carroll, R. J. Kuczmarski, et al., "Overweight and Obesity in the United States: Prevalence and Trends, 1960–1994," *International Journal of Obesity and Related Metabolic Disorders* 22 (1998): 39–47; also A. H. Mokdad, M. K. Serdula, W. H. Dietz, et al., "The Spread of the Obesity Epidemic in the United States, 1991–1998," *JAMA* 282 (1999): 1519–22.

6. NHANES identifies these ethnic groups as "Mexican American, Non-Hispanic Black, and Non-Hispanic White" but does not identify any other smaller Latino groups (the National Longitudinal Study of Youth classifies all Mexican American and Latino children as Hispanic). Because NHANES draws on a nationally representative cross-section of the U.S. population and its teams physically measure children in all sites (statistically selected by counties, blocks, and households), surveys take up to four years to analyze and accordingly have unusual date ranges.

7. Ogden, Flegal, Carroll, and Johnson, "Prevalence and Trends in Overweight among US Children and Adolescents."

8. Mei, Scanlon, Grummer-Strawn, et al., "Increasing Prevalence of Overweight among US Low-Income Preschool Children."

9. R. S. Strauss and H. A. Pollack, "Epidemic Increase in Childhood Overweight, 1986–1998," *JAMA* 286 (2001): 2845–48.

10. S. Y. S. Kimm, B. A. Barton, E. Obarzanek, et al., "Obesity Development during Adolescence; a Biracial Cohort: The NHLBI Growth and Health Study," *Pediatrics* 110 (2002): e54–e59.

11. Ogden, Flegal, Carroll, and Johnson, "Prevalence and Trends in Overweight among US Children and Adolescents."

12. M. Story, M. Evans, R. R. Fabitz, et al., "The Epidemic of Obesity in American Indian Communities and the Need for Childhood Obesity-Prevention Programs," supplement, *American Journal of Clinical Nutrition* 69 (1999): 747S–54S.

13. D. S. Lauderdale and P. J. Rathouz, "Body Mass Index in a US National Sample of Asian Americans: Effects of Nativity, Years since Immigration and Socioeconomic Status," *International Journal of Obesity and Related Metabolic Disorders* 24 (2000): 1188–94.

14. R. C. Whitaker, J. A. Wright, M. S. Pepe, et al., "Predicting Obesity in Young Adulthood from Childhood and Parental Obesity," *New England Journal of Medicine* 377 (1997): 869–73; V. A. Casey, J. J. Dwyer, K. A. Coleman, et al., "Body Mass Index from Childhood to Middle Age: A 50-Year Follow-Up," *American Journal of Clinical Nutrition* 56 (1992): 14–18. See also S. S. Guo, W. C. Chumlea, A. F. Roche, et al., "The Predictive Value of Childhood Body Mass Index Values for Overweight at Age 35 Years," *American Journal of Clinical Nutrition* 59 (1994): 810–19; S. S. Guo and W. C. Chumlea, "Tracking of Body Mass Index in Children in Relation to Overweight in Adulthood," supplement, *American Journal of Clinical Nutrition* 70 (1999): 145S–48S.

15. K. R. Foutaine, D. R. Redden, C. Wang, A. D. Westfall, and D. B. Allison, "Years of Life Lost Due to Obesity," *JAMA* 289 (2003): 187–93.

16. E. W. Karlson, "Obesity, Osteoarthritis and Hip Replacement," *American Journal of Medicine* (Feb 2003): 301–4.

17. W. H. Dietz, "Health Consequences of Obesity in Youth: Childhood Predictors of Adult Disease," *Pediatrics* 101 (1998): 518–25.

18. The diabetes rate for New York City is from J. Steinhauer, "Diabetes Rate Has Doubled, City Reports," *New York Times,* 25 Jan 2003, B1; that for San Antonio, from R. H. Epstein, "As Diabetes Strikes Younger, Children Get Lessons in Defense," *New York Times,* 20 Feb 2001, F7.

19. I. Libman and S. Arslanian, "Type 2 Diabetes in Childhood: The American Perspective," supplement, *Hormone Research* 59 (2003): 69–76, www.niddk.nih.gov/health/dmstats (accessed 1 Mar 2003).

20. Z. J. Zheng, J. B. Croft, W. H. Giles, and G. A. Mensah, "Sudden Car-

diac Death in the United States, 1989–1998," *Circulation* 105 (2002): 2158–63. Cardiovascular damage from high amounts of saturated fats (which inflame and stick to blood vessels) as well as from low physical activity and excessive weight can cause sudden cardiac death through fatal arrhythmias (alternation in electrical signals that coordinate the contraction of the left and right heart pumping chambers) or heart attacks (blockage of coronary arteries, usually by dislodged clot from buildup of plaque).

21. H. Q. Ding, D. Y. Fong, and J. Karlberg, "Blood Pressure Is Associated with Body Mass Index in Both Normal and Obese Children," *Hypertension* 36 (2000): 165–70.

22. R. M. Lauer and W. R. Clarke, "Childhood Risk Factors for High Adult Blood Pressure: The Muscatine Study," *Pediatrics* 84 (1989): 633–41.

23. An additional consequence of diabetes and hypertension worth noting is the risk of lower mental agility. A 9 Jan 2001 *New York Times* headline warned, "Diabetes, Hypertension and Slower Wits, Too: Evidence is mounting that these two conditions are leading risk factors for losing cognitive function in middle age"; also see D. Knopman, L. L. Bolund, T. Mosley, et al., "Cardiovascular Risk Factors and Cognitive Decline in Middle-aged Adults," *Neurology* 56 (2001): 42–48. In a 2003 article entitled "Big Tummies Make Men Big Dummies," another newspaper cited a study of mental abilities relating obesity to reduced intelligence in males, possibly because of its effect on blood flow in the brain (B. Hoffman, *New York Post,* 3 Mar 2003, 3). Since type 2 diabetes and high blood pressure, formerly adult diseases, are becoming more common among young people, this means that lower mental agility will threaten kids too.

24. P. F. Belamarich, E. Luder, M. Kattan, H. Mitchell, et al., "Do Obese Inner-City Children with Asthma have More Symptoms than Non-Obese Children with Asthma?" *Pediatrics* 106 (2000): 1436–41.

25. L. H. Epstein, Y. B. Wu, R. Z. Paluch, et al., "Asthma and Maternal Body Mass Index Are Related to Pediatric Body Mass Index and Obesity: Results from the Third National Health and Nutrition Examination Survey," *Obesity Research* 2 (2000): 575–81.

26. F. F. Chehab, K. Mounzih, R. Lu, et al., "Early Onset of Reproductive Function in Normal Female Mice Treated with Leptin," *Science* 275 (1997): 88–90.

27. F. J. Van Lenthe, H. C. G. Kemper, and W. van Mechelen, "Rapid Maturation in Adolescence Results in Greater Obesity in Adulthood: The Amerster Growth and Health Study," *American Journal of Clinical Nutrition* 64 (1996): 18–24.

28. Dietz, "Health Consequences of Obesity in Youth," 518.

29. R. D. Strauss, "Childhood Obesity and Self-Esteem," *Pediatrics* 105 (2000): e1–e5.

30. S. B. Schwimmer, T. M. Burwinkle, and J. M. Varni, "Health-related Quality of Life of Severely Obese Children and Adolescents," *JAMA* 289 (2003): 1813–19; also "Obese Children's Lives Found Full of Despair," *Baltimore Sun,* 9 Apr 2003, 9.

## 3. FAMILY MATTERS

Notes to chapter 3 box, "A 'Fidget Factor'?" p. 52.

*And family and twins studies estimate:* L. Perusse, A. Tremblay, C. Leblanc, and C. Bouchard, "Genetic and Environmental Influences on Level of Habitual Physical Activity and Exercise Participation," *American Journal of Epidemiology* 129 (1989): 1012–22; and L. L. Moore, D. A. Lombardi, M. J. White, and J. L. Campbell, "Influence of Parents' Physical Activity Levels on Young Children," *Journal of Pediatrics* 118 (1991): 215–19.

*One comparison of three- to five-year-old non-obese children:* M. Griffiths, P. R. Payne, A. J. Stunkard, J. P. Rivers, and M. Cox, "Metabolic Rate and Physical Development in Children at Risk of Obesity," *Lancet* 336 (1990): 76–78.

*non-exercise activity thermogenesis:* J. A. Levine, N. L. Eberhardt, and M. D. Jensen, "Role of Nonexercise Activity Thermogenesis in Resistance to Fat Gain in Humans," *Science* 283 (1999): 212–14.

*A 1988 study:* S. B. Roberts, J. Savage, W. A. Coward, B. Chew, and A. Lucas, "Energy Expenditure and Intake in Infants Born to Lean and Overweight Mothers," *New England Journal of Medicine* 318 (1988): 461–66.

*But follow-up research made quite clear:* A. J. Stunkard, R. I. Berkowitz, V. A. Stallings, and D. A. Schoeller, "Energy Intake, Not Energy Output, Is a Determinant of Body Size in Infants," *American Journal of Clinical Nutrition* 169 (1999): 524–30.

*thirty calories of excess food a day:* M. Griffiths and P. R. Payne, "Energy Expenditure in Small Children of Obese and Non-Obese Parents," *Nature* 260 (1976): 698–700.

Notes to chapter 3.

1. F. M. Cornford, ed., *The Republic of Plato* (London: Oxford University Press, 1945), 113.

2. J. V. Neel, "Diabetes Mellitus: A Thrifty Genotype Rendered Detrimental by 'Progress'?" *American Journal of Human Genetics* 14 (1962): 353–505.

3. A. E. Ravussin, M. E. Valencia, J. Esparza, P. H. Bennett, and L. O. Schulz, "Effects of a Traditional Lifestyle on Obesity in Pima Indians," *Diabetes Care* 17 (1994): 1067–74; and M. Gladwell, "The Pima Paradox," *New Yorker,* 2 Feb 1998, 42–57.

4. A. J. Stunkard, R. I. Berkowitz, V. A. Stallings, and D. A. Schoeller, "En-

ergy Intake, Not Energy Output, Is a Determinant of Body Size in Infants," *American Journal of Clinical Nutrition* 169 (1999): 524–30.

5. J. Hebebrand, H. Wulftange, T. Goerg, et al., "Epidemic Obesity: Are Genetic Factors Involved via Increased Rates of Assortative Mating?" *International Journal of Obesity and Related Metabolic Disorders* 24 (2000): 345–53.

6. T. Maratos-Flier, quoted in T. Gura, "Tracing Leptin's Partners in Regulating Body Weight," *Science* 287 (2000): 1739.

7. S. B. Roberts and A. S. Greenberg, "The New Obesity Genes," *Nutrition Reviews* 54, no. 2 (1996): 41–49.

8. Y. C. Chagnon, A. T. Rankinen, S. J. Weisnagel, L. Perusse, and C. Bouchard, "The Human Obesity Gene Map: The 2002 Update," *Obesity Research* 11 (2003): 313–67.

9. I. S. Farooqi and S. O'Rahilly, "Recent Advances in the Genetics of Severe Childhood Obesity," *Archives of Disease in Childhood* 83, no. 1 (2000): 31–34.

10. C. Bennett, *Life in the Fat Lane* (New York: Bantam Double Dell, 1998), 113.

11. J. K. Lake, C. Power, and T. J. Cole, "Child to Adult Body Mass Index Values in the 1958 British Birth Cohort: Associations with Parental Obesity," *Archives of Disease in Childhood* 77 (1997): 376–380; R. C. Whitaker, J. A. Wright, M. S. Pepe, et al., "Predicting Obesity in Young Adulthood from Childhood and Parental Obesity," *New England Journal of Medicine* 337 (1997): 869–73.

12. In M. Pena and A. Bacallao, eds., *Obesity and Poverty: A New Public Health Challenge*, Scientific pub. no. 576 (Washington, DC: Pan American Health Organization, WHO, 2000), 23–28.

13. United Parenting interview with David Ludwig, *Bay Area Parent*, April 2003, 10.

14. K. B. Horgen and K. D. Brownell, "Confronting the Toxic Environment: Environmental and Public Health Actions in a World Crisis," in *Handbook of Obesity Treatment*, ed. T. A. Wadden and A. J. Stunkard (New York: Guilford Press, 2002), 98; and K. D. Brownell and K. B. Horgen, *Food Fight* (New York: Contemporary Books, 2004).

15. D. Barboza, "Rampant Obesity, a Debilitating Reality for the Urban Poor," *New York Times*, 26 Dec 2000, F5.

16. Many of my colleagues view the USDA Food Guide Pyramid as flawed, and I agree that it could use some refinement to educate the public that certain types of fats, carbohydrates, and proteins are healthier than others. Even so, its basic recommendations remain sound advice. Chapter 7's discussion of weight reduction and management programs addresses its merits and drawbacks in greater detail.

17. CDC, President's Council on Physical Fitness and Sports, Healthy People 2010, 2000, www.health.gov/healthypeople/document/HTML/Volume2/22Physical.htm (accessed 13 Sep 2001).

18. K. A. Munoz, S. M. Krebs-Smith, R. Ballard-Barbash, and L. E. Cleveland, "Food Intakes of US Children and Adolescents Compared with Recommendations," *Pediatrics* 100 (1997): 323–29.

19. L. Young and M. Nestle, "Portion Sizes in Dietary Assessment: Issues and Policy Implications," *Nutrition Reviews* 53 (1995): 149–58; and USDA, *How Much Are You Eating? Putting the Guidelines into Practice,* CNPP Home & Garden bulletin no. 267-1 (March 2002), 4.

20. B. H. Lin, J. Guthrie, and E. Frazao, "American Children's Diets Not Making the Grade," *Food Review* 24, no. 2 (2001): 8–17.

21. L. H. Eck and R. C. Klesges, "Children at Familial Risk for Obesity: An Examination of Dietary Intake, Physical Activity and Weight Status," *International Journal of Obesity and Related Metabolic Disorders* 16 (1992): 71–78.

22. J. Putnam, "US Food Supply Providing More Food and Calories," *Food Review* 22, no. 3 (1999): 2–12.

23. Ibid.

24. M. F. Jacobson, *Liquid Candy: How Soft Drinks Are Harming America's Health* (Washington, DC: Center for Science in the Public Interest, 1998).

25. C. W. Enns, S. J. Mickle, and J. D. Goldman, "Trends in Food and Nutrients Intakes by Children in the United States," *Family Economic and Nutrition Review* 14, no. 2 (2002): 56–68.

26. Ibid.

27. C. Cavadini, A. M. Siega-Riz, and B. M. Popkin, "US Adolescent Food Intake Trends from 1965 to 1996," *Archives of Disease in Childhood* 83 (2000): 18–24.

28. Enns, Mickle, and Goldman, "Trends in Food and Nutrients Intakes."


## 4. AT HOME

1. H. Bruch, "Emotional Aspects of Obesity in Children," *Pediatric Annals* 4 (1975): 91–99.

2. R. P. Troiano and K. M. Flegal, "Overweight Children and Adolescents: Description, Epidemiology, and Demographics," supplement, *Pediatrics* 101 (1998): 497–504.

3. U.S. Department of Commerce, Bureau of the Census, "Household and Family Characteristics," *Current Population Reports,* Series no. P20-509, Mar 2001.

4. B. Kantrowitz and P. Winger, "Unmarried, with Children," *Newsweek,* 28 May 2001, 46–55.

5. K. N. Boutelle, L. A. Lytle, D. M. Murray, et al., "Perceptions of the Family Mealtime Environment and Adolescent Mealtime Behavior: Do Adults and Adolescents Agree?" *Journal of Nutrition Education* 33 (2000): 130.

6. R. C. Whitaker and W. H. Dietz, "Role of the Prenatal Environment in the Development of Obesity," *Journal of Pediatrics* 132 (1998): 768–76.

7. Underweight is a BMI (adult) less than 19.8; normal weight is a BMI of 19.8 to 26; overweight is a BMI of 26 to 29; obese is a BMI greater than 29. The National Academy of Science's subcommittee on nutritional status and weight gain during pregnancy established the weight-gain categories, and the National Heart, Lung and Blood Institute's expert panel on the identification, evaluation, and treatment of overweight and obesity in adults established the weight categories' definitions (National Academy of Science, Food and Nutrition Board, Committee on Nutritional Status during Pregnancy and Lactation, *Nutrition during Pregnancy* [Washington, DC, 1990], 10, 12).

8. G. C. Curhan, G. M. Chertow, W. C. Willett, et al., "Birth Weight and Adult Hypertension and Obesity in Women," *Circulation* 94 (1996): 1310–15; G. C. Curhan, W. C. Willett, E. B. Rimm, et al., "Birth Weight and Adult Hypertension, Diabetes, and Obesity in US Men," *Circulation* 94 (1996): 3246–50.

9. M. L. Hediger, M. D. Overpeck, A. McGlynn, et al., "Growth and Fatness at Three to Six Years of Age of Children Born Small- or Large-for-Gestational Age," *Pediatrics* 104 (1999): e33–e39; A. R. Frisancho, "Prenatal Compared with Parental Origins of Adolescent Fatness," *American Journal of Clinical Nutrition* 72 (2000): 1186–90.

10. K. K. Ong, M. L. Ahmed, P. M. Emmett, M. A. Preece, and D. B. Dunger, "Association between Postnatal Catch-up Growth and Obesity in Childhood," *British Medical Journal* 320 (2000): 967–71.

11. D. Jaquet, A. Gaboriau, P. Czernichow, et al., "Relatively Low Serum Leptin Levels in Adults Born with Intra-uterine Growth Retardation," *International Journal of Obesity and Related Metabolic Disorders* 25 (2001): 491–95; R. A. Waterland and C. Garza, "Potential Mechanisms of Metabolic Imprinting That Lead to Chronic Disease," *American Journal of Clinical Nutrition* 69 (1999): 179–97.

12. A. C. J. Ravelli, J. H. P. van der Meulen, C. Ossmond, et al., "Obesity at the Age of 50 in Men and Women Exposed to Famine Prenatally," *American Journal of Clinical Nutrition* 70 (1999): 811–16.

13. D. J. Hoffman, A. L. Sawaya, I. Verreschi, et al., "Impaired Fat Oxidation Leads to Increased Obesity in Undernourished Children: Studies of Metabolic Rate and Fat Oxidation in Shantytown Children from São Paulo, Brazil," *American Journal of Clinical Nutrition* 72 (2000): 702–7.

14. P. B. Crawford, M. Story, M. C. Wang, L. D. Ritchie, and Z. I. Sabry, "Ethnic Issues in the Epidemiology of Childhood Obesity," *Pediatric Clinics of North America* 48 (2001): 855–78.

15. J. W. Rich-Edwards, "Birth Weight and the Risk for Type 2 Diabetes Mellitus in Adult Women," *Annals of Internal Medicine* 130 (1999): 322–24.

16. R. C. Whitaker, M. S. Pepe, K. D. Seidel et al., "Gestational Diabetes and the Risk of Offspring Obesity," *Pediatrics* 101 (1998): e9.

17. Whitaker and Dietz, "Prenatal Environment in the Development of Obesity."

18. J. Diaz and E. M. Taylor, "Abnormally High Nourishment during Sensitive Periods Results in Body Weight Changes across Generations," *Obesity Research* 6 (1998): 368–74.

19. E. Oken and M. W. Gill, "Fetal Origins of Obesity," *Obesity Research* 11 (2003): 496–503.

20. D. I. Phillips and J. B. Young, "Birth Weight, Climate at Birth and the Risk of Obesity in Adult Life," *International Journal of Obesity and Related Metabolic Disorders* 24 (2000): 281–87.

21. Studies of climate's effect on obesity and metabolism note that resting metabolic rate is typically lower in people living in warm regions. Because people of African, compared to European, ancestry appear to have a lower metabolic rate, a biological response to climate was thought to be a factor in the high prevalence of obesity among African American women, inherited from warm-climate ancestors. But a well-conducted study comparing two genetically related groups, Nigerian woman living in Africa and African Americans living in the northern United States, found similar metabolic rates but large differences in obesity: African American women in the United States had an average body fat of 41 percent and average BMI of 31 (obese); African women in Nigeria had an average body fat of 29 percent and average BMI of 23 (healthy weight). An evident deduction is that many factors in the environment besides the weather, such as abundant and easy access to food, must play a powerful role in obesity (A. Luke, C. N. Rotimi, A. A. Adeyemo, et al., "Comparability of Resting Energy Expenditure in Nigerians and US Blacks," *Obesity Research* 8 [2000]: 351–59).

22. R. Eckel and L. Gartner, quoted in J. O'Neil, "In Infancy, Reducing the Odds of Obesity," *New York Times,* 20 Jun 1999, D7; also see American Academy of Pediatrics, Work Group on Breastfeeding, "Breastfeeding and the Use of Human Milk," *Pediatrics* 100 (1997): 1035–41.

23. R. van Kries, B. Koletzko, T. Sauerwaald, et al., "Breast Feeding and Obesity: Cross Sectional Study," *British Medical Journal* 319 (1999): 147–50.

24. M. W. Gillman, S. L. Rifas-Shiman, C. A. Camargo, et al., "Risk of Overweight among Adolescents Who Were Breast-fed as Infants," *JAMA* 285 (2001): 2461–67; also A. M. Toschke, J. Vignerova, L. Lbotska, K. Osancove, B. Koletzko, and R. von Kries, "Overweight and Obesity in 6- to 14-year-old Czech Children in 1991," *Journal of Pediatrics* 141 (2002): 764–69.

25. J. O. Fisher, L. L. Birch, H. Smiciklas-Wright, et al., "Breast-feeding through the First Year Predicts Maternal Control in Feeding and Subsequent Toddler Energy Intakes," *Journal of the American Dietetic Association* 100 (2000): 641–46.

26. J. A. Mennella, "Mother's Milk: A Medium for Early Flavor Experiences," *Journal of Human Lactation* 11 (1995): 39–45.

27. J. A. Mennella and G. K. Beauchamp, "The Human Infants' Responses

to Vanilla Flavors in Human Milk and Formula," *Journal of Developmental and Behavioral Pediatrics* 19 (1996): 13–19.

28. N. Stettler, B.S. Zemel, S. Kumanyika, and V.A. Stallings, "Infant Weight Gain and Childhood Overweight Status in Multicenter, Cohort Study," *Pediatrics* 109 (2002): 194–99.

29. A.C. Wilson, J.S. Forsyth, S.A. Greene, L. Irvine, C. Jau, and P.W. Howie, "Relation of Infant Diet to Childhood Health: Seven Year Follow-up of Cohort of Children in Dundee Infant Feeding Study," *British Medical Journal* 316 (1998): 21–25.

30. M.M. Zive, H. McKay, G.C. Frank-Spohrer, S.L. Broyles, J.A. Nelson, and P.R. Nader, "Infant-feeding Practices and Adiposity in 4-year-old Anglo- and Mexican-Americans," *American Journal of Clinical Nutrition* 55 (1992): 1104–8; also K.C. Mehta, B.L. Specker, S. Bartholmey, J. Giddens, and M.L. Ho, "Trial on Timing of Introduction to Solids and Food Type on Infant Growth," *Pediatrics* 102 (1998): 569–73.

31. B.A. Dennison, H.L. Rockwell, M.J. Nichols, et al., "Children's Growth Parameters Vary by Type of Fruit Juice Consumed," *Journal of the American College of Nutrition* 18 (1999): 346–52.

32. American Academy of Pediatrics, "The Use and Misuse of Fruit Juice in Pediatrics," *Pediatrics* 107 (2001): 1210–13.

33. R.C. Whitaker, C.M. Deeks, A.F. Baughcum, and B.L. Specker, "The Relationship of Childhood Adiposity to Parent Body Mass Index and Eating Behavior," *Obesity Research* 8 (2000): 234–40.

34. T.A. Nicklas, T. Baranowski, J.C. Baranowski, K. Cullen, L. Rittenberry, and N. Olvera, "Family and Child-Care Provider Influences on Preschool Children's Fruit, Juice, and Vegetable Consumption," *Nutrition Reviews* 59 (2001): 224–35.

35. J.S. Seagren and R.D. Terry, "WIC Females Parents' Behavior and Attitudes toward Their Children's Food Inter-relationship to Their Children's Relative Weight," *Journal of Nutrition Education* 23 (1991): 23–30.

36. J.O. Fisher and L.L. Birch, "Restricting Access to Foods and Children's Eating," *Appetite* 32 (1999): 405–19.

37. A.E. Baughcum, S.W. Powers, S.B. Johnson, et al., "Maternal Feeding Practices and Beliefs and Their Relationships to Overweight in Early Childhood," *Journal of Developmental and Behavioral Pediatrics* 22 (2001): 391–408.

38. T.N. Robinson, M. Kiernan, D.M. Matheson, and K.F. Haydel, "Is Parental Control over Children's Eating Associated with Childhood Obesity? Results from a Population-based Sample of Third Graders," *Obesity Research* 9 (2001): 306–12.

39. T. Tibbs, D. Haire-Joshu, K.B. Schechtman, et al., "The Relationship between Parental Modeling, Eating Patterns, and Dietary Intake among African-American Parents," *Journal of the American Dietetic Association* 101 (2001): 535–41.

40. J. B. Sherman, M. A. Alexander, A. H. Dean, et al., "Obesity in Mexican-American and Anglo Children," *Progress in Cardiovascular Nursing* 10, no. 1 (1995): 27–34.

41. D. Spruijt-Metz, C. H. Lindquist, L. L. Birch, J. O. Fisher, and M. I. Goran, "Relation between Mothers' Child-Feeding Practices and Children's Adiposity," *American Journal of Clinical Nutrition* 75 (2002): 585.

42. S. Gable and S. F. Lutz, "Nutrition Socialization Experiences of Children in the Head Start Program," *Journal of the American Dietetic Association* 101 (2001): 572; also A. E. Baughcum, K. A. Burklow, C. M. Deeks, et al., "Maternal Feeding Practices and Childhood Obesity: A Focus Group Study of Low-Income Mothers," *Archives of Pediatrics and Adolescent Medicine* 152 (1998): 1010–14.

43. J. Wardle, S. Sanderson, C. A. Guthrie, L. Rapoport, and R. Plomin, "Parental Feeding Style and the Inter-generational Transmission of Obesity Risk," *Obesity Research* 10 (2002): 453.

44. M. Cunningham, interview, *Diablo Magazine,* Mar 2003, 56.

45. M. W. Gillman, S. L. Rifas-Shiman, A. L. Frazier, et al., "Family Dinner and Diet Quality among Older Children and Adolescents," *Archives of Family Medicine* 9 (2000): 235–40.

46. Whitaker, Deeks, Baughcum, and Specker, "Relationship of Childhood Adiposity to Parent Body Mass Index"; E. A. Bergman, N. S. Buergel, E. Josseph, et al., "Time Spent by Schoolchildren to Eat Lunch," *Journal of the American Dietetic Association* 100 (2000): 696–98.

47. S. J. Nielson and B. M. Popkin, "Patterns and Trends in Food Portion Sizes, 1977–1998," *JAMA* 289 (2003): 450–53.

48. B. J. Rolls, E. L. Morris, and L. S. Roe, "Portion Size of Food Affects Energy Intake in Normal-weight and Overweight Men and Women," *American Journal of Clinical Nutrition* 76 (2002): 1207–13; and J. D. Fisher, B. J. Rolls, and L. L. Birch, "Children's Bite Size and Intake of an Entree Are Greater with Large Portions than with Age-appropriate or Self-selected Portions," *American Journal of Clinical Nutrition* 77 (2003): 1164–70.

49. Emily Nelson, "Finger Food: Marketers Push Individual Portions and Families Bite," *Wall Street Journal,* 23 Jul 2002, A1, A6.

50. J. A. Slochowar, *Excessive Eating: The Role of Emotions and Environment* (New York: Plenum, 1983), 13–14.

51. M. Y. Hood, L. L. Moore, A. Sundarajan-Ramamurti, M. Singer, L. A. Cupples, and R. C. Ellison, "Parental Eating Attitudes and the Development of Obesity in Children: the Framingham Children's Study," *International Journal of Obesity and Related Metabolic Disorders* 24 (2000): 1319–25.

52. D. F. Roberts, U. G. Foehr, V. J. Rideout, et al., *Kids and Media at the New Millennium: A Comprehensive National Analysis of Children's Media Use* (Menlo Park, CA: Henry J. Kaiser Family Foundation, 1999).

53. W. H. Dietz and S. L. Gortmaker, "Do We Fatten Our Children at the Television Set? Obesity and Television Viewing in Children and Adolescents," *Pediatrics* 75 (1985): 807–12; S. L. Gortmaker, A. Must, A. M. Sobol, et al., "Television Viewing as a Cause of Increasing Obesity among Children in the United States, 1986–1990," *Archives of Pediatrics and Adolescent Medicine* 150 (1996): 356–62; and C. J. Crespo, E. Smit, R. P. Troiano, et al., "Television Watching, Energy Intake, and Obesity in US Children: Results from the Third National Health and Nutrition Examination Survey, 1988–1994," *Archives of Pediatrics and Adolescent Medicine* 155 (2001): 360–65.

54. K. A. Coon, J. Goldberg, B. L. Rogers, et al., "Relationships between Use of Television during Meals and Children's Food Consumption Patterns," *Pediatrics* 107 (2001): e1–e9; T. N. Robinson, "Reducing Children's Television Viewing to Prevent Obesity: A Randomized Controlled Trial," *JAMA* 23 (1999): S52–57.

55. Nestle M., *Food Politics: How the Food Industry Influences Nutrition and Health* (Berkeley: University of California Press, 2002), 181.

56. Ibid.

57. C. Byrd-Bredbenner and D. Grasso, "What Is Television Trying to Make Children Swallow? Content Analysis of Nutrition Information in Prime-time Advertisements," *Journal of Nutrition Education* 32 (2000): 187–95; M. Gamble and N. Cotugna, "A Quarter Century of TV Food Advertising Targeted at Children," *American Journal of Health Behavior* 23 (1999): 261–67.

58. D. G. Borzekowski and T. N. Robinson, "The 30-Second Effect: An Experiment Revealing the Impact of Television Commercials on Food Preferences of Preschoolers," *Journal of the American Dietetic Association* 101 (2001): 42–46.

59. S. Y. S. Kimm, N. W. Glynn, A. M. Kriska, et al., "Longitudinal Changes in Physical Activity in a Biracial Cohort during Adolescence," *Medicine and Science in Sports and Exercise* 32 (2000): 1445–54.

60. C. Shufflebarger, G. Clavet, A. Wolfe, and M. Lambur, "Preventing Childhood Obesity: Identifying Barriers to Engaging in Healthy Behaviors" (program and abstracts from childhood obesity conference, "Partnerships for Research and Prevention," 3–5 May 1999, Atlanta, GA), 51.

61. J. B. Schor, *The Overworked American: The Unexpected Decline of Leisure* (New York: Basic Books, 1991).

62. R. Kuttner, "No Time to Smell the Roses Anymore," *New York Times Magazine,* 2 Feb 1992, 1.

5. BEYOND THE HOME

1. B. Weiser, "Big Macs Can Make You Fat? No Kidding, a Judge Rules," *New York Times,* 23 Jan 2003, B3; and R. W. Sweet, US District Court, Southern Dis-

trict of NY. *Pelman v. McDonald's Corporation.* 02 Civ.7821 (RWS) Opinion. New York, NY: 22 Jan 2003, www.findlaw.com (accessed 25 Jan 2003). The plaintiffs alleged five causes of action (counts) based on deceptive acts and practices and negligence in violation of the New York Consumer Protection Act: McDonald's failed to adequately disclose the ingredients and health effects of their food products; engaged in marketing to entice consumers to purchase "value meals" without disclosing their detrimental health effects; focused on marketing techniques geared to induce children to purchase and ingest their products; acted negligently in selling food high in fat, salt, and sugar when studies show that such foods cause obesity and detrimental health effects; failed to warn consumers that McDonald's products could lead to obesity and health problems and acted negligently in marketing food products that are physically and psychologically addictive. Except for the last count's implication that foods are addictive, which will keep scientists scrambling for some time, the general agreement is that all the other counts involve shared responsibility of the vendor and the person consuming the product.

2. J. L. Putnam, J. E. Allshouse, and L. S. Kantor, "U.S. Per Capita Food Supply Trends: More Calories, Refined Carbohydrates, and Fats," Economic Research Service, USDA *Food Review* 25, no. 3 (Winter 2002): 3.

3. J. K. Binkley, J. Eales, and M. Jekanowski, "The Relations between Dietary Change and Rising US Obesity," *International Journal of Obesity and Related Metabolic Disorders* 24 (2000): 1032–39.

4. A. Clausen, "Share of Food Spending for Eating Out Reaches 47 Percent," *Food Reviews* 22, no. 3 (1999): 20–22.

5. J. F. Guthrie, B. Lin, and E. Frazao, "Role of Food Prepared Away from Home in the American Diet, 1977–78 versus 1994–96: Changes and Consequences," *Journal of Nutrition Education and Behavior* 34 (2002): 140–50; C. Zoumas-Morse, C. L. Rock, E. J. Sobol, et al., "Children's Patterns of Macronutrient Intake and Associations with Restaurant and Home Eating," *Journal of the American Dietetic Association* 101 (2001): 923–25.

6. M. A. McCrory, P. J. Fuss, N. P. Hayes, et al., "Overeating in America: Association between Restaurant Food Consumption and Body Fatness in Healthy Adult Men and Women Ages 19 to 80," *Obesity Research* 7 (1999): 564–71.

7. P. LeBeau, "Fast Food Under the Gun," 4 Mar 2003, http://moneycentral.msn.com (accessed 4 Mar 2003).

8. Food Research and Action Center, "Breakfast for Learning: Recent Scientific Research on the Link between Children's Nutrition and Academic Performance, 2001 Report" (Washington, DC, 2002).

9. E. Schlosser, *Fast Food Nation* (New York: Houghton Mifflin, 2001), front cover flap.

10. Ibid., 47.

11. S. J. Nielson and B. M. Popkin, "Patterns and Trends in Food Portion Sizes, 1977–1998," *JAMA* 289 (2003): 450–53.

12. M. Nestle, quoted in B. Liebman, "Supersize Foods, Supersize People," *Nutrition Action Healthletter,* Jul–Aug 1998, 6.

13. L. R. Young and M. Nestle, "Expanding Portion Sizes in the U.S. Food Supply: Do They Contribute to the Obesity Epidemic?" *American Journal of Public Health* 92 (2002): 246–49.

14. B. Wansink, quoted in Liebman, "Supersize Foods, Supersize People," 6.

15. E. Kennedy, "Healthy Meals, Healthy Food Choices, Healthy Children: USDA's Team Nutrition," *Preventive Medicine* 25 (1996): 56–60.

16. D. Wildey, "Food Sold in School Stores," *Journal of the American Dietetic Association* 100 (2000): 301–7.

17. R. Rothstein, "For Schools' Ills, the Sugar Pill," *New York Times,* 21 Aug 2002, B7.

18. M. Nestle, "Soft Drink 'Pouring Rights' Marketing Empty Calories," *Public Health Reports* 115 (2000): 314.

19. T. Egan, "In Bid to Improve Nutrition, Schools Expel Soda and Chips," *New York Times,* 20 May 2002, A1.

20. K. L. A. Severson, "Schools to Stop Soda Sales; District Takes Cue from Oakland Ban," *San Francisco Chronicle,* 28 Aug 2002, A1.

21. "Ban on School Soda, Candy Fails," *Portland Press Herald* (Augusta, ME), 18 Mar 2003, A1.

22. M. Uhlman, "Vending at Schools: Both Sides Eye Change," *Philadelphia Inquirer,* 9 Jun 2003, C1.

23. A. E. Gallo, "Food Advertising in the United States," in *America's Eating Habits: Changes and Consequences,* ed. E. Frazao (Washington, DC: USDA, 1999), 201.

24. M. Nestle and M. F. Jacobson, "Halting the Obesity Epidemic: A Public Health Policy Approach," *Public Health Reports* 113 (2000): 19.

25. B. Steinberg, "Pepsi Is Planning Promotions to Put Some Fizz into Summer," *Wall Street Journal,* 1 May 2003, B5.

26. M. A. Tirodkar and A. Jain, "Food Messages on African American Television Shows," *Pediatric Research* 49, no. 4 (2001): 19A.

27. L. Sims, "Moving Children into the Next Century: The Federal Perspective," in *Childhood Obesity: Causes and Prevention,* CNPP-6 (Washington, DC: USDA, 1998); "GAO: School Meal Programs Face Challenges," *Food Management,* July 2003, 16; U.S. General Accounting Office, "Efforts Needed to Improve Nutrition and Encourage Healthy Eating," and "School Meal Programs: Revenue and Expense Information from Selected States," May 2003, available from www.gao.gov.

28. M. Sheridan, "Noncommercial Links," *Restaurants and Institutions* 113 (2003): 81.

29. S. D. Baxter and W. O. Thompson, "Fourth-grade Children's Consumption of Fruit and Vegetable Items Available as Part of School Lunches Is

Closely Related to Preferences," *Journal of Nutrition Education and Behavior* 34 (2002): 166–71.

30. E. Becker and M. Burros, "Eat Your Vegetables? Only at a Few Schools," *New York Times,* 13 Jan 2003, A1, A14.

31. U.S. Department of Commerce, Economics, and Statistics, "Who's Minding Our Preschoolers?" in *Current Population Reports, Household Economic Studies,* 88-00-9010 PPl-81 (Washington, DC, 1994); K. Smith, "Who's Minding the Kids? Child Care Arrangements: Spring 1997," Household Economic Studies, Bureau of the Census, U.S. Department of Commerce, July 2002, 70–86.

32. S. Gable and S. F. Lutz, "Nutrition Socialization Experiences of Children in the Head Start Program," *Journal of the American Dietetic Association* 101 (2001): 572.

33. J. Schwartz, "Is Recess On the Way Out?" *Offspring,* January 2001, 65–66; J. Wilgoren and J. Steinberg, "Even for Sixth Graders, College Looms, the Academic Pressure Is On," *New York Times,* 3 Jul 2000, A1, A12.

34. The American Association for the Child's Right to Play, www.IPAUSA.org (accessed 23 Sep 2003).

35. CDC, President's Council on Physical Fitness and Sports, "Healthy People 2010," 2000, www.health.gov/healthypeople/document/HTML/Volume2/22Physical.htm (accessed 13 Sep 2001); CDC, "Youth Behavior Surveillance System: U.S. Summary Results 2001" (Atlanta, 2001); and J. F. Sallis, "Epidemiology of Physical Activity and Fitness and Adolescents," *Critical Reviews in Food Science and Nutrition* 33, nos. 4–5 (1993): 403–8.

36. R. R. Pate, P. S. Freedson, J. F. Sallis, et al., "Compliance with Physical Activity Guidelines: Prevalence in a Population of Children and Youth," *Annals of Epidemiology* 12, no. 5 (2002): 303–8.

37. D. Wilson, "Overweight Children," *Bay Area Parent,* April 2003, 11.

38. V. J. Thompson, T. Barowski, K. W. Culllen, et al., "Influences on Diet and Physical Activity among Middle-Class African American 8- to 10-year-old Girls at Risk of Becoming Obese," *Journal of Nutrition Education and Behavior* 35 (2003): 120.

39. National Association for Sport and Physical Education, "Public Attitudes toward Physical Education, Feb 2000," www.aahperd.org/haspe/whatsnewsurvey (accessed 10 Jul 2000); P. Tyre, "Getting Physical: A New Fitness Philosophy Puts Gym Teachers on the Front Lines in the Battle against Childhood Obesity," *Newsweek,* 3 Feb 2003, 47.

40. M. S. Johnson, S. L. Herd, D. A. Fields, et al., "Aerobic Fitness, not Energy Expenditure, Influences Subsequent Increase in Adiposity in Black and White Children," *Pediatrics* 106, no. 4 (2000): e50–e56. M. Fogelholm, O. Nuutinen, M. Pasaanen, E. Myönanen, and T. Säätelä, "Parent-Child Relationship of Physical Activity Patterns and Obesity," *International Journal of Obesity and Related Metabolic Disorders* 23 (1999): 1262–68.

41. U.S. Department of Transportation, Federal Highway Administration, Research and Technical Support Center, *Nationwide Personal Transportation Survey* (Lantham, MD: Federal Highway Administration, 1977).

42. S. A. Hewlett and C. West, *The War Against Parents* (New York: Houghton Mifflin, 1998), 49.

43. U.S. Department of Health and Human Services [hereafter, DHHS], *The Surgeon General's Call to Action to Prevent and Decrease Overweight and Obesity* (Rockville, MD, 2001); also www.surgeongeneral.gov/sgoffice.

44. B. H. Lin, J. Guthrie, and E. Frazao, "American Children's Diets Not Making the Grade," *Food Review*, May–Aug 2001, 8–17.

45. C. Cavadini, A. M. Siega-Riz, and B. M. Popkin, "US Adolescent Food Intake Trends from 1965 to 1996," *Archives of Disease in Childhood* 83 (2000): 18–24.

46. M. Jacobson, "Liquid Candy: How Soft Drinks Are Harming Americans' Health," Center for Science in the Public Interest, www.cspinet.org.

47. D. S. Ludwig, K. E. Peterson, and S. L. Gortmaker, "Relation between Consumption of Sugar-Sweetened Drinks and Childhood Obesity: A Prospective, Observational Analysis," *Lancet* 357 (2001): 505–8.

48. D. Ludwig, quoted in R. Edelman, "Sweet Addiction," *Eating Well*, Fall 2002, 20.

49. G. Wyshaak, "Teenaged Girls, Carbonated Beverage Consumption, and Bone Fractures," *Archives of Pediatrics and Adolescent Medicine* 154 (2000): 612.

50. P. King, "Blaming It on Corn Syrup," *Los Angeles Times*, 24 Mar 2003, 3.

51. C. W. Enns, S. J. Mickle, and J. D. Goldman, "Trends in Food and Nutrient Intakes by Children in the United States," *Family Economics and Nutrition Review* 14, no. 2 (2002): 56–68; and A. F. Subar, S. M. Krebs-Smith, A. Cook, et al., "Dietary Sources of Nutrients among US Adults, 1989 to 1991," *Journal of the American Dietetic Association* 98 (1998): 537–47.

52. USDA, "Nutrition Insights: Report Card on the Diet Quality of Children," CNPP-9 (1998), Washington, DC.

## 6. NURTURING HEALTHY AND ACTIVE LIFESTYLES

1. W. H. Dietz, "The Obesity Epidemic in Young Children," *British Medical Journal* 322 (2001): 313–14.

2. Ibid.

3. R. S. Strauss, S. E. Barlow, and W. H. Dietz, "Prevalence of Abnormal Serum Aminotransferase Values in Overweight and Obese Adolescents," *Journal of Pediatrics* 136 (2000): 727–33.

4. R. G. Laessle, H. Uhl, and B. Lindel, "Parental Influences on Eating Behavior in Obese and Nonobese Preadolescents," *International Journal of Eating Disorders* 30 (2001): 447–53.

5. J. O. Fisher and L. L. Birch, "Restricting Access to Palatable Foods Affects Children's Behavioral Response, Food Selection and Intake," *American Journal of Clinical Nutrition* 69 (1999): 1264–72.

6. Some studies, mostly of white middle-class families, found that restricting foods interferes with children's ability to self-regulate their food consumption (J. O. Fisher and L. L. Birch, "Restricting Access to Foods and Children's Eating," *Appetite* 32 [1999]: 405–19). The most important factors affecting a child's weight, however, were the mother's concern about her own weight and her eating behavior—reflected through role modeling (L. L. Birch and J. O. Fisher, "Mothers' Child-Feeding Practices Influence Daughters' Eating and Weight," *American Journal of Clinical Nutrition* 71 [2000]: 1054–61). Both white and African American children reflect their mother's style of eating and feeding in their own body fat and eating behavior (D. Spruijt-Metz, C. H. Lindquist, L. L. Birch, J. O. Fisher, and M. I. Goran, "Relation between Mothers' Child-Feeding Practices and Children's Adiposity," *American Journal of Clinical Nutrition* 75 [2002]: 581–86), though there may be differences in the effect of parental control on weight of children in families with both overweight and normal-weight children (B. R. Saelens, M. M. Ernst, and L. H. Epstein, "Maternal Child Feeding Practices and Obesity: A Discordant Sibling Analysis," *International Journal of Eating Disorders* 27 [2000]: 459–63). In some ethnic groups, strong parental restriction may lead to under- rather than overeating among children (T. N. Robinson, M. Kiernan, D. M. Matheson, and K. F. Haydel, "Is Parental Control over Children's Eating Associated with Childhood Obesity? Results from a Population-based Sample of Third Graders," *Obesity Research* 9 [2001]: 306–12).

7. E. Satter, *Child of Mine: Feeding with Love and Good Sense* (Palto Alto: Bull, 2000), 3.

8. J. R. Hirschmann and C. Munter, *Preventing Childhood Eating Problems* (New York: Gurze Books, 1993).

9. E. Satter, *Secrets of Feeding a Healthy Family* (Madison, WI: Kelcy Press, 1999).

10. For straightforward and easy-to-follow guidelines, I use the USDA Food Guide Pyramid children's version and booklet, "Tips for Using the Food Guide Pyramid for Young Children 2 to 6 Years Old," 1999, program aid 1647, and the companion technical report of the research that supports these recommendations (USDA, "Food Guide Pyramid for Young Children 2 to 6 years old: Background and Development, 1999," CNPP-10 [2000], Washington, DC). Another scientifically grounded and "user-friendly" book with excellent detailed suggestions for early childhood feeding is *Feeding Your Child for Lifelong Health*, by nutrition scientist Susan Roberts and pediatrician Melvin Heyman (New York: Bantam, 1999).

11. M. Y. Hood, L. L. Moore, A. Sundarajan-Ramamurti, M. Singer, L. A. Cupples, and R. C. Ellison, "Parental Eating Attitudes and the Development of

Obesity in Children: The Framingham Children's Study," *International Journal of Obesity and Related Metabolic Disorders* 24 (2000): 1319–25.

12. M. Golan, M. Fainaru, and A. Weizman, "Role of Behaviour Modification in the Treatment of Childhood Obesity with the Parents as the Exclusive Agents of Change," *International Journal of Obesity and Related Metabolic Disorders* 22 (1998): 1217–24.

13. M. W. Gillman, S. L. Rifas-Shiman, A. L. Frazier, et al., "Family Dinner and Diet Quality among Older Children and Adolescents," *Archives of Family Medicine* 9 (2000): 235–40.

14. B. Rolls, E. A. Rowe, and E. T. Rolls, "How Sensory Properties of Food Affect Human Feeding Behavior," *Physiology & Behavior* 29 (1982): 409–17.

15. M. A. McCrory, P. J. Fuss, N. P. Hayes, et al., "Overeating in America: Association between Restaurant Food Consumption and Body Fatness in Healthy Adult Men and Women Ages 19 to 80," *Obesity Research* 7 (1999): 564–71.

16. S. Roberts and M. Heyman, *Feeding Your Child for Lifelong Health* (New York: Bantam, 1999).

17. L. L. Birch, L. Gunder, K. Grimm-Thomas, and D. G. Laing, "Infants Consumption of a New Food Enhances Acceptance of Similar Foods," *Appetite* 30 (1998): 283–95.

18. T. N. Robinson, "Reducing Childrens' Television Viewing to Prevent Obesity: A Randomized Trial," *JAMA* 282 (1999): 1561–67.

19. USDA, Food and Nutrition Research Briefs, "TV Eating Up Family Mealtime," Jan 2001, www.ars.gov/is/np/fnrb/fnrb101 (accessed 25 Nov 2002).

20. L. H. Epstein, "Reinforcing Value of Physical Activity as a Determinant of Child Activity Level," *Health Psychology* 18 (1999): 599–603.

21. National Heart, Lung, and Blood Institute, Star Sleeper Campaign, Feb 2001, www.nhlbi.nih.gov/health/public/sleep/starslp/about.htm.

22. M. Sekine, T. Yamagami, and K. Handa, "A Dose-Response Relationship between Short Sleeping Hours and Childhood Obesity: Results of the Toyama Birth Cohort Study," *Child Care, Health and Development* 28, no. 2 (2002): 163–70, and R. Von Kries, A. M. Toschke, H. Wurmser, et al., "Reduced Risk for Overweight and Obesity in 5- and 6-year-old Children by Duration of Sleep—a Cross-sectional Study," *International Journal of Obesity* 26 (2002): 710–16.

23. R. Brooks and S. Goldstein, *Raising Resilient Children* (Chicago: Contemporary Books, 2001).

24. D. Goleman, *Emotional Intelligence* (New York: Bantam, 1995).


7. REACHING AND KEEPING A HEALTHY WEIGHT

1. R. K. Smith, *Jelly Belly* (New York: Bantam Doubleday Dell, 1981), 17.

2. M. Nichter, *Fat Talk: What Girls and Their Parents Say about Dieting* (Cambridge, MA: Harvard University Press, 2000), 181.

3. L. Newman, *Fat Chance* (New York: Putnam and Grosset, 1996), 3–4.

4. W. H. Dietz and L. S. Stern, *American Academy of Pediatrics Guide to Your Child's Nutrition* (New York: Villard, 1999), 131.

5. S. E. Barlow and W. H. Dietz, "Obesity Evaluation and Treatment: Expert Committee Recommendations," *Pediatrics* 102 (1998): e34.

6. DHHS, Public Health Service, National Institutes of Health, "The Practical Guide: Identification, Evaluation, and Treatment of Overweight and Obesity in Adults," NIH pub. 00-4084, Oct 2000, Bethesda, MD.

7. Barlow and Dietz, "Obesity Evaluation," e32.

8. L. H. Epstein, M. D. Myers, H. A. Raynor, and B. E. Saalens, "Treatment of Pediatric Obesity," *Pediatrics* 101 (1998): 554–70.

9. M. Golan, M. Fainaru, and A. Weizman, "Role of Behaviour Modification in the Treatment of Childhood Obesity with the Parents as the Exclusive Agents of Change," *International Journal of Obesity and Related Metabolic Diseases* 22 (1998): 1217–24; M. Golan and A. Weizman, "Familial Approach to the Treatment of Childhood Obesity: Conceptual Model," *Journal of Nutrition Education* 33 (2001): 102–7; Barlow and Dietz, "Obesity Evaluation," e36.

10. F. Pescatore, *Taking the Atkins Program to the Next Generation, Feed Your Kids Well: How to Help Your Child Lose Weight and Get Healthy* (New York: Wiley, 1998).

11. D. M. Bravata, L. Sanders, J. Juang, et al., "Efficacy and Safety of Low-carbohydrate Diets: A Systematic Review," *JAMA* 289 (2003): 1837–46; F. F. Samaha, N. Iqbal, P. Seshadri, et al., "A Low-carbohydrate as Compared with a Low-fat Diet in Severe Obesity," *New England Journal of Medicine* 348 (2003): 2074–81; G. D. Foster, H. R. Wyatt, J. O. Hill, et al., "A Randomized Trial of a Low-carbohydrate Diet for Obesity," *New England Journal of Medicine* 348 (2003): 2082–90.

12. Amazon.com, customer reviews of F. Pescatore, *Feed Your Kids Well* (accessed 23 Aug 2001).

13. S. S. Andrews, M. C. Bethea, L. A. Balart, and H. L. Steward, *Sugar Busters for Kids* (New York: Ballantine, 2001).

14. J. Shaw, *Raising Low-Fat Kids in a High-Fat World* (San Franciso: Chronicle Books, 1997), 27; Amazon.com, customer reviews of J. Shaw, *Raising Low-Fat Kids* (accessed 25 Aug 2001).

15. M. R. Freedman, J. King, and E. Kennedy, "Popular Diets: A Scientific Review," supplement 1, *Obesity Research* 9 (2001): 1S–40S; National Academy of Science, Institute of Medicine, *Dietary Reference Intakes for Energy, Carbohydrate, Fiber, Fat, Fatty Acids, Cholesterol, Protein, and Amino Acids*, Food and Nutrition Board (Washington, DC: National Academy Press, 2002), www.nap.edu/books/0309085373/html.

16. Freedman, King, and Kennedy, "Popular Diets," 35.

17. USDA, "Food Guide Pyramid for Young Children: A Daily Guide for

2- to 6-Year-Olds," available at www.usda.gov/cnpp. The USDA is busy working on a redesign of the pyramid, which was first published in 1992; new guidelines are expected in 2006 (a companion for the *Dietary Guidelines for Americans,* revised by law every five years).

18. My views on commercial programs reflect recommendations of the Expert Committee on Obesity Evaluation and Treatment.

19. M. S. Sothern, H. Schumacher, T. K. von Almen, and T. K. Carlisle, "Committed to Kids: An Integrated, 4-level Team Approach to Weight Management in Adolescents," supplement, *Journal of the American Dietetic Association* 102 (2002): S81; M. S. Sothern, T. K. von Almen, and H. Schumacher, *Trim Kids* (New York: HarperCollins, 2001).

20. L. M. Mellin, L. A. Slinkard, and C. E. Irwin, "Adolescent Obesity Intervention: Validation of the Shapedown Program," *Journal of the American Dietetic Association* 87 (1987): 333–37; L. M. Mellin, L. Dickey, and S. Croughan-Minihane, "Cognitive-emotive Training: Developmental Testing of the Shapedown Method for Adults," *Journal of the American Dietetic Association* 96 (1996): A-31.

21. Shapedown contact, Balboapub@aol.com and www.just-for-kids.org.

22. S. L. Gortmaker, K. Paterson, J. Wiecha, et al., "Reducing Obesity via a School-based Interdisciplinary Intervention among Youth," *Archives of Pediatrics and Adolescent Medicine* 153 (1999): 409–18; L. W. Y. Cheung, S. L. Gortmaker, and H. Dart, *Eat Well & Keep Moving* (Champaign, IL: Human Kinetics, 2001).

23. R. J. Berkowitz and A. J. Stunkard, "Development of Childhood Obesity," in *Handbook of Obesity Treatment,* ed. T. A. Wadden and A. J. Stunkard (New York: Guilford Press, 2002), 532–55.

24. M. Ingrassia, "The Body of the Beholder," *Newsweek,* 24 Apr 1995, 66–67; S. Parker, M. Nichter, and M. Nichter, "Body Image and Weight Concerns among African American and White Adolescent Females: Differences That Make a Difference," *Human Organization* 54 (1995):103–11.

25. G. B. Schreiber, M. Robins, R. Streigel-Moore, E. Obarzanek, J. A. Morrison, and D. J. Wright, "Weight Modification Efforts Reported by Black and White Preadolescent Girls: National Heart, Lung, and Blood Institute Growth and Health Study," *Pediatrics* 98 (1996): 63–71.

26. F. M. Berg, *How to Be Slimmer, Trimmer, and Happier: An Action Plan for Young People with a Step-by-Step Guide to Losing Weight through Positive Living* (Hettinger, ND: Flying Diamond Books, 1983), quote from back cover.

27. F. M. Berg, *Afraid to Eat: Children and Teens in Weight Crisis,* 2d ed. (Hettinger, ND: Healthy Weight Pub Network, 1997), quotes from frontispiece. The 3d edition is *Children and Teens Afraid to Eat: Helping Youth in Today's Weight-obsessed World* (Hettinger, ND: Healthy Weight Pub Network, 2001).

28. G. P. Alleman, *Save Your Child from the Fat Epidemic* (Rocklin, CA: Prima Pub, 1999), 322.

29. B. A. Abramovitz and L. L. Birch, "Five-year-old Girls' Ideas about Dieting Are Predicted by Their Mothers' Dieting," *Journal of the American Dietetic Association* 100 (2000): 1157–63; K. K. Davison and L. L. Birch, "Weight Status, Parent Reaction, and Self-Concept in Five-year-old Girls," *Pediatrics* 107 (2001): 46–53.

30. In her role as the editor of *Healthy Weight Journal,* Berg describes the damage and laments of weight obsession in a review of two books, *A Waist Is a Terrible Thing to Mind* and *That Body Image Thing: Young Women Speak Out* (*Healthy Weight Journal* 15 [2001]: 31–32).

31. Nichter, *Fat Talk,* 189.

32. Ibid., 4.

33. S. S. Hall, "Bully in the Mirror," *New York Times Magazine,* 22 Aug 1999, 33.

34. Schreiber, Robins, Streigel-Moore, et al., "Weight Modification Efforts."

35. Louis Harris and Associates, eds., "The Commonwealth Fund Survey of the Health of Adolescent Girls," in *Facts on Eating Disorders and Exercise* (New York: Commonwealth Fund, 1997).

36. L. J. Neff, R. G. Sargent, R. E. McKeown, et al., "Black-White Differences in Body Size Perceptions and Weight Management Practices among Adolescent Females," *Journal of Adolescent Health* 20 (1997): 459–65.

37. D. Neumark-Sztainer, N. E. Sherwood, T. Coller, and P. J. Hannan, "Primary Prevention of Disordered Eating among Preadolescent Girls: Feasibility and Short-term Effect of a Community-based Intervention," *Journal of the American Dietetic Association* 100 (2000): 1466–73.

38. E. A. Schur, M. Sanders, and H. Steiner, "Body Dissatisfaction and Dieting in Young Children," *International Journal of Eating Disorders* 27 (2000): 74–82.

39. E. Stice, A. Trost, and A. Chase, "Healthy Weight Control and Dissonance-based Eating Disorder Prevention Programs: Results from a Controlled Trial," *International Journal of Eating Disorders* 33 (2003): 10–21.

## 8. SLOWING THE VICIOUS CYCLE OF FAT DISCRIMINATION

1. The term "fat discrimination" is coincident with the rise of the obesity epidemic in America. As in other forms of discrimination—anti-Semitism, racism, or homophobia—the attitudes fomenting it predate the term itself. Central to such attitudes is scapegoating, the perception of individuals as "the Other," with various inherent offensive characteristics of ethnicity, sexual preference, or body size. Fat people are scapegoat victims. And fat fiction written for and about kids consciously tries to communicate the torment its victims feel. In one story from a recent anthology of fiction about fat people by self-described fat authors ( J. Diaz, "The Brief Wondrous Life of Oscar Wao," in *What Are You Looking At?* ed. D. Jarrell and I. Sukrungruang [NewYork: Harcourt, 2003], 22), a fat Do-

minican child realizes his closest friends are embarrassed to associate with him and stands naked before the mirror in excruciating awareness: "The miles of stretch marks! The tumescent horribleness of his proportions! He looked straight out of a Daniel Clowes comic book." After a week of self-torment before the mirror he stops eating altogether, "starving himself dizzy," perpetuating the destructive cycle fed by fat discrimination.

Through art as well as literature, the victims are striking back. Protesting social and parental fat discrimination in the popular musical *Hairspray*, the opening number sets the tone: "Mamma, I'm a big girl now." Films are more emphatic. In *Camp* a girl arrives at camp with her jaw wired shut, an extreme weight reduction treatment arranged by her father. And *Fat Girl*, a dark French comedy, portrays an adolescent fat girl fantasizing the murder of her slim sister and nagging mother. On the scholarly front, see C. S. Crandall and K. L. Schiffhauer, "Anti-Fat Prejudice: Beliefs, Values, and American Culture," *Obesity Research* 6 (1998): 458–60; also M. E. Eisenberg, "Adolescents Teased about Their Weight May Be More Likely to Report Suicidal Thoughts and Suicide Attempts," *Archives of Pediatrics and Adolescent Medicine* 157 (2003): 733–38.

2. M. B. Schwartz, H. O. Chambliss, K. D. Brownell, S. N. Blair, and C. Billington, "Weight Bias among Health Professionals Specializing in Obesity," *Obesity Research* 11 (2003): 1033–39.

3. J. Blume, *Blubber* (New York: Bantam Doubleday Dell, 1974).

4. S. A. Richardson, A. H. Hastorf, N. Goodman, and S. M. Dornbusch, "Cultural Uniformity in Reaction to Physical Disabilities," *American Sociological Review* 90 (1961): 44–51.

5. N. Campbell, "Weighed Down," *Daily Californian*, 16 May 1995, 9.

6. J. D. Turnbull, S. Heaslip, and H. A. McLeod, "Pre-school Children's Attitudes to Fat and Normal Male and Female Stimulus Figures," *International Journal of Obesity and Related Metabolic Disorders* 24 (2000): 1705–6.

7. J. D. Latner and A. J. Stunkard, "Getting Worse: The Stigmatization of Obese Children," *Obesity Research* 11 (2003): 452–56.

8. S. Hesse-Biber, *Am I Thin Enough Yet? The Cult of Thinness and the Commercialization of Identity* (New York: Oxford University Press, 1996).

9. S. Bordo, *Unbearable Weight: Feminism, Western Culture, and the Body* (Berkeley: University of California Press, 1993), 202.

10. W. Wright, *Born That Way: Genes, Behavior, Personality* (New York: Routledge, 1999), 257–58.

11. W. Pollack, *Real Boys* (New York: Henry Holt, 1999); and *Real Boys' Voices* (New York: Random House, 2000), 108.

12. DHHS, Public Health Service, National Institutes of Health, "The Practical Guide: Identification, Evaluation, and Treatment of Overweight and Obesity in Adults," NIH pub. 00-4084, Oct 2000, Bethesda, MD.

13. J. Cloud, "Just a Routine School Shooting," *Time,* 31 May 1999, 33–43.

14. M. Faith, M. A. Leone, A. Pietrobelli, et al., "Weight-Teasing during Physical Activity: Associations with Reported Physical Activity Attitudes and Levels in a Pediatric Sample" (program and abstracts from the conference "Childhood Obesity: Partnerships for Research and Prevention," 3–5 May 1999, Atlanta, GA), 48.

15. "One Size Definitely Does Not Fit All," *New York Times,* 22 Jun 2003, C1.

16. Coles's 5-vol. work *Children of Crisis* dates from 1967 to 1977 and two others, *The Moral Life of Children* and *The Political Life of Children,* from 1986.

17. M. Miedzian, *Boys Will Be Boys: Breaking the Link between Masculinity and Violence* (New York: Anchor, 1991).

18. S. S. Hall, "Bully in the Mirror," *New York Times Magazine,* 22 Aug 1999, 32

19. C. L. Williams and S. Y. Kimm, *Prevention and Treatment of Childhood Obesity,* Annals of the New York Academy of Sciences, no. 699 (New York, 1993).

20. S. Solovay, *Tipping the Scales of Justice: Fighting Weight-based Discrimination* (Amherst, NY: Prometheus Books, 2000), 44.

21. J. K. Rowling, *Harry Potter and the Sorcerer's Stone* (New York: Scholastic Press, 1997), 1, 21.

22. J. K. Rowling, *Harry Potter and the Goblet of Fire* (New York: Scholastic Press, 2000), 25, 27, 32.

23. J. K. Rowling, *Harry Potter and the Order of the Phoenix* (New York: Scholastic Press, 2003); 1–10, 13–21.

24. W. Golding, *Lord of the Flies* (New York: Putnam, 1954), 87.

25. R. M. Lipsyte, *One Fat Summer* (New York: Harper Trophy, 1977), 126–31.

26. L. Fitzhugh, *Nobody's Family Is Going to Change* (New York: Farrar, Straus and Giroux, 1974), 55, 174–75.

27. Ibid., 55.

28. S. A. Hewlett and C. West, *The War Against Parents* (New York: Houghton Mifflin, 1998).

29. "How to Talk to Teenage Girls about Weight? Very Carefully," *New York Times,* 22 Jun 2003, C3.

30. T. Berry Brazelton, *Touchpoints 3 to 6: Your Child's Emotional and Behavioral Development* (Cambridge, MA: Perseus, 2001), 374–78.

31. Benjamin Hoff, *The Tao of Pooh* (New York: Penguin Books, 1983).

32. Barthe DeClements, *Nothing's Fair in Fifth Grade* (New York: Puffin, 1981), 49.

33. Sapphire, *Push* (New York: Vintage, 1996).

34. S. Shreve, "Writers on Writing," *New York Times,* 27 Aug 2001, E2.

35. Bennett, *Life in the Fat Lane,* 213.

36. J. Telushkin, *Words That Hurt, Words That Heal* (New York: William Morrow, 1996), 185.

## 9. MOBILIZING TO HELP OUR OVERWEIGHT CHILDREN

1. C. Stockmyer, S. Kuester, D. Ramsey, and W. H. Dietz, "Results of the Obesity Discussion Groups, National Nutrition Summit, 30 May 2000," supplement 2, *Obesity Research* 9 (2001): 41S–52S.

2. Surgeon General's office press release 13 Dec 2001, available at www .surgeongeneral.gov/news/pressreleases/pr_obesity.htm.

3. DHHS, *The Surgeon General's Call to Action to Prevent and Decrease Overweight and Obesity* (Rockville, MD, 2001); also www.surgeongeneral.gov/sgoffice.

4. Partnership to Promote Healthy Eating and Active Living, "Summit on Promoting Healthy Eating and Active Living: Developing a Framework for Progress," *Nutrition Reviews* 59, no. 3, pt. 2 (2001): 1–66.

5. J. O. Hill, J. P. Goldberg, R. R. Pate, and J. C. Peters, introduction to summit, "Promoting Healthy Eating and Active Living," *Nutrition Reviews* 59, no. 3 (2001): S5.

6. B. Yeoman, "Unhappy Meals," *Mother Jones,* Jan–Feb 2003, 81.

7. M. Story, "School-based Approaches for Preventing and Treating Obesity," supplement 2, *International Journal of Obesity* 23 (1999): S49.

8. "Junk Food Jitters," *New York Times,* 24 May 2002, A24.

9. M. Uhlman, "Vending at Schools: Both Sides Eye Change," *Philadelphia Inquirer,* 9 Jun 2003, C01; K. L. A. Severson, "Schools to Stop Soda Sales; District Takes Cue from Oakland Ban," *San Francisco Chronicle,* 28 Aug 2002, A1; and S. C. Friedman, "Sour on Sweets: Come September, Vending Machines in the City's 1,200 Public Schools Will Not Stock Soda, Gum, Candy," *New York Post,* 25 Jun 2003, 1.

10. D. Barboza, "A Warning in Expanding Waistlines; Food Makers Trim Fat as Lawsuits and New Regulations Loom," *New York Times,* 10 Jul 2003, C1, C3.

11. Editorial, *San Francisco Chronicle,* 29 Jun 2003, D5.

12. Pew Charitable Trusts, "Project 540: Students Turn for a Change, High School Students Nationwide Speak Out on Issues That Matter Most to Them," news release 28 Apr 2003, www.project540.org.

13. R. J. Trissler, "Food for Thought: New Directions for School Foodservice," *Journal of the American Dietetic Association* 100, no. 9 (2000): 997.

14. E. Becker and M. Burros, "Eat Your Vegetables? Only at a Few Schools," *New York Times,* 13 Jan 2003, A1, A14.

15. E. Lau, "Childhood Obesity Prevention in the Schools" (presentation at childhood obesity conference, "Making an Impact Now: Environmental, Family and Clinical Approaches," 6–8 Jan 2003, San Diego, CA).

16. J. Schwartz, "Is Recess On the Way Out?" *Offspring*, January 2001, 65–66.

17. International Life Sciences Institute, *Take Ten!* (Atlanta, GA, 1999); see also www.ilsi.org/activities; and T. Peregrin, "Take 10! Classroom-based Program Fights Obesity by Getting Kids Out of Their Seats," *Journal of the American Dietetic Association* 101 (2001): 1409.

18. C. B. Corbin and R. P. Pangrazi, *Physical Activity for Children: A Statement of Guidelines* (Reston, VA: National Association for Sport and Physical Education, 1998).

19. DHHS and U.S. Department of Education, "Promoting Better Health for Young People through Physical Activity and Sports: A Report to the President from the Secretary of Health and Human Services and the Secretary of Education," Dec 2000 (available from CDC at Healthy Youth, Box 8817, Silver Spring, MD 20907; www.cdc.gov/nccdphp/dash/presphysactrpt).

20. U.S. Department of Transportation, *Nationwide Personal Transportation Survey* (Lanham, MD, 1997); CDC, Division of Nutrition and Physical Activity, "Kidswalk-to-School: A Guide to Promote Walking to School," call 888-CDC-4NRG (Atlanta, GA, 2000); www.cdc.gov/nccdphp/dnpa/kidswalk.

21. The Fitnessgram is an assessment protocol created by the Cooper Institute, Dallas, TX, that measures a number of health-related aspects of a child's fitness in a multitest format. A score within the Healthy Fitness Zone indicates the person has the minimum level of fitness related to the specific test thought to provide some protection from health risks (www.humankinetics.com).

22. S. L. Gortmaker, K. Paterson, J. Wiecha, et al., "Reducing Obesity via a School-based Interdisciplinary Intervention among Youth," *Archives of Pediatrics and Adolescent Medicine* 153 (1999): 409–18. The program (first called "Planet Health") was implemented and evaluated for two years in a group of 1,300 ethnically diverse fourth- and fifth-grade students. A program guide and CD are available from Eat Well and Keep Moving, www.humankinetics.com. See also A. D. Fly and D. L. Gallahue, "Nutrition Education in the Physical Education Curriculum: Keeping the Culture with Food Pyramids, 2001," available from the Department of Applied Health Science and Kinesiology, Indiana University, Bloomington, IN, 47405. Also M. C. Burk, *Station Games, Fun and Imaginative PE Lessons* (Champaign, IL: Human Kinetics, 2002).

23. There is evidence that students who participate in service learning demonstrate improved ability to communicate, collaborate, work in teams to solve problems, and apply critical thinking skills (E. Zlotkowski, *Successful Service-Learning Programs* [Bolton, MA: Anker, 1998]). An added bonus is strong evidence that kids who develop a commitment to volunteerism (in service learning projects) are involved in significantly less binge drinking in high school and later on in college (E. Weitzman and I. Kawachi, "Giving Means Receiving: The Protective Effect of Social Capital on Binge Drinking on College Campuses," *American Journal of Public Health* 90 [2000]: 1936–39).

24. L. Belkin, "Watching Her Weight," *New York Times Magazine*, 8 Jul 2001, 30–33.

25. Z. Vahabzadeh, I. Schurmann, and D. l'Allemand, "Families of Obese Children: Problems and Needs," abstract no. 51, supplement, *International Journal of Obesity* 22 (1998).

26. K. Resnicow, A. Yaroch, A. Davis, et al., "Go Girls! Community-based Nutrition and Physical Activity Program for Overweight African-American Girls," *Journal of Nutrition Education* 31 (1999): 283C.

27. S. R. Johnson and L. M. Mellin, *Just for Kids!* (San Anselmo, CA: Balboa, 2001).

28. Channel Thirteen/WNET, *Who's Dancin' Now?* (New York: Educational Broadcasting Corp, 1999); also R. Pogrebin, "With a Push and Nudge, Young Dancers Gain Confidence," *New York Times,* 19 Jun 2001, E1, E5.

29. D. Engwicht, *Street Reclaiming: Creating Livable Streets and Vibrant Communities* (Gabriola Island, BC: New Society, 1999).

30. D. Burden, quoted in N. Macaluso, "Link Between Health and Sprawl Makes 'Smart' Growth Look Smarter," The Shape We're In, www.shapenews.com.

31. F. Bruni, "Bush Emphasizes Teaching of Values to Children," *New York Times,* 15 Aug 2001, A21.

32. J. Wisloski, "A Lake Still Beckons, But How About Those Sales? *New York Times,* 10 Aug 2003, M29.

33. B. H. Lin and R. M. Morrison, "Higher Fruit Consumption Linked with Lower Body Mass Index," *Food Review* 25, no. 3 (2002): 28–32.

34. R. J. Sokol, "The Chronic Disease of Childhood Obesity: The Sleeping Giant Has Awakened," *Journal of Pediatrics* 136 (2000): 712.

35. American Academy of Pediatrics, Committee on Nutrition, "Policy Statement: Prevention of Pediatric Overweight and Obesity," *Pediatrics* 112, no. 2 (2003): 424–30; R. Winslow, "Heart Disease Hits the Preschool Set: New Research Shows Warning Signs Begin in Early Childhood," *Wall Street Journal,* 18 Mar 2003, D1, D4.

36. M. Jacobson, quoted in L. Tanner, "Children Should Have Routine Body-Mass Checks to Prevent Obesity, Doctors Say," *Gettysburg Times,* 2 Aug 2003, A7.

37. A. Pipi, "Get Active about Physical Activity: Ask, Advise, Assist—Get Your Patients Moving," *Canadian Family Physician/Médecin de famille canadien* 48 (2002): 13–14, 21–23.

38. S. Branch, "Is Food the Next Tobacco?" *Wall Street Journal,* 13 Jun 2002, B1, B9; R. L. Rundle, "Soft-Drink Makers Say Sin-Tax Plan Is Hard to Swallow," *Wall Street Journal,* 12 Apr 2002, A17.

39. Branch, "Is Food," B9.

40. Barboza, "Expanding Waistlines."

41. W. Willett, quoted in D. Barboza, "If You Pitch It, They Will Eat; Barrage of Food Ads Takes Aim at Children," *New York Times,* 3 Aug 2003, B3, B11.

42. S. Y. Chou, H. Saffer, and M. Grossman, "An Economic Analysis of Obesity" (National Bureau of Economic Research paper no. 9247, Feb 2002), cited in D. Akst, "Belt-loosening in the Work Force," *New York Times,* 2 Mar 2002, sec. 3, p. 4.

43. *5 a Day News* [newsletter of Produce for Better Health Foundation, a founding member of National Cancer Institute's "5 a Day Program"] 2, no. 1 (2000): 3.

44. Associated Press, "Frist, Bingaman and Dodd Introduce Bill to Reduce Obesity," www.A.P.com, 4 Jun 2003.

45. Center for Consumer Freedom, www.consumerfreedom.com (accessed 20 Aug 2003).

46. M. Nestle, *Food Politics: How the Food Industry Influences Nutrition and Health* (Berkeley: University of California Press, 2002), 370.

47. S. Ahmed, "Time for a Twinkie Tax?" *US New & World Report,* 1 Jul 1998, 62–63.

48. M. F. Jacobson and K. D. Brownell, "Small Taxes on Soft Drinks and Snack Food to Promote Health," *American Journal of Public Health* 90 (2000): 854–57.

49. R. H. Frank, *Luxury Fever: Why Money Fails to Satisfy in an Era of Excess* (New York: Free Press, 1999), 277.

50. Harvard Forums on Public Health, "Public Split on Government Role in Addressing Adult Obesity; Childhood Obesity Is a Different Story," press release, www.phsi.harvard.edu (accessed 12 Jun 2003).

51. Center for Science in the Public Interest, www.cspinet.org/policy (accessed 8 Aug 2003).

52. S. Vranica, "Advertising: Critics Fault Antiobesity Ads as Not Reaching Far Enough," *Wall Street Journal,* 11 Apr 2003, B6.

53. Associated Press, "IRS Clarifies Weight Loss Tax Breaks," www.A.P.com, 28 Jul 2003.

54. C. Guthrie, "Childhood Lies Dying," *British Medical Journal* 322 (2001): 315.

55. American Health Foundation, Weight Watchers, "Getting Kids to Eat Well and Be Active" (New York, 2001).

# ACKNOWLEDGMENTS

To start, I credit my education, informal and formal. It marked my path to *Our Overweight Children*. My parents, committed community leaders in the small Idaho town where I grew up, encouraged my first cooking efforts. I learned all kinds of skills in 4-H projects and earned many blue ribbons at the Idaho State Fair with their support. My big sister, Jane, was a superb role model.

Armed with an H. J. Heinz scholarship I traveled "East" to study home economics at Iowa State University. Then for nearly four decades home economics went into a sort of "academic exile." In graduate school I studied nutrition, the status of which was rising. Both disciplines prepared me well. The importance of home economics resurfaced in an article by Jennifer Grossman, the director of the Dole Nutrition Institute (*New York Times*, 2 Sep 2003). "Want to combat the epidemic of obesity? Bring back home economics . . . teaching basic nutrition and food preparation is a far less radical remedy than gastric bypass surgery or fast-food lawsuits. And probably far more effective." Grossman cites a major finding of the U.S. Department of Education: "Since 1962, home economics has moved from the mainstream to the margins of American high school," with a dramatic decline of 67 percent. The loss of this "near universal" training, she claims, means that men and women now lack the basic domestic skills to meet "the exigencies of everyday life." I imagine my former professors at Iowa State would greet such daily domestic ignorance with incredulity. The skill and talent that go into preparing and coordinating a decent family dinner assume even greater value today. I salute especially Ersel Eppright, Margaret McKinley, and Helen leBaron.

My graduate study of obesity in low-income minority groups helped me recognize the many forces that affect food choices and the behaviors surrounding these choices. Myrtle Brown and Miriam Brush guided me well. Margaret Simko and Ruth Linke encouraged further study of "why people eat what they eat."

My students deserve high marks as teachers—I learned so much from them, here and abroad. I was inspired by extraordinary women in Nepal, during my first teaching efforts in villages. As a Fulbright scholar in Nepal years later I worked with women and men who viewed village development as much more than building roads. I learned the true meaning of their collective mantra, "It takes a village."

Sometimes fiction makes truisms compelling, so I have devoted a chapter in this book to children's literature as a guide to understanding the obesity epidemic's cost in discrimination from peers and parents. For this topic, I acknowledge the indispensable suggestions of Beth Puffer, manager of the Bank Street Bookstore in New York; the advocacy and passion of Joanne Ikeda, the Center for Weight and Health, University of California, Berkeley; the dramatic public performances and personal comments of Gareth White; and the many children, in fact and fiction, who sensitized me to the pain of fat discrimination.

During the journey of writing *Our Overweight Children* my special thanks and gratitude go to:

Marion Nestle for suggesting I undertake this project and supporting it along the way;

Stanley Holwitz for asking me in the first place and sticking with me to the final place;

Dore Brown who quietly cajoled and changed timelines while deftly uniting the pieces to become whole;

Sarah Lavender Smith for expertly coaching me and reworking my technical writing in a way that captured my voice and made it more accessible for readers;

Edith Gladstone for her incredible command of English grammar, her humor and grace when applying it to my writing;

Betsy Thorpe for adding clarity to my early manuscript;

Jenny Berg and Amy Bentley, mothers and colleagues, for reading and responding to my first draft;

All my colleagues for suppressing their disbelief that the project took "so long";

My students for their questions, interviews with child caretakers, and observations;

Fred Tripp for supplying me with news reports;

Kyle Shadix for sending constant e-mail updates;

Sheldon Watts for computer coaching;

Keith Ayoob for his reinforcement of my long-held principle "Six-year-old fat kids don't need a diet; they should eat like six-year-olds, not 6 foot football players";

All the children and their caretakers I have known and worked with for decades;

Mia, Hadley, and Sierra, my granddaughters, who refresh my child-care skills and make the challenges of raising kids in the twenty-first century crystal clear to me;

My sons, Kevin and Shaun, who taught me first and most of what I know about raising resilient children, along with their spouses, Tracy and Tammy, who manage the daily blend of careers and parenting with amazing grace;

And then—first as well as last—Dennis Dalton, DD to his many young friends and admirers. This book is dedicated to him.

# INDEX

ABCs (antecedents, behavior, and consequences), 154
activity. *See* physical activity
adiposity rebound, 19–20
Administration for Children and Families,
105–106
adolescents: diet report cards of, 113; fast
eating by, 81; fat consumption by, 59;
latchkey, 109; perception of weight
by, 24; physical education (PE) and,
107, 207–208; recommended levels of
physical activity, 207–208; resiliency
and, 142–144; sports participation
and, 108; statistics on, 30, 31–34;
sugar consumption by, 58–59; TV/
video/computer time, 86; tracking
into overweight adults, 35; voluntary/
spontaneous activity and, 52–53;
working jobs, 108. *See also* early childhood; infants; middle childhood
adults: emotional eating and, 85; overweight children becoming, 35; statistics on, 29. *See also* parental obesity
advertising: annual budget for, 101, 229;
content of, 8/; food as most heavily
advertised commodity, 229; govern-

ment standards for, 224, 227, 229–
230; public health campaign, 229–
230; recommended changes to, 223,
224, 227; research showing sensitivity
to, 201; statistics of exposure to, 86,
87, 101; student expenditures and,
101; voluntary improvements in, 222.
*See also* food industry; marketplace;
media; television
*Afraid to Eat: Children and Teens in Weight
Crisis* (Berg), 171
African Americans: advertisements and,
101; body size diversity and, 24, 170,
182; in children's fiction, 192, 193, 195,
197; diabetes and, 37; dieting and,
170, 174; fear of crime and, 56; fitness
levels of, 107; low-birth-weight/
obesity and, 70; parenting styles of,
78–79; physical activity and, 88, 182–
183; role modeling of, 262n6; socioeconomic status and, 55; statistics of,
31, 33–34; vegetable consumption of,
112. *See also* cultural differences
after-school activities, 108–109, 135, 211,
214–215. *See also* sports and athletics
age-appropriate eating, 148–151

aging, obesity and, 5
agribusiness, 105
Alabama, 104, 204
alcohol use, 41
Alleman, Gayle, 171
*Amazing Grace* (Kozol), 184
d'Amboise, Jacques, 215
American Academy of Pediatrics, 149, 152–153, 165, 219
American Association for a Child's Right to Play, 106
American College of Obstetricians and Gynecologists, 69
American Dietetic Association, 25
American Indians. *See* Native Americans
American Obesity Association, 25
America on the Move, 221
anorexia nervosa. *See* eating disorders
antecedents, behavior, and consequences (ABCs), 154
Aristotle, 7
Asia, 4–5, 32–33
Asian Americans: body image, 24; statistics of, 33. *See also* cultural differences
assortative mating, 49
asthma, 39
Atkins, Robert, 155
Atkins diets, 155–157, 160
Atkins Nutritionals, 155
authoritarian parenting style, 78–80, 105, 122, 124
authoritative parenting style, 78–80, 121–122; caregivers and, 106; control and structure provided through, 122–125, 167; raising resilient children, 137–144; theory/practice of, 125–137
autonomy, need for, 121

babies. *See* infants
balance. *See* moderation
Ballantyne, R. M., 190
Baltimore, MD, 210
Barbie dolls, 224
Bardet-Biedl syndrome, 26, 51
beauty ideal, 169–173, 174, 175
behavior, changing: environment as intrinsic to, 201; weight management and, 152. *See also* environment

behavior modeling. *See* modeling behavior
Belgium, 33
Bennett, Cherie, 53, 191, 195, 198
Berg, Frances M., 171, 172–173
bias. *See* discrimination; stigmatization
bicycling, 108, 208, 216
binging/purging, 173–175. *See also* eating disorders; eating dysfunctions
birthday parties, 136, 212
blame: moving beyond, 201, 230; of parents, 7, 59–60, 93; of working women, 225
blended-family households, 62
*Blubber* (Blume), 177, 178–179, 191, 192, 195
Blume, Judy, 177, 178–179, 191, 192, 195
Blumenthal, David, 228–229
BMI. *See* body-mass index
body image: beauty ideal and, 169–173, 174, 175; preoccupation with, 147–148, 183–184
body-mass index (BMI): adiposity (fat-gain) rebound and, 19–20; adult standards, 17; age as factor in, 17, 241; "average" growth and, 16; birth weight and later imbalance of, 69–70; calculation of, 16–17; cautions in use of, 20–21; charts for, 239–241; infant weight gain rate and, 19–20; rate of weight/height growth, 20–21; terminology and, 14–15
body shape, genetics and, 47, 48
body size: acceptance of, and fitness, 183–184; beauty ideal and, 169–173, 174, 175; cultural differences in acceptance of, 22, 24, 170, 180, 182; diversity programs and, 174; fat acceptance movement, 173, 175; literature analyzing thinness ideal, 169–170, 180; messages about, 178, 198; parental perception of, 22–24; preoccupation with, 147–148, 173–175; self-perception of, 24
Bone, Ian, 192, 195
Bordo, Susan, 180
*Born That Way: Genes, Behavior, Personality* (Wright), 180
bottle-feeding vs. breast-feeding, 72–74, 220

community environment: after-school activities and, 108–109, 135, 211, 214–215; camp programs, 217; food choices and, 109–110, 218; food programs, 218; health provider intervention, 218–221; parks, 109, 135, 214; priority of children's health in, 168; recommendations for action, 213–221; resilient children and, 139; streets, reclaiming, 215–216; surgeon general's statement on, 200; urban planning, 216, 231; volunteerism, 214; youth programs, 214–215, 217. *See also* family environment; schools

compassion, development of, 142–143

competence, 141, 143

computer/video games: amount of time spent on, 57, 86, 87; reducing time spent on, 135–136; as risk factor, 54. *See also* television

*Continuing Survey of Food Intakes by Individuals*, 111–112

control and structure, appropriate, 122–125. *See also* authoritative parenting

Cooper, Kenneth H., 165, 222

*Coral Island, The* (Ballantyne), 190

corn syrup, 111

costs. *See* economics

crime, and time spent indoors, 45, 56, 109

Crutcher, Chris, 191, 195

cultural differences: advertising targeted to, 101; binging/purging and, 174; body size acceptance and, 22, 24, 170, 180, 182; diabetes and, 37; dieting and, 170, 174; parenting style and, 78–79; socioeconomic status and; statistics of, 30–34; vegetable consumption and, 112

Cunningham, Marion, 81

Czech Republic, 73

Damiani, Charles, 100

dance, 215

Danziger, Paula, 191, 195, 196–197

day care, 105–106. *See also* early childhood; Head Start

DeClements, Barthe, 186, 191, 195, 197

depression, 5, 22

dessert: moderation guidelines for, 124–125, 133; withholding of not recommended, 132

developing countries. *See* world health

diabetes, 36–38, 71, 249n23

Dickens, Charles, 187

diet: rating of children's, 6–7, 111–113; as term, 148. *See also* dieting

dietary guidelines. *See* Food Guide Pyramid and dietary guidelines

diet industry: ethics and, 155; low-carb vs. low-fat debate, 155–160; plans compared, 155–160; prohibitions in, 157; self-esteem and, 41. *See also* food industry; marketplace

dieting: beauty ideal and, 169–173, 174, 175; cultural differences in, 170, 174; eating disorders and, 169, 171, 173–175; frequently asked questions about, 148–154; health issues and, 149; as modeled behavior, 123; negative consequences of, 169, 171–176; obsessive, 169–175, 180, 183; parental dieting, effect of, 172; pregnancy and, 70–71; restrictive diets, failure of, 148; self-esteem and, 146–147, 172, 175; societal messages and, 169–170, 171–172, 174–176; statistics on, 23; young children, not recommended for, 148–149; yo-yo (weight cycling), 41, 50. *See also* body size; diet plans; treatment; weight management

diet plans: family-oriented, 157–160; low-carb vs. low-fat debate, 155–160; obstacles to success with, 160–164; relative success rates, 156; restrictions as failure in, 157; shift to lifestyle programs, 170–172; USDA evaluation of, 160–161. *See also* weight management

Dietz, William, 3, 40

discipline, 143–144

discrimination: acceptability of, 180, 184; beauty ideal and, 172–173; comedy and, 180; fat acceptance and, 25; fiction portraying (*see* literature, children's); by medical personnel, 178; morality and, 180; as overlooked

dimension, 177–178, 184–185; overview of, 266–267n1; parenting and,
178, 182; prevention and alleviation
of, 185–186, 197–199, 232; research
illustrating, 117, 179–180; responses
to, 141; as scapegoating, 180–181,
266n1; stereotyping and, 177–178;
teaching tolerance, 196–198; vicious
cycle of, 178–184. *See also* bullying;
self-esteem problems; sensitivity;
stigmatization
disease, controversy over obesity as, 25,
230. *See also* health consequences
diversity. *See* body size
*Dr. Atkins' Diet Revolution* (Atkins), 155–
156
*Dr. Atkins' New Diet Revolution* (Atkins),
155–156
drug industry, 50, 120, 172
Dwayne. *See* case stories
dysfunctional eating, 171, 177–178, 182.
*See also* eating disorders

early childhood: BMI and, 245n7; consis-
tency of messages in, 122; dieting not
recommended during, 148–149; diet
report card of, 113; energy balance
and, 53; fat discrimination in, 179–
180; meal preparation by children
during, 130; and obesity awareness,
14; portion size and, 82; prevention
as beginning in, 121; spontaneous
activity and, 52; statistics on, 29, 31,
32; sugar consumption in, 58–59;
taste-preference development during,
74, 76–77, 132; television and, 86, 87.
*See also* adolescents; infants; middle
childhood
early maturation, 39–40
eating disorders: connection to dieting,
169, 171, 173–175; literature of, 184;
prevalence of, 173; reading aloud and
counseling about, 193
eating dysfunctions, 171, 177–178, 182
eating patterns: bullying and, 182; daily
diet as, 148; dysfunctional eating, 171;
factors influencing, 75–77; infants
and, 49, 72–75; as risk factor, 54. *See*

*also* eating disorders; eating dysfunctions; family meals; snacking
*Eating Well* magazine, 111
Eat Well and Keep Moving, 167–168, 210
economics: of diabetes, 38; fast-food
restaurants and, 225; of food industry
and obesity rates, 222; of processed
meals, 83; rising costs of epidemic,
3, 201; schools and junk-food sales,
98, 99, 100, 102; of treatment vs.
prevention, 226. *See also* marketplace
ectomorphs, 47, 48
Eddie. *See* case stories
education: fatter public in spite of, 201–
202; individualization of, 151; level
of, and obesity, 22–23, 33, 54; national
campaign for, 230–233; ongoing
coaching needed, 220–221. *See also*
environment; schools
elementary school-age children. *See* middle
childhood; schools
emotional eating, 84–85, 127, 138, 182, 214
emotional intelligence, 140. *See also*
psychological health
empathy, 139–140, 197–198
endocrine causes, 26
endomorphs, 47, 48
energy balance: genetics and, 52–53;
pregnancy and "feed forward"
effect, 71–72; small fluctuations
affecting, 53
energy bars, 156
England. *See* Great Britain
Engwicht, David, 215–216
environment: behavior patterns sensitive
to, 201; risk factors in, 53–56; "toxic,"
55–56, 138, 139. *See also* family meals;
parental obesity; parenting styles;
physical activity, lack of; socioeconomic status; television
ethic of care, 210–211
ethics, medical, 155
ethnic cuisines, 131
ethnicity. *See* cultural differences; *specific
groups*
Europe, 33
Expert Committee on Obesity Evaluation
and Treatment, 152–153

family environment: case story examples of, 62–67; division of responsibility in child feeding, 123–124, 130; emotional eating, 84–85, 127; meeting, weekly, 143; moderation and role of, 7, 126–127; nature/nurture dynamic and, 49; nontraditional, 62; obstacles to healthy eating and, 88; overview of, 61–62; reading aloud/storytelling, 193–194, 196; skills-learning vs. advice and, 220–221; taste preferences learned in, 75–77; voluntary/spontaneous activity and, 52–53; weight management support in, 151–152, 154, 166–169. *See also* family meals; genetics; parenting

family meals: breakfast, 95, 130, 131; cost vs. convenience and, 83; as endangered, 80–82; interruptions of, 142; as recommendation, 125, 129; processed meals, 82–84; refused foods, handling of, 124, 130; speed of eating, 81–82, 122, 127; staying at table, 130; theory/practice of, 129–131. *See also* eating patterns; family environment

family meetings, 143

famine, and obesity rate, 70

farmers' markets, 218, 221, 231

*Fast Food Nation* (Schlosser), 95–96

fast-food restaurants: advertising by, 87, 224; choice management and, 129–130, 223; frequency of meals at, 94–95; menu improvement by, 96–97, 223–224; moderation guidelines for consumers at, 123–124; nutrition/calorie content of food, 95; playgrounds and other enticements, 95–96; portions (*see* portions); proposed national campaign and, 231, 232; school lunch improvements vs., 204, 205; speed of eating and, 224; statistics of obesity rise from, 225; suits against, 92–93, 96, 222, 223; upscale development of, 224; working mothers and, 225. *See also* food industry; soft drinks

fat, as term, 15

fat acceptance movement, 173, 175

*Fat Boy Saves the World* (Bone), 192, 195

fat cells, infancy and, 74

*Fat Chance* (Newman), 147, 191, 195

fat discrimination. *See* discrimination

fat-free foods, 155

fats: consumption statistics, 59; debate on balance in diet, 155–160; recommended amounts, 159; table of types and recommendations, 158–159

*Fat Talk: What Girls and Their Parents Say* (Nichter), 147, 173

"feed forward" effect, 72

*Feeding Your Child for Lifelong Health* (Roberts and Heyman), 130

feminism, 170

fiction. *See* literature, children's

fidget factor, 52–53

*Fit Kids: Getting Kids Hooked on Fitness Fun!* (Laderer), 165

*Fit Kids: The Complete Shape-Up Program from Birth through High School* (Cooper et al.), 165

fitness: body acceptance and increase in, 183; declining levels of, 107, 108; as health indicator, vs. BMI, 209; recommendations for, 164–165. *See also* physical activity

Fitnessgram, 209, 270n21

Fitzhugh, Louise, 191, 192, 193, 195

flavor bridge, 74

food. *See* family meals; fast-food restaurants; portions; school meal programs; taste preferences; variety of food

Food Guide Pyramid and dietary guidelines: alternative versions of, 163; Atkins diet vs., 156; children's, 161, 162, 163, 262n10; confusion over, 155; diet plans evaluated in light of, 160–161; juice consumption and, 74–75; pregnancy and, 68–69; reality compared to, 56–59, 111–113, 132; serving sizes recommended, 162–163; "servings" vs. "portions," 57–58, 128, 162–163; vegetables and fruits in, 131–132; weight management and use of, 149, 150

food industry: annual per capita calorie

production, 94; consumer pressure on, 222; fat content of meals, 59; government regulation of, 222; healthier choices from, 96–97; portion size (*see* portions); promotions by, 224; proposed national campaign and, 231–232; recommendations for action, 222–225; research supported by, 201; sales figures, 95; school lunches and, 103–104, 203; school vending machines and, 98, 99–101; statistics on away-from-home meals, 94–95; strategies to effect change in, 225; suits against, 92–93, 96, 222, 223; voluntary change by, 222. *See also* advertising; fast-food restaurants

*Food Politics* (Nestle), 87, 227

Forster, Thomas, 104

Forward, Toby, 191, 195

Frank, Robert, 228

"Freeze My TV," 168, 210

Fresh Air Fund, 217

Friendly Town program, 217

friendship: body size and, 24, 179; play activity and, 165; reduction of television and, 135, 136

fruits and vegetables: Atkins diet restricting, 156, 157; availability of, 109–110, 218; consumption rates, 111–112; farmers' markets, 218; home delivery, 218; juice drinking, 59, 74–75, 112; modeling behavior to enjoy, 106, 132; recommendations to increase consumption, 131–133; repeated exposure to, 124, 132–133; school lunch programs and, 104, 204–206; subsidizing of, 218, 227, 231; tasting ceremony, 133; weight lowering through consumption of, 218

fullness, feeling of. *See* satiety

"FunFit" events, 214

Gaines, Isabel, 196

gall bladder problems, 36

Gandhi, Mahatma, 144

Gartner, Lawrence, 73

gay-parent households, 62

gender differences: BMI differences and, 17;

body size preoccupation and, 173; physical activity and, 107; school-based weight management programs and, 168; self-esteem and, 13; soda consumption and, 110

genetics: asthma and, 39; in causes of obesity, 26, 46–53; fidget factor, 52–53. *See also* environment

genotypes: defined, 47; thrifty, 47–49, 70

gestational diabetes, 71

"Getting Kids to Eat Well and Be Active" (Weight Watchers), 236

"Getting Worse: The Stigmatization of Obese Children" (Latner and Stunkard), 179–180

Gilligan, Carol, 210–211

globalization, 4–5, 32–33

Go Girls!, 214

Golding, William, 187, 190–191, 194, 195

Goldstein, Sam, 137–144

Goleman, Daniel, 140

Gortmaker, Steven, 167–168

government: priority of children's health in, 168, 201–202; produce availability and, 218; recommendations for action, 226–230, 231, 233–235; strategies and steps recommended by, 200–201. *See also* taxes; U.S. Department of Agriculture (USDA)

grandparents as storytellers, 196

Great Britain: diets in, 7; overweight increasing in, 33, 235; weather-related metabolic rates, 72

Grocery Manufacturers of America, 222

grocery shopping: division of responsibility and, 123–124; recommendations for, 131; weight management and, 151

grocery stores: socioeconomic status and choices in, 109–110, 218, 221; super sizes and, 97

*Growing Up Today Study*, 73

growth charts, 16, 17

growth curve, dip in, 19–20

growth rate, 20–21, 219

*Guidelines for Collecting Heights and Weights on Children and Adolescents in School Settings*, 18

Hamilton, Charles, 187
*Handbook of Obesity Treatment* (Wadden and Stunkard, eds.), 168–169
Harry Potter stories (Rowling), 187–190, 194, 195
Haverford, PA, 100
headaches, 36
Head Start, 93, 105–106, 234
health consequences, 35–40; adult diseases in children, 35; breathing difficulties, 39, 149; diabetes, 36–38, 71; early maturation, 39–40; heart disease, 38, 248–249n20; hypertension, 38–39, 149, 161; less common problems, 36. *See also* psychological consequences
health insurance, 25, 230
Healthy Eating Index, 112–113
heart disease, 38
HeartSmart, 107
Hearts N' Parks, 214
Hewlett, Sylvia, 89, 193
Heyman, Melvin, 130
high blood pressure (hypertension), 38–39, 149, 163
high school. *See* adolescents; schools
Hill, James O., 201
Hirschmann, Jane, 124
Hispanics. *See* Latinos
HMOs. *See* health insurance
Hoff, Benjamin, 196
*Holes* (Sachar), 191, 195
Holt, Connie, 202
home. *See* family environment; parents
home delivery of produce, 218
homework, 137
hopscotch, 135, 216
*How to Be Slimmer, Trimmer and Happier* (Berg), 171
*Human Obesity Gene Map* (Chagnon et al.), 51
hydrogenated oils, 158, 159. *See also* fats
hypertension, 38–39, 149, 163

ideal, as term, 17
ideal of beauty, 169–173, 174, 175
Igo, Shirley, 99
Improved Nutrition and Physical Activity Act (IMPACT), proposed, 226

India, 32
Indians. *See* Native Americans
infants: birth weight of, 67, 69–70; BMI and, 245n7; breast- vs. bottle-feeding of, 72–74, 220; eating patterns of, 49, 72–75; fat cells of, 74; juice drinking by, 74–75; physical activity and, 52; solid foods and, 74; statistics on, 28, 29, 31; taste-preference development and, 74, 76–77, 132; teachable moments of, 221; weight gain rate of, 20. *See also* adolescents; early childhood; middle childhood
insurance, health, 25, 230
Internal Revenue Service, 25, 230
international health. *See* world health

Jacobson, Marc, 219
*Jane Eyre* (Brontë), 187
*Jelly Belly* (Smith), 146, 195
juice and juice drinks, 59, 74–75, 112
jump rope, 182–183, 216
junk food, 8; media promotion of, 56, 88; proposed tax on ("Twinkie Tax"), 55, 227–229, 231; in schools, 98, 100, 127, 202; weaning children from, 131, 132, 134, 153, 164. *See also* fast-food restaurants; vending machines
Just for Kids, 214–215

Kidswalk-to-School, 208
kindergarten age children. *See* early childhood
Kindlon, Daniel, 89
Kozol, Jonathan, 184
Kraft Foods, 83, 222

labeling. *See* name calling; stigmatization
labeling of restaurant foods, 223
Laderer, Mandy, 165
language: measurement of children and, 18; stigmatization and, 13–14. *See also* name calling; sensitivity
latchkey children, 109
Latinos: body size diversity and, 24, 170; diabetes and, 37; parenting styles of, 79; statistics of, 31, 33–34. *See also* cultural differences

middle childhood *(continued)*
122–123; statistics on, 29–33; sugar
consumption during, 58–59; television and, 86. *See also* adolescents;
early childhood; infants
Miedzian, Myriam, 184
military service, alternative to, 234
milk consumption, 59, 75, 100
Milne, A. A., 196
minority groups. *See* cultural differences;
*specific groups*
mistakes, learning from, 141–142
modeling behavior: dieting, 123, 171–172;
emotional eating, 85, 127; influence
of, 126–127, 144–145, 262n6; moderation, 126–127, 175; physical
activity and, 88, 135; restaurant alternatives and, 223; style of parenting/
caregiving and, 80, 105–106; taste
preferences and, 76–77, 130, 132,
164; by teachers, 105–106; vegetables,
enjoyment of, 106, 132; worksite
wellness and, 224–225
moderation: authoritative parenting style
and development of, 123–125; of consumer response, 222; defined, 7; diet
plans and, 171; modeling of, 126–127,
175; as practice, 126–128, 176; as sensitive understanding, 178
monounsaturated fats, 158. *See also* fats
morality, 180
Munter, Carol, 124

name calling: empathy vs., 139–140; stigma-
tization and, 41, 141, 146, 178–179,
191–192
NASH (non-alcoholic steatohepatitis), 36,
120
National Association for Acceptance of Fat
People, 25
National Association for Sport and
Physical Education, 207
National Health and Nutrition Examina-
tion Study (NHANES), 31
National Institutes of Health, 17, 25, 163, 174
National Longitudinal Survey of Youth, 31,
41

National School Lunch Program, 101–105
National Soft Drink Association, 203
Native Americans: diabetes and, 37;
movement programs and, 215; Pima
Indians, 37, 49; statistics of, 33; thrifty
genotype and, 49. *See also* cultural
differences
nature and nurture, 46–47. *See also*
environment; genetics
Neel, J. V., 48
negative scripts, 141
Nepal, 4
Nestle, Marion, 87, 97, 227
Newman, Leslea, 147, 191, 195
New Mexico, 215
New York: camp programs, 217; causes of
overweight, 45; health consequences
in, 37; junk food restrictions, 203;
McDonald's suits, 92, 96; physical
activities, 135, 182; school activities,
107; school food service, 104, 205–
206; statistics on overweight, 34
Nichter, Mimi, 173
*Nick Jr.,* 87
*Nobody's Family is Going to Change*
(Fitzhugh), 191, 192, 193, 195
non-alcoholic steatohepatitis (NASH),
36, 120
non-exercise activity thermogenesis, 52
normalization, rebellion against, 180
North Carolina, 216
*Nothing's Fair in Fifth Grade* (DeClements),
186, 191, 195, 197
novels. *See* literature, children's
nurture and nature, 46–47. *See also*
environment; genetics
nutrition. *See* diet; malnutrition;
undernutrition
*Nutrition Action Healthletter,* 97
nutrition education. *See* education

Oakland, CA, 100, 204–205
obesity: diagnosis of, 13–14, 26; as disease,
controversy of, 25–26, 230; as term,
14–16, 45. *See also* overweight
obstructive sleep apnea, 39
*Oliver Twist* (Dickens), 187

*One Fat Summer* (Lipsyte), 191, 192, 195
Opelika, AL, 204
*Ophelia Speaks* (Shandler), 184
*Ordinary Resurrections* (Kozol), 184
organic produce, 218
Ornish, Dean, diet plan, 159, 160
orthopedic problems, 36
overweight: as condition of immoderation,
    26; rate of increase, 28; at risk of
    becoming, 15, 16, 17, 26, 29, 31, 57;
    risk factors for, 53–54; statistics of,
    29–34; as term, 14–15; various causes
    of (*see* fast-food restaurants; genetics;
    parenting; physical activity, lack of;
    soft drinks)
*Overworked American, The* (Schor),
    89–90

parental obesity: dietary guidelines and,
    58; dieting culture and, 172; genetics
    and, 52; parenting skills and, 167;
    parenting style and, 79–80; percep-
    tion of children's weight and, 22–23;
    pregnancy and, 69, 70, 71; as risk
    factor, 54
parenting: breast- vs. bottle-feeding, 72–
    74, 220; Caring About Children
    Corps in support of, 233–235; custody
    of children issue, 213; fat discrimina-
    tion and, 178, 182; limit setting and,
    122–125, 130; prenatal care and nutri-
    tion, 67–72, 221; recommendations
    for overweight prevention, 125–137;
    resilient children, raising, 137–144;
    taste-preference development and,
    75–77; time pressure and, 89–90;
    weight management support, 152–
    154, 167; Weight Watchers advice
    for, 236. *See also* family environment;
    modeling behavior; parental obesity;
    parenting styles; parents
parenting styles: authoritarian, 78–80, 105,
    122, 124; permissive, 78–80, 121–122,
    124; as risk factor, 54, 77–80. *See also*
    authoritative parenting style
parents: as advocates for change in schools,
    212; blaming of, 7, 59–60, 61, 93, 225;

communication by (*see* communica-
    tion); empathy of, 139–140; fictional
    portrayals of, 193; influence of, 23, 122;
    perception of children's weight by,
    22–24; prevention as dependent on,
    121; responses to overweight, 213;
    time pressures and, 56; "war against,"
    193; worksite wellness and, 224–225.
    *See also* family environment; model-
    ing behavior; parental obesity;
    parenting; parenting styles; pregnancy
Parent Teacher Association (PTA), 99
parks, 109, 135, 214
Payne, Melanie, 104
Peace Corps, 233
*Pediatrics*, 15
pedometers, 208
Pennsylvania, 100
PepsiCo, 101, 222
perception of weight, 22–24
permissive parenting style, 78–80, 121–122,
    124
pharmaceutical industry, 50, 120, 172
physical activity: bicycling, 108, 208, 216;
    mild levels of as effective, 108; public
    health messages for, 229–230; recom-
    mendations for increasing, 133–136,
    164–165, 206–212; schools and im-
    provement of, 206–212; spontaneous
    play as, 119, 165, 207; street reclaim-
    ing and, 215–216; television reduction
    and, 119, 134–136; USDA guidelines
    for, 208. *See also* physical education
    (PE); play; sports and athletics;
    walking
physical activity, lack of: after school,
    108–109, 135, 211, 214–215; asthma
    and, 39; declining as children get
    older, 87–88; fidget factor, 52–53;
    genetics and, 52–53; hypertension
    and, 39; recess, 106–107, 206–207;
    safety concerns and, 45, 106–107, 108–
    109, 200; schools and, 106–108; size
    as factor in, 182; socioeconomic status
    and, 119; statistics, 4, 57; television/
    computer/video games and, 85–88.
    *See also* physical activity

physical education (PE), 107–108; guidelines for time spent, 207–208; Fitnessgram, 209; New PE, 108, 207;
recess distinguished from, 207; rein-
statement of, 206–208; statistics of
participation in, 57, 107; stigmatization and, 181–182
*Pickwick Papers* (Dickens), 187
*Pie Magic* (Forward), 191, 195
Pima Indians, 37, 49
Pipher, Mary, 184
pizza, school lunch programs and, 103–
104, 203
"pizza effect," 49
Pizza Hut, 103, 203
Planet Health, 270n22. *See also* Eat Well
and Keep Moving
Plato, 46
play: creating more opportunities for, 119,
165; dates for, 136, 140–141; fast-food
promotions and, 95–96; and recess,
lack of, 106–107, 207; street reclaiming and, 215–216; structured activities
vs., 215–216
PMO (psychosomatic model of obesity),
85
Pollack, William S., 181, 184
polyunsaturated fats, 158. *See also* fats
portions: defined, 57; limiting, 127–128;
"reality-size," 223, 229, 230; vs. recommended servings, 57–58, 128,
162–163; serving one's self, 82; super
size, 82–84, 96, 97, 128, 223
potatoes, 112
Potter, Harry, stories, 187–190, 194, 195
poverty, perception of overweight and,
22–23. *See also* socioeconomic status
Prader-Willi syndrome, 26, 51
pregnancy: early maturation and, 40; fat
discrimination research and, 180;
prenatal care and nutrition during,
67–72, 221; teen, 40, 72; weather-
related birth conditions and, 72
prenatal care and nutrition, 67–72, 221
preschool-age children. *See* early childhood
*Preventing Childhood Eating Problems*
(Hirschmann and Munter), 124
prevention: anti-smoking campaign as

example of, 8–9, 222, 226–227, 232,
236; autonomy and, 121; campaigns
for, and risk of obsession with weight,
172–173, 174–176; Caring About
Children Corps (CACC) proposed
for, 233–235; choice and, 121; eating
disorders, 174; family environment
and recommendations for, 121–125,
126–137; funding for, 226, 229, 230;
ideal program for, 176; moderate
eating and, 126–128; overview of,
7–9, 120–121; parents as key to, 121;
proposed national campaign for, 230–
235; and resilient children, 137–144;
responsibility-sharing, 123–125, 130;
treatment vs., 7–8, 120–121, 226. *See
also* self-regulation; treatment; weight
management
problem solving, teaching, 143
processed meals, 82–84
protein, balance in diet, 155–160
psychological consequences: depression,
5, 22; overview of, 40–41. *See also*
self-esteem problems; stigmatization
psychological health: authoritative parenting and, 121–125; emotional intelligence, 140; recommendations to
parents, 125–137; resilient children
and, 137–144
psychosomatic model of obesity (PMO),
85
PTA (Parent Teacher Association), 99
purging/binging, 173–175. *See also* eating
disorders; eating dysfunctions
*Push* (Sapphire), 195, 197

quick fixes: as harmful, 50; and healthy
diets, 164; as nonexistent, 7–8;
question of effectiveness of diets
and, 164

*Raising Low-Fat Kids in a High-Fat World*
(Shaw), 157, 159–160
*Raising Resilient Children* (Brooks and
Goldstein), 137–144
reading aloud/storytelling, 193–194, 196
*Real Boys* (Pollack), 181
*Real Boys' Voices* (Pollack), 181, 184

scripts, negative, 141

*Secrets of Feeding a Healthy Family* (Satter), 125

self-esteem problems: diagnosis of obesity and, 13; dieting and, 146–147, 172, 175; drug use and, 41; fighting fat discrimination as solution to, 186; overview of, 41; resilience building and, 142; stigmatization and, 41, 179; weight loss and, 41

self-monitoring, 154

self-regulation: authoritative parenting and, 122–125; breast- vs. bottle-feeding and, 73–74; choice management, 122–125, 129–130, 178, 223; discipline and, 143–144; family meals as fostering, 129; as prevention, 8

sensitivity: in collecting heights and weights, 18; diagnostic terms and, 13, 14–16; moderation and, 178

servings: recommended, 162–163; vs. portions, 57–58, 128, 162–163

set point, 47, 50

sexuality, early maturation and, 39–40

Shalala, Donna E., 20

Shandler, Sara, 184

Shapedown, 166–167

Shaw, Judith, 157, 159–160

shopping, as leisure activity, 90; safety concerns and, 109. *See also* grocery shopping

short stature, 74, 173

Shreve, Susan Richards, 197

single-parent households, 62

skin growths, 36

sleep, importance of, 136–137

sleep apnea, 39, 149

slenderness. *See* beauty ideal

slowing down, 127, 224, 232

smell, sense of, 49

Smith, Robert Kimmel, 146, 195

smoking, 41

smoking regulation, 8–9, 222, 226–227, 232, 236

snacking: alternatives to, 127, 128, 131, 160; forbidding, as unworkable, 127; refrigerator, management of, 131, 160; as

standard accompaniment to activities, 94, 203, 232. *See also* eating patterns; family meals

social conscience, development of, 142–143

socioeconomic status: and cost of treatment, 31; effective parenting and, 89–90, 213; fruit/vegetable subsidies and, 227; grocery store choices and, 109–110, 218, 221; health consequences and, 37; obesity rates and, 31, 32–33, 247n3; parenting styles and, 78–79; perception of child's weight and, 22–24; resilient children and, 138–139; as risk factor, 54–55, 121; weight management programs and, 169

soda. *See* soft drinks

soft drinks: family control of, 81, 160; juice as preferable to, 75; manufacturers' response to epidemic, 222; obesity risk and consumption of, 110–111; recommended limits to, 223; school vending machine sales of, 99–101; statistics of consumption, 58–59, 75, 110. *See also* water

Sokol, Ronald J., 8, 218–219

Solovay, Sondra, 185

*Solution, The: Six Winning Ways to Permanent Weight Loss* (Mellin), 167

Sothern, Melinda, 166

South Carolina, 174

SPARK (Sports, Play, and Active Recreation for Kids), 211

"Speak No Evil Day," 199

speed of eating, 81–82, 122, 224

sports and athletics: fundraising for, 99, 212; participation in, 108, 211; snacks and treats integral to, 94. *See also* physical activity; physical education (PE)

*Staying Fat for Sarah Byrnes* (Crutcher), 191, 195

Step Test Exercise Prescription, 219

stereotyping, 177–178. *See also* discrimination; stigmatization

stigmatization: assortative mating and, 49; depression and, 22; diagnosis and,

13–14; fiction illustrating, 178–179; genetic explanation for obesity and, 51; medical care and avoidance of, 219; name calling and threats, 41, 141, 146, 178–179, 191–192; school lunch programs and, 103, 206; self-esteem problems and, 41, 179; as stimulus for seeking help, 22; weight management and, 167. *See also* discrimination; sensitivity

storytelling/reading aloud, 193–194, 196

street reclaiming, 215–216

*Street Reclaiming* (Engwicht), 215–216

Stunkard, Albert, 168–169, 179–180

sucrose, 111

*Sugar Busters for Kids* (Andrews, ed.), 157

sugar intake: corn syrup, 111; recommendation, 58; statistics on, 58–59

surgeon general, 110, 200–201, 205, 206

*Surgeon General's Call to Action to Prevent and Decrease Overweight and Obesity*, 110, 201, 205

surgical procedures, 172

Take 10! program, 207

*Taking the Atkins Program to the Next Generation* (Atkins), 156

*Tao of Pooh, The* (Hoff), 196

taste preferences: factors affecting, 75–77; infant feeding and development of, 74, 76–77, 132; juice drinking and, 74; marketplace competition for, 164; repeated exposures and, 104, 124, 132; television commercials and, 87. *See also* variety of foods

taxes: on junk foods ("Twinkie Tax"), 55, 227–229, 231; on luxury items, 228; obesity as disease and, 25, 230

Teach for America, 233

teaching. *See* schools

teasing, 181–182. *See also* bullying; discrimination

teenagers. *See* adolescents

Teen Lifestyle Project, 170

teen pregnancy, 40, 72

telephone, as interruption, 133, 134

Teletubbies, 87, 224

television: Channel One, 98, 212, 229, eating as co-activity with, 90; exploitation of children, 87; reading aloud as alternative to, 194; reducing viewing time, 119, 134–136, 152, 165, 168, 194; as risk factor, 54; statistics of viewing time, 57, 86. *See also* advertising; media

Telushkin, Joseph, 199

10,000 Steps a Day program, 208

Texas, 107

Thailand, 32–33

thinness. *See* beauty ideal

Thomas, Clarence, 228

time pressure, 89–90

*Tipping the Scales of Justice* (Solovay), 185

tobacco regulation, 8–9, 222, 226–227, 232, 236

Tolkien, J. R. R., 194

*Too Much of a Good Thing* (Kindlon), 89

toxic environment, 55–56, 138, 139

trans-fats, 155, 158, 159, 164. *See also* fats

treatment: effectiveness, question of, 148, 149, 153–154; ideal program for, 176; preoccupation with weight and, 147–148; prevention vs., 7–8, 120–121, 226; quick, as harmful, 50; self-esteem and, 41; surgical/pharmaceutical, 172; weight management as goal of (*see* weight management). *See also* diet plans; prevention

*Trim Kids*, 166

"Twinkie Tax," 55, 227–229, 231

unconditional love, 142

undernutrition, 32, 33; during pregnancy, 69

urban planning, 216. *See also* community environment

U.S. Department of Agriculture (USDA): Child and Adult Care Food Program, 105; Healthy Eating Index, 112–113; physical activity recommendations by, 208; School Breakfast Program, 101; School Lunch Program, 101–105; weight-loss plans reviewed by, 160–161. *See also* Food Guide Pyramid and dietary guidelines

Vanderbilt, Gloria, 180
variety of foods: as hallmark of better diet, 129, 164; infant feeding and taste for, 74, 76–77, 132; learning to manage choice, 129–130; recommendations for, 129, 131. *See also* taste preferences
vegetables. *See* fruits and vegetables
vehicles, dependence on: reclaiming streets and, 215; regulating use of, 208–209; urban planning and, 216, 231
vending machines: healthy alternatives stocked in, 100, 203; in schools, 98, 99–101, 202–203, 205; ubiquity of, 110
VERB: It's What You Do, 229–230
video games. *See* computer/video games
Vietnam, 32
violence. *See* bullying
voluntary vs. involuntary activity, 52–53
vomiting, 174. *See also* eating disorders; eating dysfunctions

Wadden, T. A., 168–169
walking: decline in, 108; encouragement of, 208–209, 212; lack of fitness for, 107; safety in, 208; urban planning and, 216, 231; variations on, as family activity, 136; vehicle regulation and, 208–209. *See also* physical activity
walking trains, 208, 212
Wall Street, 84, 222
Wansink, Brian, 97
*War Against Parents, The* (Hewlett and West), 89, 193
water: fountains, provision of, 100–101; free, at fast-food restaurants, 223; habit of drinking, 75; modeling drinking of, 77; public health messages for, 229; quenching thirst with, 128; in vending machines, 100, 203
weather-related birth conditions, 72
weight cycling (yo-yo dieting), 41, 50
weight-loss treatment. *See* diet plans; treatment; weight management
weight management: calorie intake appropriate to age, 148–151; campaigns

for, and risk of obsession with weight, 172–173, 174–176; defined as goal, 148; dieting vs., 148–149; family support for, 151–152, 154, 166–169; goal-setting and, 152; ideal program for, 176; recommendations for programs, 166–169; research evaluating plans for, 160–161, 168–169; school-based programs, 167–168, 169; self-monitoring (record keeping) and, 154. *See also* diet plans; treatment
weight measurement, sensitivity in, 18
Weight Watchers, 160, 236
West, Cornel, 193
*Whale Talk* (Crutcher), 191, 195
"white" carbs, 164
whites: beauty ideal and, 170, 180; dieting and, 169, 170, 174; physical activity and, 88; socioeconomic status and, 55; statistics of, 31; unhealthy dieting behaviors, 24, 170; vegetable consumption, 112
*Who's Dancin' Now?*, 215
WIC (Women, Infants and Children) program, 218
Willett, Walter, 161, 224
Windsor, duchess of, 180
Winfrey, Oprah, 3, 50, 167
*Winnie the Pooh First Readers* (Gaines), 196
Winnie the Pooh series (Milne), 196
Women, Infants and Children (WIC) program, 218
worksite wellness, 224–225
world health: globalization and, 4–5, 32–33; poverty link and, 55; statistics of overweight, 32–33
World Health Organization (WHO), 32
Wright, William, 180

YMCA, 217
"You Can Only Demonstrate" (Martin), 144–145
yo-yo dieting (weight cycling), 41, 50

Zolkowski, George, 18

DESIGNER: Victoria Kuskowski
COMPOSITOR: Integrated Composition Systems
INDEXER: Victoria Baker
ILLUSTRATOR: Bill Nelson
TEXT: 11.25/13.5 Adobe Garamond
DISPLAY: Adobe Garamond, Futura
PRINTER AND BINDER: Maple-Vail Manufacturing Group